INSTITUTE OF PSYCHIATRY

THE LATER
PAPERS OF
SIR AUBREY LEWIS

INSTITUTE OF PSYCHIATRY

THE LATER
PAPERS OF
SIR AUBREY LEWIS

LL.D., D.Sc., M.D., F.R.C.P., F.R.C.Psych.

Lately Emeritus Professor of Psychiatry
University of London
formerly of the
Institute of Psychiatry

OXFORD UNIVERSITY PRESS
1979

Oxford University Press, Walton Street, Oxford OX2 6DP

OXFORD LONDON GLASGOW
NEW YORK TORONTO MELBOURNE WELLINGTON
KUALA LUMPUR SINGAPORE JAKARTA HONG KONG TOKYO
DELHI BOMBAY CALCUTTA MADRAS KARACHI
NAIROBI DAR ES SALAAM CAPE TOWN

British Library Cataloguing in Publication Data
Lewis, *Sir* Aubrey
　The later papers of Sir Aubrey Lewis.
　1. Psychiatry
　I. Institute of Psychiatry
　616.8'9'008　RC458　79-40186

ISBN 0-19-712150-0

*Printed in Great Britain by Spottiswoode Ballantyne Ltd.
Colchester and London*

CONTENTS

ACKNOWLEDGEMENTS

The articles reprinted here first appeared in the following publications and we should like to thank the Editors and Publishers for permission to reproduce:

Acta Psychiatrica Scandinavica; Biological Council; British Journal of Psychiatry; Confrontations Psychiatriques; Evolution Psychiatrique; Israel Annals of Psychiatry and Related Disciplines; Librairie de l'Université, Georg et Cie, Geneva; Proceedings of the Royal Society of Medicine; Psychological Medicine (Cambridge University Press); The Lancet; The Listener; The New York Review of Books; The Times Literary Supplement; University of Glasgow, Maurice Bloch Lectures; Wellcome Institute of Historical Medicine: The Wellcome Trustees.

INTRODUCTION

From 1966, the year of his retirement, up to the time of his death in 1975 Sir Aubrey Lewis continued to work part-time as emeritus professor at the Institute of Psychiatry. Free of the burdens of administration and teaching, he was then able to concentrate on some of the topics in which he had long maintained a special interest. Prominent among these were the fundamental issues relating to the definition and classification of mental disorders and the relevance of an historical perspective to the theory and practice of psychiatry.

Sir Aubrey's best-known activities during this decade are probably represented by the British and the World Health Organization Glossaries of Mental Disorders which he steered successfully through their various stages and which have already been widely adopted as the basis of a common language among psychiatrists throughout the world. A comparable achievement was the group of papers which have been brought together to make up the bulk of this volume. Several are about words, for no one was more aware than Sir Aubrey of how much psychiatry is bound up with the use of words and their associated concepts and how much of the history of the discipline is embodied in them. His searching analysis of the evolution of some of the basic terms employed by practising psychiatrists demonstrates clearly his remarkable capacity for combining the historically important with the clinically significant. The other papers also display this sense of continuity in various ways, and all of them bear witness to the breadth of his scholarship and to the esprit de finesse which characterizes so many of his writings. As he once wrote: 'The humanities cannot, by definition, be classed as sciences but history and ethics and, in the long run, philosophy are branches of knowledge from which medicine draws sustenance. This is particularly true of their relation to psychiatry'. No one was better able to illustrate the truth of this assertion.

Sir Aubrey's own place in the history of psychiatry is secure. It is entirely fitting that this collection of late papers should appear under the auspices of the Institute of Psychiatry, of which he was for so long the moving spirit.

MICHAEL SHEPHERD

Institute of Psychiatry
1978

Amnesic Syndromes

Sir Aubrey Lewis (*London*)
The Psychopathological Aspect

Many of those who made notable contributions to the psychopathology of amnesia have begun with an affirmation of the importance of memory function, using some such phrase as Janet (1898), who said at the opening of his report to the London Congress of Experimental Psychology: 'The part played by memory is of paramount importance in the functioning of the mind, and its smallest alterations have grave pathological consequences'. Such aggrandizement of memory is now out of fashion: psychologists concern themselves more with applying the theory of learning and of communication to its experimental study than with observation of its disorders, and clinicians are apt to look more closely at the limbic system than at dissection of the elements of retention and recall that seem to depend on the integrity of that system.

Consequently there has come about some confusion of terms. Whereas for clinicians the consummation of the memory process is the reappearance in consciousness of a former precept, for the psychologist the reappearance in consciousness is unimportant: what is significant is decay of inhibition, transfer, retroaction and other characteristics of change in performance over a period of time; these can be as well, or better, investigated on some motor task than on verbal reports of conscious recall. The psychologist is therefore ready to study memory in animal experiments; but the psychiatrist, and I think the neurologist, would have to re-examine his concept of remembering before he could comfortably follow suit. The psychiatrist finds it particularly difficult to dismiss consciousness from his concept of memory because he usually thinks of the active process of forgetting on Freudian lines, whether he is a psychoanalyst or not; and he is furthermore reluctant to extend the concept of memory because he knows how Semon and Bleuler and other clever men came to grief when they enlarged memory till it was almost coextensive with biology or psychology. Indeed the predominant state of mind of the psychiatrist in dealing with memory and its disorders is one of hopeful caution: he does not want to trip up over engrams, or premature localization, or screen memories, or any of the other traps for the unwary which he knows about, and he is disappointed at the relatively meagre advances made in the psycho-logical study of this field during the last twenty or thirty years. But he is in no doubt of its importance – he would say, with Locke, that 'memory is an intellectual creature, is necessary in the next degree to perception. It is of so great moment, that where it is wanting, all the rest of our faculties are in great measure useless; and we, in our thoughts, reasonings, and knowledge, could not proceed beyond present objects, were it not for the assistance of our memories . . .'.

The Korsakoff Syndrome

In a consideration of amnesic syndromes the first question must be 'How many are there?' and the second 'What are their characteristics?' To this the psychiatrist has a short answer: 'There is one, and its typical features are those known by Korsakoff's name – severe defect of retention and other functions of memory, time disorder, disorientation and confabulation, without any corresponding impairment of consciousness or intellectual deterioration' (Korsakoff 1890). This, according to common usage, is the amnesic syndrome. There are, of course, disturbances of memory, sometimes startling and total, in other conditions, but the amnesia in them is not so central and conspicuous, and it does not so regularly concur with other psychological features as to constitute a clinical pattern deserving to be known as an amnesic syndrome. It may be urged that hysterical loss of memory has a strong claim to be so termed, but the manifestations of this condition are too varied and dependent on accidents of circumstance to make up a syndrome. Still, since syndromes are not handed down to us from on high and are merely provisional constructs it will do no harm if hysterical and other conditions in which memory fails are called amnesic syndromes. I shall, however, describe mainly what for the last sixty years has been the amnesic syndrome *par excellence*.

There are two familiar points which it is well to restate before any discussion of the Korsakoff syndrome: First that it may follow an extraordinarily wide variety of forms of cerebral damage or decay – general paralysis, Wernicke's encephalopathy, senile dementia, cerebral trauma, anoxia from strangulation, tumour, arteriosclerosis, encephalitis, poisoning by carbon monoxide, lead and other noxæ, artificially induced convulsions, epileptic states and many more diseases of the brain. Secondly, it centres on a function which has been dissected and redistributed

1

almost out of existence. As Bartlett (1932) put it 'It is perfectly true that nobody can put a ring around memory and explain it from within itself. The dissolving power of modern research seems to have split memory into a number of variously related functions. The functions may be many and yet, acting together, they issue in a specific process demanding its own name, and its own special modes of study'.

Nature of the Disturbance

The commonest division of memory is into the four stages – registration of impressions, retention, recall and recognition. The first of these, the learning phase, is that which was chiefly incriminated in the amnesic syndrome by the old masters – Wernicke, Bonhoeffer and Kraepelin. But though they regarded defect of registration as the chief, and perhaps the fundamental and essential, anomaly, they were aware of the indirect nature of their evidence: they inferred this defect because the patient had grossly inadequate immediate recall. Thus in Brodmann's investigation (1902, 1904) because the patients could not reproduce a sequence of eight or twelve nonsense syllables even after innumerable repetitions, he assumed that the repeated impressions had not been recorded fully. But he also satisfied himself, by Ebbinghaus's sparing method, that traces were left – traces which could only have been derived from impressions made during the learning process. Similar observations were made, in careful experiments by Gregor (1909), Schneider (1912), and Köppen & Kutzinski (1910), using words, series of pictures and incomplete sentences and figures. The choice of material to be remembered and the manner in which it is represented are of more importance than the earlier workers realized. André Rey (1959) has recently demonstrated that in dysmnesic patients concrete objects visually presented are recalled better than single words spoken aloud to the subjects: this difference is evident also in normal persons, but in the patients it may go so far that words are apparently not registered at all, while objects are.

A somewhat similar observation was lately made by Nyssen (1957): he found that Korsakovians (as he pleasantly calls them), even when very severely amnesic, can acquire, recall and recognize to some extent simple figures and words with concrete meaning if given sufficient opportunity to learn them through daily presentation and copying, but that figures are more easily recognized than words.

There is now abundant reason to conclude that although in the Korsakoff syndrome the immediate reproduction of recent impressions can be very defective, their subsequent recall or recognition may give clear proof that registration did

occur, at any rate partially. The disorder must therefore be investigated also in other stages of the memory function or in other functions closely connected with memory, of which the most obvious is perception.

Pick (1915) and Grünthal (1924) were the first to conclude that thinking is the psychological area basically affected in this disorder and that the patient's prime difficulty lies in forming a mental set (*Einstellung*): his past perceptions are not available to him, he cannot relate them to a present situation. This finding was much elaborated by Bürger-Prinz & Kaila (1930) in the light of their experimental studies, and has been lately explored again in the thorough Boston inquiries (Talland 1958, Talland & Miller 1959) which showed the patients to have an inflexibility of perceptual set, a reduced capacity to shift attention, what might be called a dysdiadochokinesia of perceptual attitude. Tied, as it were, to the first object-stimulus he receives the Korsakoff patient cannot check and revise his subsequent percepts and interpret them successfully. This militates, of course, against their utilization in recall and may favour confabulation. Nevertheless, the perceptual disorder must be considered a minor and separate aspect of the amnesic syndrome: it is not sufficient explanation of the disorder of memory to postulate as its essence a disturbance of 'set', faulty perception and incapacity to grasp orientating events and relate them to one another.

Disturbance of Time

The second most striking anomaly in the Korsakoff syndrome is the disturbance of time. This invariable feature can be most readily recognized in the patient's temporal disorientation and in his jumbling of remembered events: he cannot order the succession in which they occurred. Though recognized by Korsakoff (1890) and Bonhoeffer (1904), this characteristic did not come into its own until thirty years ago. With the little burst of philosophical and psychological studies in time-experience that took place about that time, the Korsakoff disturbance was closely looked into, notably by van der Horst (1932, 1956) and by Ehrenwald (1931) and Krauss (1930). It was put forward as the basic disturbance. Van der Horst (1956) has maintained that the deficit is in respect of events that have once had personal meaning: whereas impersonal experience (for example, learning an algebraic formula or nonsense syllables) does not have a temporal sign attached to it and may not be demonstrably at fault when the customary psychological tests of registration and retention are applied, quite striking incapacity will be evinced in the same patient when he is questioned about the events of his personal life, *la vie vécue*. Personal events cannot be recalled with normal sharpness and clarity unless they can be placed in time: but the Korsakoff patient, says van der Horst, has an impairment in his ability to place events plucked from the continuity of past experience, and all else that occurs in the Korsakoff syndrome is a secondary effect of his temporal incapacity. 'Time is the psychological category that enables us to distinguish between perceptions which are otherwise identical.' From this supposedly primary defect in temporal organization, van der Horst also ingeniously, but not quite plausibly, derived the retrograde amnesia, the reduplicative paramnesia, the confabulations and disorientation of Korsakoff patients.

The abnormality in temporal location, which van der Horst linked so closely to personal experience, has been formulated differently by other investigators such as Ehrenwald (1931), Krauss (1930), Lidz (1942) and, recently, Mouren & Felician (1958) in France, and Whitty & Lewin (1960) in this country. They rested their conclusions partly on experimental data. A good example of such a study is in the report by Williams & Zangwill (1950), who found that if a series of pictures had been exposed to moderately amnesic patients, the order was retained better when the consecutive exposures could be perceived as building a related sequence (e.g. the numbers 8, 9, 10) than when they consisted of disconnected items; they also noted a tendency to antedate recent events by pushing them further back into the past. They inclined to the view that disturbance of sequence-relation is a consequence of the retention-defect, and not the basic or primary disorder. Since the point at issue does not at present lend itself to decisive experimental inquiry, it is sufficient to recognize that the aspect of memory-function which deals with temporal order and relation is invariably disturbed in the amnesic syndrome, and that, as Bartlett (1932) pointed out, the capacity to pick out events from the series in which they occurred is probably a late acquisition, demanding 'special devices' for reconstructing schemata; these devices will be among the first to go when the neural substrate is damaged.

Confabulation

Confabulation is so picturesque a feature of the amnesic syndrome that it has received a good deal of attention, especially from the earlier writers. They explained it, rather too readily, as a defensive effort to hide failures of recollection: Bonhoeffer (1904) called it 'embarrassment-confabulation' (*Verlegenheits-konfabulation*), while admitting that the fantasies produced could take a wider scope than this interpretation would account for. We have to ask why these patients do not simply answer 'I don't remember', and why they accept their false memories as correct; also why some patients produce their confabulations spontaneously and in plenty, while others have to be prodded with suggestions and leading questions. There are clearly considerable differences between individuals in these perversions of memory, just as there are differences in normal activities of memory between one person and another.

There is in some confabulations a dream-like quality, suggesting that they may have had their origin in a preceding delirious state or in the hallucinations of nocturnal confusion, or even in actual dreams: in such patients the confabulations are less likely to be changed in response to suggestion. Long ago Wernicke pointed out that confabulations might originate thus out of a confusional state: they are not, then, strictly products of disturbed memory. Nor is confabulation a distinctively morbid activity. Bartlett (1932) showed in his classical monograph that normal remembering is not a mechanical affair of literal, exact reduplication: we do not summon and reproduce memories in the way that we repeat nonsense syllables, by rote; our memories are subjected to a constructive process in which condensation, elaboration, and invention play a leading part. Similarly in the Korsakoff state inventive fantasy plays a more important part in determining composite fabrications than does the need to compensate for defective recall. If we examine the content of the false memories we find, as Russell (1959) and Russell & Nathan (1946) pointed out, that fragments of past experiences have been dislocated from their proper temporal sequence and their context; they are mingled with perceptual data drawn from recent events or from the situation in which the patient is being examined at the moment.

Closer examination of the content of false memories suggests that much of what is remembered, and even more of what is forgotten, depends on emotional forces, such as psychoanalytic studies have elucidated (Flament 1957). Whereas Ebbinghaus, G E Müller and other pioneers in the study of memory ignored these affective influences, Bartlett stressed them in his vigorous revolt against the depersonalized analysis of memory, based on artificial situations. The catathymic influence of feeling-tone has been well demonstrated in systematic tests of patients with the amnesic syndrome. When, for example, they have to repeat the gist of short narrative passages that have been read to them, there is appreciably less distortion of affectively neutral passages than of disagreeable ones (Hartmann 1930, Talland & Ekdahl 1959). In Lindberg's (1946) thoroughly investigated patient, who had a very severe and typical Korsakoff syndrome attributable to prolonged alcoholism, his amnesia was most striking

3

and complete in matters referring to his fiancée, whose death had been a profoundly distressing event for him: in a word-association test, his reaction-time was most delayed when the stimulus word touched on the painful circumstances of their relationship. It follows from findings such as these that some at any rate of the forgotten memories may be difficult or impossible to recall, not because of damage to the neural substrate but because repressive or other emotionally determined forces hinder the appearance of the memories in consciousness. This is only to bring the amnesia of pathological states into line with normal remembering: cf. Darwin's reason for noting down adverse observations 'I had also, during many years, followed a golden rule, namely that whenever a published fact, a new observation or thought came across me, which was opposed to my general results, to make a memorandum of it without fail and at once; for I had found by experience that such facts and thoughts were far more apt to escape from the memory than favourable ones'. A catathymic explanation for some of the Korsakoff amnesia is consistent with the well-known fact that although such a patient cannot recall or recognize something once well within his knowledge, he may be able to reproduce it under hypnosis or in other facilitating circumstances: it may appear in his confabulations, or serve to shorten materially the time required to relearn it. An emotionally shattering experience can either distort (as in confabulation) or have the effect of repressing (as in amnesia) the recall of the event as a historical occurrence, and can operate outside consciousness to exaggerate or build upon those disturbances of memory which are the direct result of damage to cerebral structures. Striking instances of this have been reported in the Korsakoff syndrome after a suicidal attempt at strangulation: and it is, of course, a well-known aspect of retrograde amnesia after head injury.

Forgetting

But these catathymic influences are by no means the whole story. No one would now dispute that forgetting is an active process, not a mere passive fading with the lapse of time. There is, it is true, a curve of forgetting in which, as Ebbinghaus showed us, a rapid fall immediately after learning is succeeded by a general flattening out as the interval is extended. But the matter is more complex than this – and certainly more complex than our clinical methods of examination allow for. Although retention declines generally in proportion to the log of time, there can be considerable differences in the rate of decline, which will depend on the initial strength of the memory trace and of the factors which annul it. The latter

are what chiefly concern us in pathological disturbances of memory. The strength of trace, however, will, both in normal and in Korsakoff subjects, itself depend on the success of the initial learning or perception, on the amount of repetition, i.e. relearning, on the kind of thing learnt or perceived, and the vividness of the initial experience to be remembered. It may also be reinforced by verbal formulation on the patient's part.

Among the factors which can annul the traces of a past experience and so prevent its recall, interference from a succeeding event has had the most attention from psychologists. This retroactive inhibition is most clearly in evidence when the two events are tasks in which the subject has to learn different responses to the same, or similar, stimuli: it is a laboratory phenomenon, which may or may not occur also when the casual events of daily life succeed one another. Whether it could be accountable for the amnesia of Korsakoff states was experimentally tested by Talland (1959) in the elaborate studies he has made in Professor Raymond Adams' department. The subjects were 14 women and 6 men with well-established alcoholic Korsakoff states: there was a control series of 23 alcoholic and neurological patients. The subjects were asked to learn words – 15 nonsense syllables and 20 real words – printed on cards and shown to them for three minutes each: they were then asked to recall as many of the words as they could. Then they were either given the same list to relearn or they were given a matched series of words and the procedure repeated for this list, after which they were tested with the first list again, to see whether the second learning task had interfered with the first. A similar procedure was followed in tests of recognition. The control group showed an increase in the number of syllables or words correctly recalled when they had had to relearn the same list, but this gain was reduced when a second, matched list had been interposed and the subject required to memorize it: in other words, in the control subjects there was clear evidence of retroactive inhibition. But the Korsakoff patients showed no gain in relearning, and no retroactive interference effects, whether tested by reproduction or recognition. It can be concluded that in Korsakoff patients who have a residual though poor, capacity for learning and retention, there is no evidence to suggest that their forgetting can be attributed to retroactive inhibition. Whether the converse phenomenon of reminiscence – improved recall after an interval of rest – occurs in Korsakoff patients has not, as far as I know, been investigated.

Another approach to the problem of forgetting has been by relating it to extinction (Woodworth & Schlosberg 1954). There are conspicuous differences between the two processes, of course,

4

but there are also similarities, notable in the way that an extinguished conditioned response can be spontaneously recovered after an interval. Without entering into a controversial field, it is worth recalling that in eyelid response conditioning to a buzzer, with a puff of air as the unconditioned stimulus, Korsakoff patients have shown abnormally rapid extinction; they also, as one would expect, were much less able to form conditioned responses in the first place. This was demonstrated in the study made by Horsley Gantt & Muncie (1942) of a series of Korsakoff patients. The unconditioned stimulus was a painful faradic shock, the conditioned stimulus a light or sound. The experiments confirmed the importance of 'set', especially when reinforced by the patient's verbal formulation of what is happening, and they showed that a Korsakoff patient's ability to form conditioned responses is roughly proportionate to the severity of his clinical condition.

Distinctiveness of the Syndrome
In any survey of the problems of the amnesic syndrome, it is paradoxically evident that, remarkable and characteristic as are the clinical anomalies in this condition – the contrast, for instance, between the patients' retained verbal facility and his profound disturbance of memory – yet systematic examination of his memory reveals only quantitative differences between him and a healthy person of the same age. The extent of the quantitative differences can indeed be enormous, but still it is possible to detect in normal people the same essential phenomena occurring sporadically: we all have unexpected and unexplained lapses of memory, we all develop paramnesias, we all confabulate and have occasional disturbances in our time-attribution and sequence; even retrograde amnesia can be observed in healthy people after a severe emotional upheaval. The cognate similarity in quality, in spite of coarse and obtrusive differences in pattern and corrigibility, may be found between hysterical amnesia and some features of the organic amnesic syndrome. I do not mean to say anything so absurd as that a patient with hysterical amnesia exhibits the typical phenomena of a Korsakoff patient, but I suggest that there is nothing in the known psychopathology of hysterical amnesia which has not been observed in the organic cerebral syndrome. A dramatic instance was supplied by my patient (Lewis 1953) with partly arrested G.P.I. and a severe amnesic syndrome, periodically aggravated. He had developed, while in the United States, such apparently psychogenic dissociation that his amnesia was wholly attributed to this by an experienced observer, an authority on the psychological effects of brain damage, who wrote a book about this patient's symptoms and

psychopathology; they were there interpreted as wholly hysterical (Franz 1933).

If we concede these points of close similarity between the psychopathology of the organic amnesic syndrome and that of the hysterical-dissociative dysmnesia, as well as between these and the psychology of normal forgetting, we will want to examine what is known, or theorized, about the substrate of the amnesic syndrome and of normal remembering and forgetting. It would be in the hope, not that precise correspondence would emerge, but that a terra firma would be established on which the data of behaviour and process could be securely placed. A psychopathology that does not take full account of related physiological and pathological neural phenomena is riskily unmoored and unballasted. But there is also a notorious danger in trying to pass from psychological to physiological and anatomical data. Lashley said that 'we seem little nearer to an understanding of the nature of memory trace than was Descartes'. It is startling, after that, to turn to what Descartes actually wrote about his understanding of the nature of the memory trace: 'When the soul wills to recall something, this volition, by causing the pineal gland to bend successively now to one side and now to another, impels the spirit towards this and that region of the brain, until they come upon the part where the traces left by the object we will to recall are found. These traces consist in the manner in which the animal spirits, owing to the paths they have taken on the presence of that object, have so modified the pores of the brain that these have acquired a greater facility than the others of being opened in that same fashion when the spirits again come towards them'. If in truth we are little nearer than Descartes was to understanding the nature of memory trace, we had better be rather cautious in our conjectures about what has happened in the brain to make memory traces as scanty and inaccessible as they are in the amnesic syndrome.

Cerebral Substrate
There is now a consensus of opinion that in the Korsakoff syndrome, as in Wernicke's encephalopathy, degenerative changes are regularly and primarily found in the pericentricular and periaqueductal grey matter, the corpora mamillaria, the dorsal medial nucleus of the thalamus and to some extent in the brain-stem and cerebellum. Essential connexions between these areas, the cornu ammonis and the cingulate cortex, have been postulated and given functional significance, on the lines which Papez (1937) and, more recently, MacLean (1958) and others have emphasized. But the discrepancies between the results of ablation in human beings and animals, and the

diverse functions which these systems are believed to subserve – motivation, emotion, memory, execution of complex sequences of action – impose caution. It seems premature to assume that because the corpora mamillaria and other rhinencephalic structures show degenerative changes in the Korsakoff state, we can therefore assign to these cell-aggregates and their connexions a direct responsibility for serving the functions of memory. Brierley (1961) in his recent review of the correspondence between neuropathological findings and defect of recent memory, concluded that there are two groups of cells, not necessarily acting in unison, which are essential for remembering – the cortical group in the hippocampi and a hypothalamic group in the mamillary bodies: and he drew attention, as others have, to the extensive pathways entering and leaving these areas and linking them to the fornix. What features of the memory function depend on the integrity of either of these areas and projections it is scarcely possible to say. Penfield (1958) is sometimes invoked in support of the view that retention and recall are located in the mesial temporal cortex. His observations are very well known but it is only fair to remark that he disavows knowing how and where the recording of memory impressions takes place: he goes no further than to say that somewhere in the brain there is a 'pathway of synaptic and ganglionic facilitations which linger on after a present experience has faded into the past' leaving a record of experience which has been activated in certain of his patients by rhythmic electrical impulses delivered to the superior and lateral surfaces of the temporal cortex: he suspects that the 'ganglionic patterns of experience' are in the hippocampi. That is probably as far as anyone might go in localizing memory, at present.

I have referred to these anatomical and physiological aspects of memory only because psychopathology, however boldly independent, has to modify its formulations whenever some clear correspondence is established between physical events and psychological events. But such clear correspondence has not yet been demonstrated and the seeker after truth is confronted by a rapidly changing array of concepts borrowed from information – theory and biology. There are curious and ironical similarities between some of the recent attempts to interpret the memory process in terms of synaptic facilitation (Burns 1958) and the speculations of Freud in 1895 on the same subject. Freud postulated two sorts of neurons – 'permeable' neurons, which subserve perception, and 'impermeable' neurons, i.e. neurons in which excitation does not pass readily across the 'contact-barriers' and which subserve memory. The latter neurons are permanently

affected by an excitation, so that facilitation occurs, making their 'contact-barriers' more permeable to the spread of such excitation (Freud 1954). Interesting and ingenious as was Freud's development of this neurologizing theory, I shall not quote it further; it serves, however, as a reminder of the perennial fascination of conjectures about the substrate of normal and disturbed memory.

Hysterical Amnesia
It would seem odd for a psychiatrist to finish even a very brief talk about amnesia without a further word on hysteria. Hysterical amnesia can be such a spectacular affair, and the instances of 'multiple personality' due to it are so arresting – when well told – that it gets more attention than its frequency warrants. Out of 1,259 patients admitted between April 1959 and March 1960 to a hospital receiving psychiatric emergencies in London, 58 had the organic-amnesic syndrome, but there were only 2 patients admitted during the year because of hysterical amnesia for the details of their personal identity and experience. During the last five years only 12 such patients were admitted to the hospital in question. Gross hysterical amnesia is in fact rather a rare condition. But there is a stronger reason than rarity for dealing with it summarily in a discussion of amnesic syndromes: it hardly belongs there. It is in a sense misleading to call it amnesia, for in these people, as Henri Ey (1950) has rightly said, we are dealing not with a circumscribed disorder of memory, but with a disturbance of synthesis which engages the whole personality. The War provided crude examples of the phenomenon, less spectacular than the dramatic cases reported in the last century and again lately, but clearly demonstrating that a personality-reaction rather than an isolated amnesia was here evident. The treatment was correspondingly distinct in its aims and effect. It is true that in the organic-amnesic syndrome the characteristic disorder of memory is associated with other anomalies of mental function; it is not really an isolated amnesia and nothing more. But there is, as Korsakoff so strongly emphasized, a startling contrast between the severity of the memory deficit in this condition and the excellence of other cognitive functions, especially those concerned with the use of words. The contrasts which obtrude in the mental state of hysterical dissociation are of another order and they can be abolished.

I am sorry that this brief review is inconclusive. Experimental psychology, neurophysiology, psychiatry, neurology and neurosurgery have all been depositing offerings, large and small, towards the solution of the fascinating, perplexing problems of psychopathology which the amnesic syndrome

6

presents. But these contributions are still far removed from synthesis or certainty. There is enough stir and movement around the subject to make a propitious turmoil: not so lively a turmoil perhaps as Freud once made with his exploration of the arcana of forgetting, but stimulating and suggestive enough to promise real advances.

REFERENCES

Bartlett F C (1932) Remembering. Cambridge

Bonhoeffer K (1904) *Allg. Z. Psychiat.* **61**, 744

Brierley J B (1961) *Gerontol. clin.* **3**, 97

Brodmann K
    (1902) *J. Psychol. Neurol., Lpz.* **1**, 225
    (1904) *J. Psychol. Neurol., Lpz.* **3**, 1

Bürger-Prinz H & Kaila M (1930) *Z. ges. Neurol. Psychiat.* **124**, 553

Burns B D (1958) The Mammalian Cerebral Cortex. London

Ehrenwald H (1931) *Z. ges. Neurol. Psychiat.* **134**, 512

Ey H (1950) Les Troubles de la Mémoire. (Études Psychiatriques: Étude No 9); Paris

Flament J (1957) *Acta Neurol. belg.* **57**, 119

Franz S I (1933) Persons One and Three. A Study in Multiple Personalities. New York.

Freud S (1954) The Origins of Psychoanalysis: Project for a Scientific Psychology. London

Gantt W H & Muncie W
    (1942) *Bull. Johns Hopk. Hosp.* **70**, 467

Gregor A (1909) *Mschr. Psychiat. Neurol.* **25**, 218, 330

Grünthal E (1924) *Z. ges. Neurol. Psychiat.* **92**, 255

Hartmann H (1930) *Z. ges. Neurol. Psychiat.* **126**, 496

Janet P (1898) Névroses et Idées Fixes. Paris. Vol 1, Ch 3

Köppen M & Kutzinski A (1910) Systematische Beobachtungen über die Wiedergabe kleiner Erzählungen durch Geisteskranke. Berlin

Korsakoff S S (1890) *Rev. psychol.* **21**, 669

Krauss S (1930) *Arch. ges. Psychol.* **77**, 469

Lewis A J (1953) *Mschr. Psychiat. Neurol.* **125**, 589

Lidz T (1942) *Arch. Neurol. Psychiat.*, Chicago **47**, 588

Lindberg B J (1946) *Acta psychiat., Kbh.* **21**, 497

MacLean P D (1958) *J. nerv. ment. Dis.* **127**, 1

Mouren P P & Felician J (1958) *Ann. méd.-psychol.* **116**, 664

Nyssen R (1957) *Acta neurol. belg.* **57**, 639

Papez J W (1937) *Arch. Neurol. Psychiat.*, Chicago **38**, 725

Penfield W (1958) In: Ciba Foundation Symposium on the Neurological Basis of Behaviour. Ed. G E W Wolstenholme & M O'Connor. London; p 149

Pick A (1915) *Z. ges. Neurol. Psychiat.* **28**, 344

Rey A (1959) *Arch. Psychol.*, Genève **37**, 126

Russell W R (1959) Brain, Memory, Learning. Oxford

Russell W R & Nathan P (1946) *Brain* **69**, 280

Schneider K (1912) *Z. ges. Neurol. Psychiat.* **8**, 553

Talland G A
    (1958) *J. nerv. ment. Dis.* **127**, 197
    (1959) *J. abnorm. (soc.) Psychol.* **59**, 10

Talland G A & Ekdahl M (1959) *J. nerv. ment. Dis.* **129**, 391

Talland G A & Miller A (1959) *J. abnorm. (soc.) Psychol.* **58**, 235

van der Horst L (1932) *Mschr. Psychiat. Neurol.* **83**, 65
    (1956) *Evolut. Psychiat.* **1**, 189

Whitty C W M & Lewin W (1960) *Brain* **83**, 648

Williams M & Zangwill O L (1950) *J. ment. Sci.* **96**, 484

Woodworth R S & Schlosberg H
    (1954) Experimental Psychology. London

RESEARCH AND ITS APPLICATION
IN PSYCHIATRY

I appreciate the honour of delivering the Maurice Bloch Lecture in this University, and I would like to take as my text a passage from the lectures of William Cullen, who taught medicine here in Glasgow two hundred years ago. He said: ' I am persuaded that diligent inquiry and a cautious collation of facts will bring out some instruction from the most dark and intricate subjects; and in particular on the Vesaniae (or disorders of the mind) I think we have obtained something to relieve us in part from the random empirical practice which has hitherto prevailed.' Psychiatry has advanced a good deal since then, and it has been furthered by two main influences—first by diligent enquiry, as Cullen said, and secondly by the spread of humane regard for the mentally ill. During long stretches of history there was little or no research into mental disorder, and instead of humane understanding there was fear and the cruelty that grows out of fear. But in the last two centuries progress has been achieved that is impressive when viewed against the background of preceding ignorance and superstition, though it is still inadequate, and meagre in comparison with some other medical advances. I shall not attempt to review its achievements but rather outline the varieties of approach in psychiatric research, and the

8

factors that seem to have favoured, or hindered, the progress of psychiatric knowledge and its application in daily life.

Research, as everyone knows, is the expression of controlled and perceptive curiosity, using every means available to it, but ultimately resting on some assumptions about the verifiability of data and the logic of refutation. It is the outcome of a habit of mind (Darwin said it was a method of ' habitually searching for the causes and meaning of everything which occurs ') and is not the monopoly of professional scientists. The distinction between fundamental research and applied research is not a satisfactory one : often it means no more than that the bearing of the so-called fundamental research on practical problems is not yet apparent, or is not apparent to inexpert observers. There is no research finding so fundamental or so remote that it cannot be used for human purposes : sometimes it looks as though the more abstract and the more isolated from practical affairs it is, the more effective will it be in eventual usefulness or harm. It is convenient, therefore, to think in terms not of fundamental research and applied research, but of knowledge gained through research, and the application of such knowledge to meet specific needs. In psychiatry the final application will be the prevention and the treatment of specific forms of mental illness.

These are very general considerations. It will be as well to pass from them to some detailed instances which illustrate the stages of psychiatric research and, more particularly, of its application to meet the

9

medical needs of individuals and of the community.

I hope you will allow me to recapitulate briefly the history of two efficacious methods of treatment.

Early in the 19th century a disease was described in which impairment of memory, disturbance of speech, incomplete general paralysis and final dementia were prominent features. Many authorities disputed that this was an independent disease and preferred to regard it as a complication of other forms of mental disorder. Demonstration of inflammatory changes in the brain and meninges of these patients, however, established its identity. Then psychiatrists turned their attention to its causes ; constitution, heredity, mental stress, excessive drinking, violent passions, debauchery, and sustained intellectual effort were all blamed. There were, however, a few men who from the 'sixties insisted that syphilis was the indispensable cause of this disease : the much greater frequency of a history of syphilis in those who had the disease than in other psychotic patients was their main argument. A subsidiary argument was provided by a hardy investigator in Vienna who inoculated syphilitic material into nine patients who had general paralysis, and as they did not develop syphilis he inferred that they all had an immunity to it conferred by a previous infection. The authorities did not like his experiment and he nearly went to gaol. By the beginning of the twentieth century syphilis was generally credited with being the main but not the indispensable cause of this disease. Sir Thomas Clouston, for example, in his Clinical Lectures in 1904, said

10

there was one cause above all others, viz. syphilis, and two exciting or contributory causes, viz. sexual excess and alcoholic intemperance. ' If hard work, muscular or mental, with a stimulating diet of flesh, are combined with these, then we have an additional liability.' But in his next sentence he went on to declare: ' I cannot agree that syphilis is the sole cause always, because I have had many cases in which the existence of personal syphilis was excluded by every sort of reliable evidence. Mental shocks and strains of all sorts will of themselves cause the disease. There is a certain temperament that predisposes to it—the intensely sanguine ', and he adduced the story of two identical twins with the disease, which, he said, showed conclusively that heredity may predispose to it.

The Wassermann test for syphilis, discovered in 1906, proved positive in the blood and cerebro-spinal fluid of such a very high proportion of persons with general paralysis that it became a criterion of correct diagnosis. The case for regarding general paralysis as a consequence of syphilis was by now almost irresistible, but there were many who argued that it was what they called a metasyphilitic or parasyphilitic condition, by which they meant that it was a complication or sequel to syphilis rather than a straightforward syphilitic affection of the central nervous system. The evidence for the latter view was, as you will recognise, a statistically confirmed association between syphilis and this psychiatric disease: and those who questioned the conclusion said that they must have direct evidence of the

11

infection being active in the brain before they would concede any causal nexus. Their attitude was, in essentials, very like that of the people who today refuse to believe in the causal nexus between cigarette smoking and cancer of the lung.

In 1913 Noguchi supplied the desired link in the chain of testimony: he found the spirochaete, the organism responsible for syphilis, in the brain of patients who had died of general paralysis of the insane.

So far so good. The disease had been defined, its characteristics and pathology demonstrated, its diagnosis made certain, and its essential cause pinned down. All this had taken a century to accomplish. But the course of illness was still inevitably tragic, reducing the patient's mental and physical powers until he died of the disease. It could not be arrested or improved, nor could it be prevented by medical means. It was very doubtful whether prompt treatment of the original infection could avert the development of general paralysis; indeed many investigators suspected that early treatment might have promoted the location of the spirochaete in the relatively inaccessible fastnesses of the central nervous system. There was, obviously, a great gap in our knowledge. Besides the outstanding need to know how to treat and how to prevent the disease, there was ignorance as to the other elements in causation, particularly those responsible for the fact that of the people who contracted syphilis only a minority developed general paralysis, and for the evident differences in form and frequency of the

12

disease at different times or in different countries.

Once it had been established that general paralysis is a syphilitic condition, treatment by methods effective in treating systematic syphilis were vigorously applied to it. When they failed, ingenious modifications, designed to meet the special anatomical and physiological conditions of the central nervous system, were tried, but the results were again disappointing. Success came by following another, less logical road.

Long before general paralysis had been recognised as a disease, careful observers had noted that mental illnesses sometimes cleared up dramatically when the sufferer developed some infectious fever: among those recorded in the nineteenth century were patients with paralysis who improved after they had contracted erysipelas. Then a Russian psychiatrist, to oblige a bacteriological colleague, between 1864 and 1875 inoculated with relapsing fever twenty-two patients suffering from various psychoses; several of them recovered from their psychoses. He reported this in a prominent German psychiatric journal but took the precaution of using an assumed name. Not long after, a young Austrian psychiatrist called Wagner Jauregg wrote, while still in his twenties, a comprehensive review of all the published instances in which an intercurrent infection had caused improvement or recovery from a psychosis, and he affirmed that the evidence warranted the artificial production of fever as treatment for psychotic illness. Accordingly, in 1888 he tried using erysipelas, but the infection did not take. He next employed other means of producing fever, and, persisting through the years, he gradually came to depend on tuberculin, especially in general paralysis—the psychosis on which he concentrated his efforts from 1900 onwards. His results were not regarded by psychiatrists elsewhere as good enough to justify systematic adoption of this method of treatment, and he had to put up with some vilification in his own country. Convinced nevertheless that he was on the right track, he seized the opportunity afforded by the First World War to inoculate with benign tertian malaria nine patients who had general paralysis. This was in 1917. The results were good, and in spite of some misfortunes the malarial treatment was thereafter adopted on a large scale and in many countries : Wagner Jauregg received the Nobel Prize. One may ask why a method that had been advocated by him for so long but little regarded by others was now so speedily accepted. I think the main factors were two : (1) Influential and energetic support was given by Weygandt and Nonne, very prominent German psychiatrists, who promptly tried the method out, found it effectual, and proclaimed it *urbi et orbi*, so that it was quickly taken up also by psychiatrists in Frankfurt and Munich and then in other countries. (2) The second factor was the success which two other investigators reported in 1919 from the use of relapsing fever, which they had tried for quite different reasons from those that actuated Wagner Jauregg. Their theoretical assumption was that immunity produced against one spirochaetal infection (relapsing fever) might prevent the spread or

14

continued activity of the syphilitic spirochaete in the brain, much as cowpox protects against smallpox.

There was, further, an atmosphere immediately after the war which seemed more adventurous and receptive to these drastic attempts to drive out one disease with another than that which prevailed in the calmer days before 1914. Many other lines of research into general paralysis have been followed besides those I have mentioned, and research in quite other fields led to the superseding of malaria by penicillin : but the historical sequence I have outlined provides a telling example of how tributaries and confluents feed the stream of psychiatric research, and how such research can in the long run promote the health of the community.

The first stage was entirely clinical : a disease was recognised and delineated : out of the poorly differentiated mass of conditions called melancholia, mania, phrenitis and dementia a particular disorder was enucleated, and its course, its clinical features and its macroscopic pathology defined. We are so accustomed to look to the laboratory for advances in knowledge that the contribution of clinical observers, men like Sydenham and Boerhaave and Cullen, is often underrated. If general paralysis had not been delimited, the other advances I have sketched out would have been delayed, and we might have floundered among a confusing medley of heterogeneous conditions, grouped in one huge class : that is, unfortunately, to some extent still the case with schizophrenia. The abilities required for genuine nosological discoveries are very considerable, and a great physician-philosopher, John Locke, recognised this. ' I see it is easier ', he wrote, ' and more natural for men to build castles in the air of their own, than to survey well those that are to be found standing. Nicely to observe the History of Diseases, in all their changes and circumstances, is a work of Time, accurateness, Attention and Judgement."

But although the disease general paralysis had been clinically delimited, its recognition in the early stages remained difficult. This obstacle was sur-mounted by contributions from the laboratory—in particular the discovery of the Wassermann test for syphilis. The pathology of the disease was illumin-ated by the findings of microscopic morbid anatomy, and the microscope also played the major part in putting the syphilitic nature of the disease beyond doubt. The application of the new knowledge acquired by research up to this stage had been confined to diagnosis and prognosis. A pragmatist —the sort of man of whom Bacon said ' When men build any science and theory upon Experiment, they almost always turn with premature and hasty zeal to practice. . . . Hence, like Atalanta, they leave the course to pick up the golden apple, interrupting their speed, and giving up the victory '—such a man might have urged that until the new knowledge could be applied to treatment or prevention of the disease, it must be regarded as barren knowledge, the product of an intellectually satisfying set of exercises which had no discernible bearing on human well-being.

Wagner Jauregg's discovery disposed of this. But

16

he stood on his predecessors' shoulders. If all their research had not been accomplished, his original inference and his insight into the therapeutic possibilities of artificial fever might have led to nothing conclusive : it would have been shipwrecked, as the efforts of other have been shipwrecked, on the shoals of uncertain diagnosis and alternative explanations. Thirty years lay between his formulation of the therapeutic plan and its fulfilment: during those thirty years the way was being prepared for him to define his aim so narrowly that he could succeed— and not only succeed, but succeed in a way that left no room for doubt.

It is clear that the time had to be ripe; his intuition based on clinical observations had been correct, but premature attempts to apply it gave results which, though they confirmed him in his conviction and his hope, did not avail to convince others.

That the time was ripe between 1917 and 1920 is attested not only by his success but by other signs. There was intense interest in diverse efforts to treat general paralysis. A different artificial fever treatment was developed—viz. inoculation with relapsing fever—based on quite a different theoretical assumption. Prominent neuropsychiatrists, forsaking their reserved attitude, approved Wagner Jauregg's method enthusiastically: it was being adopted all over the world within two or three years after the report of his successes in 1917. This receptiveness bespeaks both the force of the evidence and the readiness of the times to receive it. This need not be

17

attributed to some mysterious force, the Zeitgeist or Kairos, but rather to the social circumstances, the researches that had gone before, and the technological advances that created a social and scientific setting propitious for making such a discovery. The American sociologist, R. K. Merton, has put forward with much cogency his reasons for believing that the prevailing social conditions, as well as the presence of a man of genius, are responsible for a scientific discovery being made at a particular time or in a particular country. It is through this sociological approach (rather than through the customary psychological approach, which concentrates on the mental equipment of the discoverer) that he explains the well known fact of multiple discovery, i.e. two, or more, scientists making the same discovery, quite independently and possibly working from very different premises and observations. Darwin and Alfred Russell Wallace, Le Verrier and Adams, Newton and Leibnitz—the list of co-discoveries is very long and makes it hard to deny the force of Professor Merton's argument. It holds good, I think, for the sequence of researches which culminated in effective treatment of general paralysis.

Malarial treatment was not, of course, the last word in that story: penicillin supplanted artificial fever, and must be given the credit not only for the modern method of treating the disease but also for preventing it, since from a scourge general paralysis has within a generation become a rare disease.

I should like to pass now to a shorter history, the development of a method of treatment more recent than the use of artificial fever. The method is the induction of seizures, often called 'electric shock treatment'. Early in the 1930's a few psychiatrists in Germany and Hungary were interested in a rather abstract problem: when schizophrenics have epileptiform attacks, does this indicate the accidental concurrence of two diseases, epilepsy and schizophrenia, or is there some closer intrinsic or 'biological' connection between the two seemingly distinct diseases? Their inquiries led them to conclude that the concurrence of epilepsy and schizophrenia was decidedly rare, and that when a schizophrenic patient began to have fits, it improved his chances of improving or recovering. Pursuing this line of thought, and connecting it with some observations he had made in the laboratory, a young Hungarian, Meduna, arrived at the idea, not very remote in kind from Wagner Jauregg's, that there was an inherent or, as he called it, biological antagonism between schizophrenia and epilepsy, such that if fits were induced in the schizophrenic patient metabolic changes would occur which might reduce the schizophrenic disturbance greatly. On this theoretical, decidedly shaky, foundation he built his therapeutic plan, which depended on the intravenous injection of a convulsive drug. He was obliged to consider first the moral justifications of his proposed experiment. Having come to terms with his conscience, he carried out, in 1934, the treatment of 25 schizophrenic patients: by 1937 he had treated 110, of whom 54 had completely recovered from their mental illness. The first report of his work in 1935

19

excited little attention but, by 1938, when his monograph had appeared and been discussed at an international conference in Berne, it was being widely tried out ; and it soon vied with insulin coma treatment for schizophrenia, which had been developed at about the same time but along an entirely different line of thought and experiment.

While this was going on, in Genoa the Professor of Neuropsychiatry, Cerletti, was interested in an academic problem in pathology : are the known changes in the Ammon's horn region of the brain in epileptics the pathological basis of repeated convulsions or merely the consequence of the convulsions? To determine the point he induced fits in dogs by passing an electric current through the brain, without otherwise harming the dog or endangering its life. In due course he was appointed Professor in Rome, and there he introduced into his clinic Meduna's method of bringing about convulsions in schizophrenic patients by the injection of a drug, cardiazol. It occurred to him that instead of the injection of cardiazol the passage of an electric current, with proper safeguards, would be a better method. But he decided that the risk of accidental electrocution ruled it out as unjustifiable. Some further experiments, however, were made possible—by what he called a lucky accident—at the Rome abattoirs, and in the course of these he satisfied himself that passage of the electric current across the head of large animals, for example pigs, could be made quite safely. He therefore substituted this method— without ill effects—for the cardiazol method in

20

treating schizophrenic patients, and it was rapidly adopted elsewhere so that from 1938 or 1939 it largely replaced the cardiazol procedure, being equally effective and technically preferable. Electric convulsive therapy has had a conspicuous place ever since in the therapeutics of mental disorder : it has, however, become clear that its optimum field of action is not schizophrenia but depressive conditions, and that the hypothesised antagonism between epilepsy and schizophrenia cannot be substantiated.

Here, then, we have what sounds like a comedy of errors, diversified by lucky accidents and with a happy paradox as its epilogue. But, at bottom, it is a consecutive tale. Meduna began his experiments by using camphor as the convulsant drug, for which he later substituted cardiazol. In the eighteenth and even the nineteenth centuries, camphor was one of the drugs most recommended for its beneficial effect upon mental disorder, especially when pushed to the point of causing convulsions. This method was particularly favoured in Central Europe, but was also advocated in France and England : thus Samuel Simmons, the much travelled physician who looked after George III for a time during the later phases of his psychosis, advised that camphor should be pushed to the point where the patients would fall to the ground in a convulsion, after which their reason would be mostly restored; in some this happened only after the second paroxysm had been thus brought about. So Meduna's method was not as revolutionary as it seemed, and in Hungary lingering traditions of the camphor treatment could have obscurely influenced Meduna. At all events, the absorbing local concern with epilepsy in the Budapest Clinic ensured ready interest in such an experiment as Meduna's, which might have been very difficult to undertake in a less propitious environment. The chain of events that led Professor Cerletti in Rome to switch to the electrical technique was also more consequent than it seemed : his own spirited account divides it very fairly into the three stages—a preparatory period, devoted to study of the conditions for producing safe convulsions in dogs by means of electrical stimulation of the brain ; a second period in which he was aided by contact with some colleagues who provided him with other animals than dogs on whom to test the margin of safety ; and a final period during which he applied to human beings the idea that had been maturing and given shape during the earlier phases. Its application was not for Professor Cerletti the end of a road, but a passage opening the way to further research.

It is tempting to multiply examples of the very diverse routes followed in psychiatric research, and to see how social and psychological factors were at work in particular studies, determining their course and the vicissitudes of their application to medical practice. But the two examples I have mentioned are, I think, sufficient to indicate that no single approach can be recognised in the processes of psychiatric research. If I had taken instances from psychopathology or psychotherapy, or from genetics, it would have been still more evident.

Certain favourable conditions for advance can be

discerned. Technological advances, as Ogburn has taught us, can be immensely powerful stimuli to innovation and progress. When psychiatrists are closely in touch with people conducting research in other medical or scientific fields, and are not isolated in groups wholly engaged in clinical routine, and when they are men whose training and interests are of a kind to make them ready to consider new information and to see old information in a new light, the chances that a train of discovery will be fired are high. A man's education, the facilities available to him, adequate economic support, advances in other branches of science, and informed criticism are as valuable, or indispensable, in the advancement of psychiatry as of any other field of knowledge. In psychiatry just criticism is perhaps even more valuable than in older, solidly established subjects like the natural sciences. By criticism I do not mean fault-finding but expert judgment and appraisal. It is perhaps true, as Bacon wrote, that ' by far the greatest obstacle to the advancement of the sciences and the undertaking of any new attempt or department is to be found in men's despair and the idea of Impossibility. For men of a prudent and exact turn of thought are altogether diffident in matters of this nature, considering the obscurity of Nature, the shortness of Life, the deception of the Senses, and weakness of the Judgement. They think therefore that . . . when (the Sciences) have attained a certain degree and condition they can proceed no further.' Clearly such a frame of mind is inimical to research : but in the history of psychiatry the harm and waste that can be laid at the door of pessimistic nihilists, such as Bacon has in mind, is not more, I believe, than that attributable to the uncriticised extravagances of mistaken enthusiasts.

This has sometimes been painfully evident when a new idea or a new finding was applied to the treatment of mentally ill patients. The stumbling-blocks in the way of evaluating the success of a new method of treatment are great ; often in psychiatry the course which a disease would have followed if untreated is hard to determine in the individual case, the correct measurement of significant changes in the patient's mental health is difficult, and the conduct of a therapeutic experiment faces ethical and practical dilemmas. It is therefore now widely recognised that a poorly controlled trial of a new method of psychiatric treatment, or a confident claim based only on clinical impressions, demands severe criticism.

In science generally the application of new knowledge has over most of recorded history been a tardy process. Innovations have been subject to a cultural lag, which could extend over as much as a century or two. However, as we come closer to our time, the lag in applying scientific discoveries has become steadily shorter, and now the interval, in some technological fields, has become frighteningly short. Lord Stamp in 1937 proposed that there should be a moratorium on invention until the lag had been overcome and society had caught up with the inventions already available. In 1962 we might wish to impose such a moratorium for the opposite reason ; for some inventions are developed and

24

applied to practical ends much too quickly for our peace of mind, and we would like to see the social sciences advancing and being applied, to keep pace with the physical sciences and to cope with the destructive possibilities that the application of the physical sciences to warfare has disclosed.

In psychiatry, however, as in medicine as a whole, no serious lag now occurs in the application of new methods of treatment. On the contrary, new techniques are promptly espoused, unless there are social or administrative hindrances. We have seen this in the case of prefrontal leucotomy, widely employed for some years—except in Russia, where its use was forbidden. Prompt use of new treatment is likewise evident as new varieties of ' tranquilliser ' or ' anti-depressant ' are steadily brought forward and widely prescribed. If a new therapeutic procedure is complicated, or has disadvantages in the form of undesired side-effects, it will of course take longer to get into general use, or will be kept in the hands of those who are expert in it, until it has been modified so that its administration no longer calls for special skill or precautions. The use of induced malaria was more restricted, for this reason, than that of penicillin ; the induction of convulsions by intravenous injection of cardiazol was a more exacting procedure than the electrical method ; and among the many factors that have militated against the general use of psychoanalysis must be reckoned the complexity of the method, which puts it outside the scope of those who have not had appropriate special training.

When a research finding has been applied widely

25

in treatment and found efficacious, the subsequent fate of the new procedure will often depend on whether a simpler or a more effective method becomes available to supersede it. Its fate may also be influenced by extraneous social factors such as have been responsible for the extraordinary waxing and waning of the popularity of hypnosis as a form of treatment during the two hundred years it has been before the world. As Pierre Janet put it in 1925, the rapid rise and precipitous decline of hypnotism, which has been witnessed more than once, has had very little to do with its efficacy as a form of psychotherapy; it has had a great deal to do with transient medical and other fashions, social unrest, and swings towards the romantic or the sceptical approach to life and literature.

Other influences that may retard the application of research in psychiatry are familiar in the history of science: there may be collision with accepted religious, moral or philosophical ideas, or exposure to the incredulity of other scientists when they are faced with a conclusion that is at variance with their strongest preconceptions. We have only to recall the opposition Darwin's theory encountered, or the storm aroused by Freud's theory. A further ground of repudiation is that the propounder of some new idea is ill-qualified to speak on the subject because he is not properly trained or fit to intrude into the expert field in question: this may, of course, be true, but there are occasions when it is an irrelevant, though none the less damaging, accusation. Philippe Pinel, one of the greatest of psychiatrists, expressed himself well on this matter. 'Il importe en médecine, comme dans les autres sciences, de compter pour beaucoup un jugement sain, une sagacité naturelle, un esprit inventif dépouillé de tout autre privilège. Il ne faut pas s'informer si tel homme a fait certaines études d'usage, ou rempli certaines formalités, mais seulement s'il a approfondi quelques parties de la science médicale ou s'il a decouvert quelques vérités utiles.'

Because of the harm done by irrational resistance and the delay in the application of discoveries, we have come to regard receptiveness to new ideas and promptitude in applying them as a virtue. For the most part this may well be so, but, as the example of leucotomy reminds us, excessive zeal can be worse than wary hesitancy, and enthusiasm can once more show itself as the friend of action but the enemy of wisdom. Moreover the propagation of a new set of ideas can exert a disturbing and even disruptive effect on social standards and on the equilibrium of an established order of society : adjustment may then be painful and protracted, and not unlike adjustment to the clash of cultures which occurs when a preliterate society is exposed to Western ways and values. Philosophy and literature have on occasion influenced society drastically in the past : today science and medicine can do so. It is generally believed that psychoanalysis, as a theory of human behaviour, has exercised a powerful influence on the general outlook and personal conduct of contemporary people. He would be a confident student of human affairs who ventured to say where this effect could be traced most clearly, and whether it had been beneficial or baneful :

I suggest only that the introduction of a new system of ideas—and their zealous application in psychiatric or other treatment—may carry implications that go far beyond the medical sphere.

Advances in medical treatment are not a benefit to be proffered or withheld from the public by medical decision alone. Obviously the research worker who makes a discovery publishes it, unless there are some very special reasons why he should not; and its application to therapeutic purposes is for the most part a technical matter on which the clinical scientist is the person best qualified to pass judgement. Equally obviously the individual patient, or his relatives, are entitled to refuse the new treatment, no matter how enticing it is, or to accept it, no matter how daunting it may be. The decision is theirs, and is often surprising. As Oliver Wendell Holmes colourfully put it 'There is nothing men will not do, there is nothing they have not done, to recover their health and save their lives. They have submitted to be half-drowned in water and half-choked with gases, to be buried up to their chins in earth, to be seared with hot irons like galley-slaves, to be crimped with knives like cod-fish, to have needles stuck into their flesh and bonfires kindled on their skin, to swallow all sorts of abominations, and to pay for all this, as if to be singed and scalded were a costly privilege, as if blisters were a blessing and leeches were a luxury.' Most of the items in that list are obsolete now, but we have replaced them with some others almost as redoubtable.

But treatment is not solely a matter that lies

between the individual patient and his doctor, nor is it limited to therapeutic measures directly applied to the individual. Least of all is this the case in psychiatry. The social causes and social effects of mental illness ramify widely : the treatment of a patient may depend more on his family, his employer, and the community's attitude towards him than on the drugs or the psychotherapy he receives. For this reason the social aspects of psychiatry are the object of increasing research, and the social sciences —what are now often called the behavioural sciences —play a large part in psychiatric inquiries. Telling evidence of this is supplied by the World Health Organization's list, published last year, of what they considered 'areas of high priority for mental health research'. First came brain function, or neurophysiology and neurochemistry—traditional and central themes. Then epidemiology, in which mental disorders would be investigated as infectious diseases had been and chronic diseases of every sort now are. Next 'health and social study of communities undergoing rapid change', followed by 'social study of the hospital milieu' and the 'ecology of mental illness'. Among further areas of research were 'effect of nutrition on mental health', 'problems of ageing', genetics, 'education of the public about mental health' and 'child development'.

Among these areas of inquiry are some, e.g. the effect of malnutrition on mental health, which are, partly, matters of biochemical and other somatic research, but which also require social studies, e.g.

into food habits, customs in bringing up children, dietary taboos, etc.

Social studies are particularly needed when the prevention of mental disorder is considered. It is convenient here to think of primary, secondary and tertiary prevention : primary where the development of a morbid condition is directly prevented ; secondary where an incipient illness is nipped in the bud or arrested before it has become inveterate ; and tertiary where the amount of disability and distress from a chronic or persistent condition is reduced. The term ' prevention ' is appropriate to the secondary and tertiary sorts of activity because they prevent the total amount of morbidity and disability in the community from being as much as it would have been. In a stricter sense, primary prevention is the only true prevention, which depends on recognition and control of causes.

Prevention is never a simple matter, in the field of psychiatry. There are forms of mental illness and mental defect that might be thought easily preventable because they are due to specific damage to the brain. Many of the causes of such damage are identified and some can be controlled. Inheritable diseases such as amaurotic family idiocy ; infections transmitted from the mother during pregnancy (such as syphilis and perhaps German measles) ; infections acquired during post-natal life, e.g. syphilis and toxoplasmosis ; injury and asphyxia during birth ; iodine deficiency causing myxoedema ; other nutritional deficiencies, as in pellagra ; some kinds of poisoning : there is a long array of indications for the prevention of some forms of mental abnormality. Control would, however, entail administrative and social measures, as well as purely medical ones. Among these measures would be efforts at persuading the public and various local authorities and institutions of the advantages to be derived from preventive action : this would be the modern equivalent of those efforts at popular education in matters of health which were made in many countries in the eighteenth century, not least by that energetic Scot, William Buchan. It is now being painfully realised that to change the outlook of individuals and of the community at large, even when the aim is the prevention of illness, cannot be surely or quickly achieved by simply imparting knowledge and making a rational appeal.

Despite these difficulties, however, it can be said that some of the causes of mental incapacity associated with disease or faulty development of the brain have been brought under control and their harmful psychiatric effects greatly reduced. The outlook is less cheering when we come to the prevention of those mental affections which are not dependent on cerebral disease.

There is no unanimity as to their causes : consequently there is no clear line of prevention. To illustrate the present position let me take one of the most widely accepted hypotheses, viz. that certain experiences in early childhood can have a harmful effect upon the development of personality. Some emphasize the damage done by letting a child be separated from his mother during the first year of life : it is urged that this will conduce to delinquency, incapacity for forming affectionate ties, and other departures from mental health. The hypothesis has earned very wide general acceptance, but critical studies and further evidence have shown that the issues are much more complex, that the effects of separating a young child from his mother need not be detrimental, and that much anxiety has been needlessly caused in mothers, temporarily separated from their baby, because they had heard or seen over-confident, simplified accounts, in films and articles and books, of the risks this entailed. Similarly much research has been devoted to studying the family relationship and upbringing of people who develop mental illnesses, especially schizophrenia, and it has been concluded by some that various harmful experiences to which these people were exposed during their childhood have been responsible for their subsequent illness. There has been a general readiness to assume that the personality of children is extremely plastic, and can take a shape which leads to mental illness of various sorts if mistakes are made in bringing them up as members of a family and ' socializing ' them. But here, too, evidence is conflicting, and the most thorough and sober investigations now available do not confirm these inferences about damage in childhood. It is not surprising, nor discreditable to the investigators, that there should be conflicts of opinion and evidence in these matters, for the definition of the problem, the collection of a suitable sample of subjects, and the collection of trustworthy data which must stretch over ten or twenty years, present formidable difficulties. It would be a crude mistake to infer that how a child is brought up is of little consequence to his later happiness and mental stability : but we do not know the exact relationship. I mention the unsettled state of our present knowledge as an explanation of why there are as yet few serious programmes of preventive psychiatry touching on family life and child rearing, though there is no dearth of vague generalisations.

Improvements in the mental health services provided for a community should, of course, lead to a reduction in the total amount of psychiatric morbidity in that community. The effectiveness of the services, whether therapeutic or preventive in intention, must therefore be gauged from those changes for the better in the incidence or the prevalence of such disorders which follow the introduction of the new services and can be attributed to them. But to measure the amount of psychiatric morbidity in a community is a difficult undertaking, not least because many people with neurotic troubles do not consult a doctor since they do not regard these as a form of illness. The technical and other obstacles are, fortunately, now being overcome, and much more regard than formerly is paid to the measurement of psychiatric disability in specified populations, both in order to check and confirm the effect of preventive measures and to make comparisons from which we can estimate the impact of various social and cultural influences upon mental morbidity. This is one of the areas in which the methods of epidemiological research are now being applied on a wide scale.

Less extensive investigations are sufficient to determine the effectiveness of secondary prevention. In the same way as the amount of ill health due to physical diseases like diabetes, epilepsy, tuberculosis and syphilis has been strikingly reduced by early diagnosis and prompt and efficacious treatment, the amount of mental ill health due to depressive conditions, or cretinism, toxic deliria, or general paralysis has been curtailed by early diagnosis and treatment: individual cases provide cumulative evidence which cannot be gainsaid.

When we come to tertiary prevention, and examine measures which, though they cannot wholly prevent nor appreciably shorten the duration of mental illness, nevertheless can make it less disabling, we are very close to what, in a slightly different context, is called rehabilitation. This too has become an active field of research. Its scope is wide. It is concerned with the training and potentialities of the patient, with the social circumstances in which he can most happily live and work either inside hospital or from a hostel, or in the normal community. It is concerned with the education of the public so that they come to understand and tolerate disabilities, e.g. in the epileptic, which once alienated them. There is also the application of drugs and other measures to minimize those symptoms which are likely to antagonize and frighten others, or to lessen the patient's capacity because of, say, insomnia, or inertia.

Chronic schizophrenia has outstanding importance

in this connection. Schizophrenic patients occupy about three-quarters of the mental hospital beds in this country, and a sizeable proportion of them are patients who have a poor prospect of recovery. The official policy of the Ministry of Health aims at restoration of the majority of these ' long-stay ' patients to life in the community, and in many hospitals now most vigorous efforts are made to discharge as many as possible to the care of their families or friends. ' Community care ' might almost be said to have become the watchword of progressive psychiatrists. But to implement such a policy, without detriment to the patients or hardship to their families and associates, demands more than energy, good will and clinical experience. One of the first desiderata is knowledge of how the mental hospital as a social institution helps, and how it may hinder, the patients' adjustment and fitness for ordinary life, bearing in mind that the schizophrenic patient is particularly prone to withdraw from social contacts into a private and isolated world. The longer such a patient stays in hospital, it has been shown in one investigation, the less does he want to leave, and the more nebulous and unrealistic do his plans for living and working outside hospital become. If, however, such patients are admitted to a course at an Industrial Rehabilitation Unit, alongside the mentally healthy men who are also referred, their attitude to work and their plans may be considerably improved ; for example in one such experiment it was found that of the moderately handicapped chronic schizophrenic men under 45 who went to the I.R.U. more than

35

half were supporting themselves by ordinary remunerative work a year later. In an experiment of the same type with 45 older men, also chronic schizophrenics who had been in the mental hospital for years, twenty were satisfactorily employed outside the hospital a year after the course at the I.R.U. had ended. This result was obtained because of constant supervision during the follow-up year; it was also demonstrated that if such patients had had special preparation in a workshop and rehabilitation villa within the hospital before they went to the I.R.U., they were likely to do better than if they went straight to the I.R.U. Some of this may seem self-evident. But that it is not really so is attested by the fact that many such patients in mental hospitals are, so to speak, written off as far as rehabilitation is concerned. The virtue of planned experiments, such as these were, with controls in the form of matched groups of patients cared for according to the customary hospital regime, lies in their objective and reproducible evidence that the working capacity of schizophrenics who have spent many years in a mental hospital is much greater than textbooks and many psychiatrists and mental nurses assume, and that a considerable proportion of these chronic schizophrenics can, by suitable measures of rehabilitation, be as effectively dealt with and enabled to live tolerably normal lives outside hospital as men with correspondingly severe physical handicaps. Similar experiments are being carried out to determine how far community services can effect tertiary prevention for chronic schizophrenics who have left hospital.

There are other valuable approaches to this matter of rehabilitation. The successful treatment centre for chronic schizophrenics at Glasgow Royal Mental Hospital described by Dr. Freeman, Dr. Cameron and Dr. McGhie was a kindred effort, carried out within the hospital and with a different theoretical background from the experiments I have mentioned : it demonstrated what can be accomplished in the way of reactivation and the reduction of disability when chronic schizophrenics are treated with hopeful understanding.

I would not like it to be thought that I am making all progress dependent on research. There have been notable advances in psychiatry which were not based on research but on clinical experience and conviction: for example, the reforms instituted at the end of the eighteenth century in England, France and Italy were humanitarian measures, in keeping with the spirit of the time, and owing little to the method of systematic inquiry which characterises scientific research. It would be stupid to maintain dogmatically that this intensely human branch of knowledge will progress only as fast as the fruits of research permit : there may be men of genius whose insight will run ahead of experiment and demonstration, and get them to the heart of some crucial obscurity. But in the main we will continue to look to research (of which the hypotheses and approaches also derive from creative imagination and insight) for the furtherance of this abstruse subject. The social sciences, as well as the biological and physical sciences, will be essential to this end. But it is a commonplace that the divisions between sciences are not hard and fast ; it is certainly often difficult or pointless today to try to distinguish whether a particular investigation is in the province of the psychologist or the physiologist, or whether an inquiry has been epidemiological or genetic.

Whenever the welfare of the whole community is furthered through the application of research findings it is very unlikely that the exponents of one discipline will alone have effected it ; the more it is of general advantage to the community at large, the more likely that collaborative effort, by individuals and agencies, will have been required to translate knowledge into effective action. When zeal has outrun discretion—as has happened, I think, in the recent legislation providing for the compulsory treatment of psychopaths—there has usually been too little knowledge to build on, or too little collaboration with experts in the behavioural sciences, among which I include psychiatry. The application of the fruits of research is itself a piece of research : if it is not, it should be. The truths disclosed by research are never absolute and final : in applying them to so complex a business as human behaviour in health and disease it is to be expected that relevant factors may be overlooked and the results be other than those intended. It is not enough to wait until errors or miscalculations are flagrantly evident, whether we are dealing with the introduction of a new anxiety-allaying drug or the hospital policy of early discharge and ready re-admission : there is imperative need in these things for the alert, controlled research outlook

38

from the outset. It is legitimate to ask, wherever new knowledge is deliberately applied to the treatment and prevention of mental illness, that provision should be made for it to be planned as an experiment, designed in advance to yield data from which in due course observers will judge objectively whether the desired goal has been attained. In a few fields of application this may not be practicable; in others the success of the therapeutic measure is so dramatic that it needs no special design to prove it quickly; but these situations are rare. The United States Report on the Behavioural Sciences, issued last month by the President's Scientific Advisory Committee, put the need strongly. ' Expanding (social) programmes at state and national levels . . . have created a demand for applied research. This demand has been largely unmet, or met in piecemeal, after-the-fact ways. . . . Although the few such studies that have been conducted have clearly proved to be valuable, large-scale action programmes have seldom been accompanied or preceded by pilot studies. . . . The need is especially great in those areas where an action taken now has consequences that continue far into the future. . . . At the very least, research on action programmes should be undertaken simultaneously with the initiation of action, and used to guide further development.'

In this address I have spoken frankly of the deficiencies in psychiatric knowledge and of the need for research in overcoming them. In research it is true that the wind bloweth where it listeth; and so long as enough men with the right qualities of mind

39

can be brought into touch with the problems of psychiatry and given adequate facilities and support, I do not think there will be need for others to worry about whether the right problems are being tackled. However, as I have tried to stress, social and cultural forces mould the shape of research, serving to concentrate interest and promote particular sorts of discovery. What happens in research, whether we call it fundamental or applied, will reflect the state of our society, its values and its overriding concerns. If our society regards the improved mental health of its members as a major object of endeavour, this will have its effect on psychiatric research. Enough has been achieved by such research already to warrant hope about a larger mastery than we now have, and surer prospects of control.

3

MAN AND BEAST

WHEN DOLLARD and his pleiad of collaborating psychologists at Yale wrote their notable monograph on Frustration and Aggression, they concerned themselves only with the behaviour of man. Now, twenty years later, a recorded symposium, *The Natural History of Aggression*, devotes two-fifths of its space to the behaviour of non-human animals, and its editors, introducing the lucid, many-sided and authoritative papers and discussion, proclaim their faith that biological studies provide scale and perspective against which the origin, history and future of man may be viewed. It is a matter of temperament and training whether the similarities between human and animal behaviour are chiefly studied, or the differences; but an exclusive stress on differences is no longer the hallmark of the theologian insistent on the dignity and spirituality of man, or of the biologist alarmed at the possible charge of anthropomorphic thinking. Human aggression, in particular, has become too serious a subject to leave to the humanists: and animal aggression has turned out to be too controlled to fit the picture of Nature red in tooth and claw.

The notion of a world of ravening animals seeking whom they may destroy is chiefly attributable to the neglect of two distinctions—first, between attacks upon prey for food and non-predatory attacks that seem to bespeak an instinct of pure pugnacity; and secondly, between the behaviour of animals in their wild natural state and that of animals in captivity. The difference between predation and aggression is blurred for us by the compassion we feel for the victim, whatever the biological purpose or necessity of the attack upon him. Predation apart, vertebrates, and indeed many other animals, are remarkably tolerant and peaceful in their behaviour towards other species in the wild. As until recently the closest and commonest observation was of animals living under the abnormal conditions of zoos and labora-tories, misleading inferences were readily drawn, especially about aggressive behaviour towards animals of the same species.

In their normal setting, mammals do not engage in overt, uninhi-bited fighting against others of their own species. Fighting is restrained and controlled, it stops short of actual injury, and conforms to strict rules; evolutionary forces have anticipated the Marquess of

Queensberry. The ritualized, intra-specific fights are trials of strength, not fights to the death. Threats take the place of physical contact; submission and flight conclude the contest, so far as the weaker participant is concerned. The stronger has asserted his dominance and maintained his territory inviolate. In the circumstances of captivity, it is quite otherwise: escape from the aggressor is impossible, territorial rights cannot be maintained without bloodshed. Overcrowding may have the same effect, as Verheyen found in the hippopotamuses of Lake Edward and Wood Jones in the bandicoots of South Australia.

Nowhere is the falsity of popular belief about ravening ferocity better shown than in wolves. They fight, it is true, but in such ritualized fashion that when the weaker has been worsted he does not run away but throws himself on his back, exposing his most vulnerable surface; his opponent takes no advantage of this opening for lethal attack. Similarly the common shrew, when it forages in a neighbour's feeding area and blunders into collision with him, screams and bites but presently one of them breaks away and throws itself on its back, giving the victor opportunity for a deadly onslaught: he does nothing of the kind but runs off leaving his opponent vanquished but unhurt.

The evolutionary benefits of this peripeteia could hardly have been attained unless the loser was permanently subdued: in practice the losers long retain their memory of the superiority of their former antagonist, just as they would continue to avoid traps and painful situations from which they had once suffered and escaped.

Aggression is closely related to joint action; attack may be conducted by a group in alliance against an intruder and attachments between individuals or groups can be, as in ducks and geese, the outcome of ritualized aggression that has been redirected away from 'friends' and mates.

The adaptive nature of aggression is strikingly evident in primates other than ourselves. Under natural conditions of breeding, feeding and defence, the ritualized displays express redirected attack or preparation for defence against a predator, and vary with the ecological conditions: baboons show a controlled aggressiveness in keeping with their size and ranging habits and their need for group cohesion, whereas the langurs of India and the light-weight Patas monkeys of West Africa behave as though dominance had little importance in their social relations.

Chimpanzees show little aggression towards each other, or towards outsiders of the same species. They pass from one group to another peacefully, there is little evidence of a hierarchy of dominance causing individual males to concede priority in taking food to another male: and even during mating they display mutual tolerance. Gorillas, too, so unjustly credited with extreme ferocity, live in relative peace with their neighbour groups and within the group they maintain a dominance order between young and mature males with minimum fighting. This is the general rule among non-human primates; changes in dominance rank, when they occur, are effected by a policy of steady harassment, and the successful male achieves his aim by threatening behaviour rather than by physical combat. Between groups (apart perhaps from rhesus) there is, in wild conditions, mutual tolerance or mutual avoidance. But in the restricted conditions of captivity, monkeys can be violently aggressive and bring about the death of an intruder. The potential aggressiveness of primates is, in normal ecological conditions, effectively inhibited; change these conditions so that the equilibrium arrived at through appropriate distribution of population and social learning is upset, and their aggression is released to a savage degree.

Enormously varied though the patterns of aggressive behaviour are, they have in common a purposefulness and survival value which extends all the way from insects and cichlids to the higher apes. It can take harmless or 'sublimated' forms, but it may, of course, in certain circumstances, appear as naked attack. The lobster's claws are vicious weapons. The wasp and the bee use their sting. The female spider may eat her husband. Reptiles give each other no quarter. The Siamese fighting fish is a redoubtable warrior. The cock asserts his barnyard rights against all comers. And in mammals it is not only the carnivore who is aggressive; witness the herbivorous bull. Many species fight over the possession of females. Aggression is evidently necessary, and possibly adaptive and salutary, so long as it is balanced and tempered by inhibitory, ritualizing and redirecting forces.

McDougall was not the first to call pugnacity or aggressiveness an instinct. Since his day the concept of instinct has had some rough handling, but it stoutly persists and can legitimately be applied to the aggressive mechanism. The old antithesis between innate genetically transmitted patterns of behaviour and social learning has been replaced by a more comprehensive view of the combined, complex influences which go on moulding behaviour that has been genetically coded in the first place. The patterns or systems of instinctive behaviour have to be released by appropriate sign-stimuli before they can come into action. The receptors an animal has for such stimuli will be important in determining its adaptive relation to its environment.

Neurophysiology and endocrinology have their quota to offer in the understanding of how the aggressive instinct works. Perhaps the most immediately telling instance of this is in the wild Norway rat, a notoriously savage customer: the average weight of his adrenal glands is three or four times that of the domesticated Norway rat, which can be handled without risk. Forty years ago Cannon demonstrated the cardinal role of the adrenal medulla in mediating some gross emotional disturbances, including rage: the medullary products—adrenaline and noradrenaline—appear in raised concentration when an animal is excited to an aggressive or other emotional outburst.

Surgical removal of parts of the brain and electrical stimulation of cells or groups of cells in the hypothalamic region of the brain have shown that there is in some animals an evident balance between regions which are concerned with exciting aggression and others which inhibit it. The hypothalamus is an important area for the production of a visible rage reaction but not the 'centre' for it, and there are differences between different animals; whereas in cats interference with certain areas (the amygdala and hippocampus) will produce fury, it makes rhesus monkeys tractable and placid. The network of connexions involved in expressing hostility is so complex that what seemed to be clear about the neural basis of 'sham rage' in experimental animals has been much modified, and it is necessary not only to determine very cautiously the area affected by surgical or electrical intervention, but also to distinguish between the evoked patterns of aggression. The most striking feature is that the behaviour of an animal that has had its cortex removed is much more determined by a limited external stimulus than is that of the intact animal exposed to many environmental stimuli: the behaviour of the decorticate animal is consequently more predictable and stereotyped.

There is beyond doubt an innate mechanism in animals which can be provoked into action by appropriate stimuli from outside; but what anatomical or biochemical events underlie the ritualized sequence of behaviour that then ensues is still unknown. For human beings the patterns and stages of aggressive response to a wide range of situations are anything but stereotyped.

Experimental studies in man are barely practicable: the nearest approach is afforded by localized disease causing damage to cerebral functions, and by the effects of neurosurgical intervention. A large proportion of those who have lesions in the limbic system (which includes the amygdala and the hippocampus) become more irritable and easily stirred to aggression. But the chief interest in human aggression does not lie in its physiological or anatomical basis but in the psychological and social complexities it only too plainly exhibits. Man's aggression can take such strange forms, appear at the call of such peculiarly individual challenges and frustrations, that any analogy with the set instinctual behaviour of a social insect or a cichlid fish seems to wear very thin.

44

Dollard and his colleagues made a brave case for frustration as the essential condition for aggression, but even in animals frustration is by no means the whole story. The frustrated stickleback, as Tinbergen found, did not attack the enemy approaching its nest but started digging a new nest; mice do likewise. Rats frustrated in getting access to food fought less in Seward's experiments than when they were not being frustrated. But in human behaviour there are countless examples of aggression serving to relieve the emotional tension of frustration or to end the frustration by driving away the frustrator. The attack in such circumstances may, however, be redirected upon another individual, or be restricted to abuse and fantasies of revenge and destruction.

Freud's instinctual theory of aggression, which has commanded much attention, passed through several phases. He differentiated the sexual from the aggressive drive, then postulated a compulsion to repeat unpleasant experiences which run counter to the 'pleasure principle'. When there is obstruction to the search for pleasure or the avoidance of pain, he supposed that aggression comes into play—an aggression directed outward, towards the people apparently responsible for the impediment, or inward towards oneself. The next stage in his speculation, in 1920, centred on the notion of a death-instinct, wholly destructive in its intent, which would work towards reinstating the inorganic condition that has preceded each individual life. Freud reversed his previous conception of primacy: instead of self-destructive tendencies being the displaced or redirected form of an externally directed aggressive drive, the attack upon others (equated to a large extent with sadism) was seen as secondary to the self-injury tendency.

Freud's conception of the death-instinct has met with less acceptance among psychoanalysts than any other part of his theory, but he clung to it. In the exchange of letters with Albert Einstein which took place in 1933 he wrote:

I would like to dwell a little longer on this Destructive Instinct. . . . With the least of speculative efforts we are led to conclude that this instinct functions in every living being, striving to work its ruin and reduce life to its primal state of inert matter. Indeed it might well be called the 'Death Instinct'; whereas the Erotic Instincts vouch for the struggle to live on. The Death Instinct becomes an impulse to destruction when, with the aid of certain organs, it directs its action outwards, against external objects. . . . The diversion of the destructive impulse towards the external world must have beneficial effects. Here is then the biological justification for all those vile, pernicious propensities which we now are combating.

This is the view which he expressed again in the last book he wrote, the *Outline of Psycho-Analysis*.

The Yale group's emphasis on frustration and Freud's on a destructive instinct have had much effect on subsequent investigators and theorists but have been modified and superseded. Contemporary studies of aggression in man have been directed mainly on the influences in childhood that intensify or minimize aggressive behaviour; the special conditions and psycho-social determinants of war; and the ways aggression is manifested in small groups.

In a small group hostility may take the form of direct aggression, or the hostile member may withdraw from the group. Paradoxically the more cohesive the group, the quicker the readiness to express hostility within it. The collective attitude of the group may concentrate on one member who becomes a scapegoat, an overt target for hostility, which he may have aroused because he expected it and behaved accordingly. The vicious circle interplay in such a setting is a psychiatric common-place, especially when group psychotherapy is used. Sociologists see it as a special case of 'autistic hostility'; the conditions are such that hostile impulses develop into persistent attitudes, and a false defini-tion of the situation by a participant evokes new behaviour in himself and others which makes the false definition come true.

The hostility that can be directed towards an outsider, especially a non-conforming outsider, is as discernible among children as in adult communities. Children are, on many matters, more tolerant than their elders, and the diversity of their attitudes of friendliness or aggression bespeaks the plasticity enabling them to be moulded by their upbringing. Their social learning powers are considerable for good and ill. Where parents have shown hostility to the child, especially by severe punishments, his aggressive tendencies are fortified; but so are they if the child's acts of aggression are often repeated and are rein-forced by some gratification that they bring with them. Unfortunately relationships of this sort can bear alternative explanation. Punitive and hostile attitudes in the parents may be not the cause but the conse-quence of hostile or other unwelcome attitudes in the child; and the gratification a child gets from aggressive behaviour may be of the sort that is sanctioned by a competitive society which puts a high value on courage, physical endurance, and success. There is similar uncertainty in interpreting studies showing that aggressive behaviour in children is prone to occur when there is an aggressive model in the home or school.

The disposition to war is the gravest aspect which aggression now wears.

As the nature of Foule weather lyeth not in a showre of two of rain; but in an inclination thereto of many dayes together; So the nature of War, consisteth not in actuall fighting; but in the known disposition thereto, during all the time there is no assurance to the contrary.

46

So wrote Hobbes in 1651. The disposition to war is no longer openly avowed or consciously nourished. But it remains true that, in the words of William James, man is is many respects the most ruthlessly ferocious of beasts, and the cruellest: his propensity stretches from trivial hates to impersonal holocausts, and it was reasonable for the authors of a book on aggression to say that they were endeavouring to place within a common discourse such diverse phenomena as race prejudice and suicide, sibling jealousy and lynching, satire and crime, wife-beating and war.

When war was on the horizon in 1935 psychiatrists from many countries addressed a manifesto 'to the statesmen of the world' in which they pointed to the seeming contradiction 'between the conscious individual aversion to war and the collective preparedness to wage war' and they went on to assert that

our science is sufficiently advanced for us to distinguish between real, pretended, and unconscious motives. . . . International organization is now sufficiently advanced to enable statesmen to prevent war by concerted action.

The claims were overbold, the degree of ignorance underrated. We are still far being able to discriminate motives, and must be modest about our ability to lay down principles of concerted action. It is only necessary to examine Lewis Richardson's mathematical analysis of the causes of wars—a strangely neglected work of signal thoroughness and originality—to appreciate the complexity of the problem and the inadequacy of current knowledge.

Nobody knows how far we can apply to human beings the principles detected in the aggressive behaviour of other animals. At one extreme stands an expert like Zing Yang Kuo who, after many years of experimental study of fighting crickets, Siamese fighting fish, chickens, dogs, cats, rats, rabbits, guinea pigs, Japanese grey quails and a Noah's ark of other birds and fishes, expressly disavows any intention to apply the results of animal experiments to human conduct: the behaviour patterns of animal fighting are too complex and variable, and human behaviour can be made to fit in with the results of animal studies only by oversimplifying it. At the other extreme there is Konrad Lorenz asserting that from the study of behaviour we have come to know so much already about the natural history of aggression that we can make pronouncements regarding its deviations in man.

To whichever of these positions individual judgment inclines, the risks of wholesale transfer from other animals to man are plain enough to impose caution. 'Territory' as a defended region is not a concept that can be safely carried across to man from other species: his diversified behaviour regarding property has to be learnt because it is culturally determined: it is not a standardized response to a common system of signals. Similar objections preclude the ready application to human society of the concepts of dominance and submission. The findings of ethology and comparative sociology give rise to stimulating hypotheses about the causation and sequences of human aggressive behaviour, but they leave us with very little guidance about how to control our aggression. Its power and our failure to cope with it where it works to the detriment of our happiness and survival have been the theme of many a jeremiad; the sad argument is rehearsed, briefly but conclusively, by an anthropologist in the Institute of Biology Symposium—*The Natural History of Aggression*—who concludes (as William James did) that 'the extreme nature of human destructiveness and cruelty is one of the principal characteristics which marks off man, behaviourally, from other animals'. The same topic led Voltaire to exclaim: 'Manichéens, voilà votre excuse!'

Much of men's shameful preeminence in destroying has been put down to their possession of weapons. So far from being handicapped because they were 'not armed with horns of arbitrary might, or claws to seize their furry spoils in flight', men devised weapons which could operate from a distance: they did not develop the inhibiting submissive rituals which depend on close confrontation. This depersonalized remoteness has become ever more characteristic: in atomic war it would reach its apogee. Other social causes—the pressure of population (producing the overcrowding which in caged animals can lead to murder), the frustrations of poverty and despotism, the deliberate fostering of hate, the aggrandisement of warlike virtues—have been often enough recognized as enhancing the more lethal forms of human aggression. When the hostility is less than lethal and bitterer than gall—when, for example, we consider Housman consigning lesser Latinists to the pit, or Pope giving Lord Hervey his quietus—the analysis of causes has to be more subtle.

The search for ways of limiting or reshaping human aggressiveness so that war is improbable is pursued, in deceptively objective and dispassionate form, in such symposia as that of the Institute of Biology, or the American Academy of Psycho-Analysis in 1963. The participants soberly review the possibilities of prevention, suggested by study of the behaviour of animals, of young children, of the mentally ill, of psychopathic and delinquent people, and they suggest remedies for our danger, but they state their argument with an emotional undertone or an unscientific emphasis that bespeaks their concern—like that of all of us.

Hopes which are akin to fantasies here demand as attentive a

48

hearing as discriminating analogies drawn from biology. Margaret Mead recently put forward a suggestion with something of both these elements. She reminded the members of the psycho-analytical symposium that it is the plain fact that human beings are all of one species, whatever their colour or nationality, and it is also the plain fact that animals do not habitually destroy other animals of their own species. No matter whether these facts are stated as moral principles or biological generalizations, let men's attitude towards any act that infringes them be as prompt and unreasoning an abhorrence as their attitude to incest, and we shall be safer. But will we be within sight of as peaceful a world as that of the monkeys or the wolves? As yet we do not know how to inculcate the taboo, nor can we be sure it would hit the right target.

It is often urged that man's innate aggressiveness cannot be abolished, but can be diverted into harmless substitutive channels—tournaments, sports, space exploration, scientific and artistic rivalry. Easier said than done; and still to be demonstrated convincingly. Sublimation is a good psycho-analytical concept, but sublimation of the sexual impulse does not abolish libidinal desire; it only changes its goal to one that will not meet with resistance from the environment. The process of sublimation, moreover, is not one that is deliberately set in motion in adult life, but is a product of earlier development. Its success depends on the child's environment and upbringing: its alternative is the production of neurosis. 'The question whether aggressive impulses can be sublimated is *sub judice*', wrote Edward Glover in 1948. It still is.

One of the most distinguished students of animal behaviour, John Paul Scott, has expressed his agreement with the suggestion put forward in 1910 by William James, in his essay on 'The Moral Equivalent of War', that young men be given the opportunity to find a substitute for group aggression by joining a 'peace-army' which would be occupied with public works, doing away with manifest social evils, and helping in disasters. Various modifications of this project are, of course, in being: perhaps the general idea would seem familiar to Ignatius Loyola, and to William Booth.

A bolder proposal has been made by American sociologist, Anthony Leeds, who regards war as a cultural system that has multiple social functions—creating an equilibrium, welding the people together, sloughing off outworn institutions, revitalizing neglected ideological values, permitting reallocation of resources, forming new economic or political alliances, redistributing rewards within the society, fostering cultural diffusion. Mr. Leeds would substitute for war a vast comparable institution which would have equivalent functions, and so serve the mostly unrecognized purposes which have made war ubiquitous; it is a corollary of his thesis that the psychological or biological concepts of an innate aggressiveness in individual human beings, acting in sum as the main cause of war, are fallacious and inadequate: they cannot be the basis of prevention.

Football games or international contests will not do: changing infancy experiences or revolutions in the education of children to achieve new motivations are irrelevant, as are virtually all the multitudes of such suggestions appearing with ever-increasing frequency even from professional scientists.

Instead he proposes using existing multifunctional institutions—the family, the state, the church—to take over the functions subserved by war. The conclusion is less arresting than the exordium. If we are engaged, now as onlookers, some day as winners or losers, in a race between knowledge and destruction, we need more to encourage us than this.

Perhaps simple comfort can be derived from Konrad Lorenz's fervent optimism in *Das Sogenannte Böse*—a book written with his characteristic mixture of gusto, intimacy and confident biological detail, so that it is no wonder there have been six editions since it appeared in 1963.

I am honestly convinced that in the near future very many men—indeed perhaps the majority of mankind— will regard as obvious and banal truth all that I have written in this book about intraspecific aggression and the dangers which its perversions entail for humanity.

And, discarding any hope of avoiding the dangers by removing the occasions of hostility, imposing moral vetoes, or trying to breed out pugnacity by eugenic means Lorenz, like many others, advocates letting off aggressive steam, 'abreacting' on substitute objects such as sport; and then, with an unexpected change of direction, he bids us take lessons from the demagogues who know so well how to whip up desired feelings, attitudes and actions; they have an understanding of instinctual drives and how to direct them which has been turned mostly to evil ends but could be learnt and used for controlling aggression to the advantage of society. Broadly Lorenz asks for psychological and social research. The programme is eloquently set out, but, as he says, it is subject to the general rule that to apply the results of research creatively and well demands no less acuteness and painstaking work on detail than were required to obtain these results in the first place. Erudition, whether in biological or social sciences, is not enough: how to apply in good time such knowledge as we have to the better control of aggression is among the most urgent problems facing us but also among the least adequately tackled as yet by systematic investigation.

REFERENCES

The Natural History of Aggression. Edited by J. D. Carthy and F. J. Ebling. 159pp. Academic Press.

KONRAD LORENZ: *Das Sogenannte Böse.* Zur Naturgeschichte der Aggression. 391pp. Vienna: Dr. G. Borotha-Schoeler.

4

CANCER COUNTRY

Smoking, Health, and Personality

by H. J. Eysenck.

Basic Books, 166 pp., $4.95

AUBREY LEWIS

When tobacco was first introduced into Europe and Asia, potentates saw harm in it and some enacted the death penalty for those of their subjects who persisted in smoking. But only a proportion of the culprits were in fact put to death for the widespread crime, and the potentates soon substituted taxes for excommunications and executions. After three hundred years the death penalty is still linked to smoking, though not now by due process of law, and taxes on tobacco are still levied by governments: neither the risk of a shortened life, nor expense, nor alternative pleasures have eliminated smoking, nor is it less profitable for the revenue. Why the habit should have spread so fast and so far, and proved so tenacious, is a matter for conjecture. Other problems which it offers have not been left to conjecture, but made the subject of very active research. These are the problems raised by the association of smoking with disease, or, more specifically, by the association of cigarette smoking with cancer of the lung. Two impressive reports, from the Royal College of Physicians in England and the Surgeon General's Advisory Committee in the United States, documented and reviewed the present state of knowledge about this threatening aspect of public health. Both reports concluded that cigarette smoking is an important cause of lung cancer, far outweighing all other factors.

Although the consensus of informed opinion is powerfully to this effect, there are dissenters whose criticisms have demanded close scrutiny—people like Dr. Berkson of the Mayo Clinic who have been voicing their misgivings for a good many years, and others more recent, like Professor Eysenck, the author of this book.

Professor Eysenck is a psychologist well known for his many valuable contributions to the study of personality in its varied aspects, and for his lively polemical writing, as spirited and forthright in defense as in attack, and firmly based on the principle of tit for tat. His powers of lucid exposition have been evident in a large number of publications, describing the psychological experiments and arguments on which his views rest. In this book, characteristically readable, he lays an axe to the generally accepted conclusion about the role of cigarette smoking, and he links the association between smoking and cancer to certain features of his study of personality. His survey and his assertions are broadly on the following lines.

Epidemiological methods of investigation can suggest causal relation but cannot confirm or ensure it: Only experiment can do that. The association between smoking and lung cancer is not specific; other diseases also are related to cigarette smoking. The populations on whom the observations have been made were not selected in such a way that they can each be accepted as a representative sample, nor did a sufficiently large proportion of the people to be studied agree to take part in the inquiries. Measurement of the amount of smoking was unduly crude. The samples of population studied were self-selected. These and other objections, mainly derived from Berkson and another biostatistician, Yerushalmy, are given in considerable detail, but they are followed by chapters expounding the more novel explanation which Professor Eysenck offers to account for the association between cigarette smoking and mortality from lung cancer, which he does not dispute.

His thesis is in keeping with the suggestion advanced by the late R. A. Fisher, that the practice of cigarette smoking and the development of cancer of the lung might be largely influenced by a common cause, the genotype or hereditary make-up of the individual. Fisher considered that the genotype exercises a considerable influence on smoking and on the particular habit of smoking adopted; groups classified according to their smoking habits would furthermore differ in their genetic predisposition to develop cancer. Eysenck carries this line of thought further.

He had found that, by appropriate inquiries (chiefly questionnaires, experimental tests, and study of twins) we can recognize two dimensions of personality—extraversion and neuroticism—which are determined to some extent by heredity. In large surveys carried out under his supervision by Mass Observation Ltd. on behalf of the Tobacco Manufacturers' Standing Committee, he found that cigarette smoking was related to extraversion and pipe-smoking to introversion; neuroticism was not related to smoking. The relation between extraversion and cigarette smoking was stronger in those who smoked heavily than in the light smokers and the ex-smokers. Therefore, he argues, a constitutional factor may be presumed which is responsible for the extraverted personality and the predisposition to cancer: This makes it unnecessary, in his view, to attribute to cigarette smoking the main causal role in lung cancer. He accounts for the rapid growth in the incidence of the disease in recent years by incriminating air pollution. In brief, he holds it is justifiable, on the available evidence, to say that persons of an extraverted temperament are, because of their hereditary endowment, more likely than introverts to smoke cigarettes and more likely to develop cancer: hence the strong association.

Eysenck is too familiar with the uncertainties of psychological and genetic inquiries into causation to make dogmatic assertions for or against the hypotheses he examines (though the blurb on the jacket intemperately declares that he 'rejects as unproved, exaggerated, or full of paradoxes, riddles, and contradictions the assertion that smoking *causes* lung cancer'). His chief concern is first to demonstrate to the reader the weakness of the accepted view, and then to indicate the superior cogency of his claim for a commom inherited predisposition. He reiterates his destructive arguments lucidly and for the most part with studied moderation; occasionally, however, partisan fervor gets the better of him, and the advocate elbows the judge out of the way. In the end, however, he gives us his pacific credo about the smoking hypothesis and his own: 'I believe (although I cannot at the moment prove) that both the hypotheses under discussion will be found to be true'—but he promptly adds that the direct deleterious effects of smoking are, he believes, 'less important than suggested by the calculations in the British and the American Report.'

There are weaknesses in his grounds of objection to the accepted view. The chief of these lies in the differing rigor with which the evidence is scrutinized. A striking example of this is afforded by Eysenck's reference to Poche in the controversy that followed publication of Eysenck's book: It is worth detailing at a little length. Professor Poche and his two colleagues examined the smoking history of 1229 people in the North Rhineland and Westphalia who had histologically verified bronchial cancers. They concluded that there was no relation between cigarette smoking and the development of the cancer. Professor Eysenck calls this 'an extremely careful study' and says that it 'was methodologically far superior to the studies usually cited.' In fact the defects of the study, for which it has been arraigned by several authorities on medical statistics, are gross. The selection of cases studied was biased in that it depended on whether doctors had filled out answers to a questionnaire about the patients' habits; the participation of the pathological institutes which supplied the material was uneven and arbitrary; and Poche himself characterizes the

54

selection as casual (*Zufallsauswahl*). The specific questions about smoking were very crude: All the information about this that the doctors were asked to provide was a bare statement whether the patient was a smoker and, if so, how many cigarettes, cigars, or pipes he smoked per day and per week. No intimation was given as to what period the question referred to: It might have been the last few months before the patient came into hospital with advanced disease or it might have been his last few years. The avowed purpose of the investigators was to determine the complex of possible part-causes of carcinoma, but they did not include a control group of non-affected persons such as is needed for a retrospective study of causes; instead they compared patients who had a particular type of cancer known to be mainly responsible for the increase in prevalence of cancer of the lung, with others who had a different form of bronchial new growth. Poche and his colleagues accepted the diagnoses made in the participating institutes of pathology; but from internal evidence it is plain that the institutes differed very sharply in their criteria and diagnostic practice, so much so that it is impossible to accept the diagnoses in the absence of any organized exchange of histological preparations and without dual or multiple assessment by experienced pathologists in order to check 'observer-error.' Professor Koller, of Mainz, who has hauled Poche and his colleagues drastically over the coals, points to several other departures from sound statistical or clinical procedure, and declares roundly that Poche's failure to discover any significant evidence of a relation beteween cigarette smoking and cancer is of no scientific importance, because of the crass methodological defects. Nevertheless Professor Eysenck acclaims it as methodologically far superior to the studies usually cited, i.e., those by Bradford Hill and Doll, Hammond and Horn, Dorn, and others who earn his strictures on one count or another.

Similarly he devotes considerable space to the findings and speculations of Beffinger, and declares that 'the neglect of Beffinger's hypothesis by the authorities is curious': The explanation is that Beffinger's hypothesis met the fate of Belshazzar—weighed in the balance and found wanting.

Eysenck reviews the evidence provided by studies of twins that the extravert type of personality is inherited, and that the tendency to smoking likewise has a hereditary determinant. He does not refer, however, to the mainly negative findings in what should be the third limb of his argument—twin studies of the inheritance of cancer, such as those by Clemmesen and his colleagues in Copenhagen. Nor does he give the statistical data on which he no doubt bases his rejection of the view that extraverts develop lung cancer more readily than introverts simply because they smoke more: 'a very small proportion of the relationship may possibly be due to this factor, but it cannot by any stretch of the imagination be held responsible for the total effect.' Whose imagination? And what evidence?

Arguments about the etiology of particular diseases used to be centered on 'the cause,' as if only one cause was operative. Putting aside philosophic or semantic issues, it is now commonly recognized that multiple causes are responsible, through in very different degrees: Delirium tremens, for example, and cirrhosis of the liver have alcoholism as a cause, indeed as the commonest cause, but alcoholism is not a necessary cause nor a sufficient cause of either condition. The Surgeon General's Advisory Committee underlined the point:

No member of this Committee used the word 'cause' in an absolute sense in the area of this study. Although various disciplines and fields of scientific knowledge were represented among the membership, all members shared a common conception of the multiple etiology of biological processes. No member was so naive as to insist upon mono-etiology in pathological processes or in vital phenomena. All were throughly aware of the fact that there are series of events in occurrences and developments in these fields, and that the end results are the net effect of many actions and counteractions.

By a regrettable slip Professor Eysenck in quoting the Royal College of Physicians' conclusion that 'cigarette smoking is a cause of cancer,' substitutes 'the' for 'a'. This alters the statement significantly and runs counter to the explicit reminder in the College Report: 'It is important to recognize that the hypothesis is not that cigarette smoking is the *only* cause of lung cancer. The fact that the disease does, rarely, occur in non-smokers and the effects of air pollution and various industrial hazards clearly indicate that other factors are concerned.'

Eysenck's illustrative analogies are somewhat inaccurate. He tells us, apropos of the limited efficacy of epidemiological methods, that John Snow 'finally removed the handle from the Broad Street pump and brought the cholera epidemic to a conclusion.' This well-worn dramatic tale has been exploded: The number of fatal attacks of cholera commencing each day in the area served by the Broad Street pump in 1854 had been falling rapidly, from 143 on September 1st to 12 on September 8th, the day on which the handle was removed from the peccant pump. In another analogy, Eysenck takes the inherited metabolic abnormality, phenylketonuria (consistently mispelled in text and index as 'phenylcatonuria') as an example of how by 'understanding the precise way in which heredity works we can arrange a rational method of therapy which makes use of the forces of nature...' But so far from understanding the precise way heredity works in this instance, it is unfortunately still true that there are many obscurities in the matter. As Harris and others have emphasized, we do not know the nature and role of the factors that decide when and where the crucial enzyme is formed, nor how it is that the metabolic upset leads to a failure in mental development.

Professor Eysenck believes that atmospheric pollution is a more important agent upsetting 'the delicate balance between carcinogenic and carcinoprotective factors' than it is credited with being in the British and the American Reports. It is true that the high urban mortality from lung cancer at first blush invites such an assumption, but against it are the very high death rate from this disease in Finland (where air pollution is slight and cigarette smoking very prevalent), the fact that the mortality is not higher in people exposed by their work to petrol and diesel fumes, and the finding that when the urban-rural residence factor has been controlled, there remains a large difference in mortality risk from cancer of the lung between smokers and non-smokers. It is not possible to agree with Eysenck that atmospheric pollution is probably a more important factor than cigarette smoking.

There is however much common ground between those who have satisfied themselves that cigarette smoking is the most important cause of cancer of the lung and those who dispute this, with or without an alternative explanation. The strong association between cigarette smoking and lung cancer is hardly any longer in serious dispute; by common consent the causes of lung cancer are multiple, the smoking habit depends in part on personality factors which are probably transmitted, and there is—who questions it?—much need for further research. Whether research should be concentrated particularly on the topics which Professor Eysenck prescribes—those bearing on the interaction between smoking, personality, and constitution—is a proposal likely to be judged according to our opinion of the strength of the case for the genetic hypothesis which he puts forward.

The most telling objections to a genetic explanation of why cigarette smoking and cancer of the lung are so closely associated all over the world, are those brought out by Doll and Bradford Hill in their report on ten years' observations of British doctors. They found that a fall in mortality rapidly followed the cessation of cigarette smoking, and that it continued to fall step by step the longer smoking had been given up: This they justly urge 'can be explained in terms of a diminishing risk from the previously operative environmental agent, but not in terms of genetic selection of those who choose to give up.' They also found that whereas the death rate from cancer of the lung in all men over twenty-five in England and Wales increased by 22 per cent during the ten years of their inquiry, among the male doctors as a whole whom they studied it fell by 7 per cent: This can easily be accounted for in terms of the great change in doctors' smoking habits, but it runs counter to the implications of the genetic hypothesis. A further difficulty for anyone who regards inherited predisposition as a major factor is the recency of the enormous rise in the incidence of cancer of the lung: It is highly improbable that the genetic endowment of the population has changed correspondingly in the last forty years, but it is certain that the smoking of cigarettes has increased correspondingly during that period.

Eysenck's quarrel with the medical conclusion on this matter is about the cogency of the evidence pointing to cigarette smoking as the main agent of death from cancer of the lung. The issue is not academic. The medical view is that we know enough to warrant doing all we can to discourage cigarette smoking. This would not preclude other measures directed, say, at reducing atmospheric pollution, nor would it lessen the need for research; but it would brand the main criminal. The genetic standpoint, as advanced by Eysenck, would not oppose such preventive methods, but would play down the role of cigarette smoking. He declares: 'What we think we know is largely surmised, and even if most of it were true it would not help us to take any practical steps to overcome the menace of lung cancer...' Apart from some forms of psychological treatment by conditioning which he has espoused or developed, he sees very little prospect of dissuading people from smoking. He refers to 'the possible exception of doctors who seem to have stopped smoking to a significant extent.' The phrasing is unduly cautious: Doll and Hill found that in their population of 31,000 male doctors, 19 per cent had given up the habit between 1951 and 1958. The consumption of cigarettes by men in the United Kingdom has declined by about 10 per cent since the Royal College of Physicians published their Report. There is, then, some hope that more vigorous action, combining educational and fiscal influences, might have more preventive effect than Eysenck supposes, especially in certain sections of the population. 'One lifetime, nine lifetimes are not long enough for the task of blocking every cranny through which calamity may enter'; but cigarette smoking is, by a great consensus, such a cranny, which could, and should, be blocked. Medical critics consequently find it hard to give Professor Eysenck's book, which would delay such action, the praise which its clarity and competence might otherwise earn.

5

ANALYSING THE ANALYST

More than once Freud ranged himself alongside Copernicus and Darwin. Bold as the claim was, it has been conceded by many besides psychoanalysts: Dr. Stafford Clark, for example, asserts roundly that Freud's name will always rank with those of Darwin, Copernicus, Newton, Marx and Einstein. It is not easy to reconcile this apotheosis with the summary appraisal by a recent critic:

there is no conclusive evidence that, as a method of therapy, psychoanalysis is more effective than others, and it is costly beyond its merits; as a philosophy it is chaotic, contradictory and circular; as a science it is unestablished; and as a religion it is inadequate, appealing only to a small section of the intelligentsia with a special background.

Between these extremes of exaltation and dismissal, there is a huge and repetitive body of controversial argument, tedious to read but attesting the vitality of psychoanalysis and its unsettled status in spite of its having been before the world for more than half a century.

Its history is less like that of a therapeutic method or a scientific theory than of a cult—a cult, moreover, which spread to many countries, satisfied many needs and stimulated inquiry. Though, like hypnotism and phrenology, and the malarial treatment of general paralysis, it began in Vienna, its triumphs were reserved for the United States, so that a prominent sociologist could write in 1960 that in America today Freud's intellectual influence is greater than that of any other modern thinker.

The most tangible aspect of psychoanalysis is its use as a method of treatment. Developed at a time when clinical research was very rarely supported by academic or public funds, it is likely that if psycho-analysis had proved to be clearly ineffectual as treatment Freud would have had no private patients on whom to work, and his sources of information would have dried up. Fortunately he did not get into this predicament. But he was a man of few illusions; he did not regard the therapeutic power of psychoanalysis as its most interesting or most important feature. Still he was able with a good conscience to treat neurotic patients in the honest belief that we have—or had during his lifetime—nothing better at our disposal for the treatment of neuroses than the technique of psychoanalysis 'and for that reason, in spite of its limitations, it is not to be despised'. Since then the therapeutic scene has changed. Drugs have been synthesized which, as he conjectured, might exercise a direct influence on the activities of the mind, alternative methods of psychological treatment have been devised or refurbished, psychoses (which Freud believed impregnable to psychoanalytical treatment) have been tackled, and the climate of opinion about the effectiveness of the method has changed greatly.

Psychoanalysts have become aware of the dispiriting nature of their results, and ashamed that their services are at the disposal only of a comparatively small and affluent section of society. Analytic group therapy, which seemed to promise wider scope than individual treatment, has likewise turned out to be expensive and restricted. A current view justifies the limitations by saying that the aim of psychoanalytic treatment is not to remove symptoms but to let the patient assume responsibility and freedom for his own conduct, and 'the kind of personal freedom psychoanalysis promises can have meaning only for persons who enjoy a large measure of economic, political and social freedom'. It is on that showing no wonder that analysis flourished in America and was viewed with strong disfavour in the Soviet Union.

It is hardly credible that there is still no verified and dependable information on whether psychoanalytic treatment works. Personal convictions abound but systematic therapeutic experiments are almost unknown in this field. The weighty overt reasons for this gap are the difficulty of getting full data about private patients, the lack of objective measures of improvement, the ill-defined aims of treatment, the dropping out of patients on financial or psychological grounds, the lack of uniformity in the techniques used by analysts, and the disparity in their skill. In spite of these obstacles, some figures have been published. One psychoanalyst recently reported his results with thirty-seven patients: each of them had had on the average 527 hours of treatment, 38 per cent of them improved. Results obtained by the same psychoanalyst in patients receiving shorter periods of treatment, ranging from twenty hours to 300 hours, were equally good. This has to be read against the background of two statements by Freud in his paper on the termination of analysis: that to fulfil the demands made on analysis, its duration must not be shortened, and that we have no means of predicting what will happen later to a patient who has been 'cured'. As to the former of these dicta Jules Masserman tells us that when he lectured before the British Psychoanalytical Society he was asked why in America an analysis lasts only two to three years whereas in England 'a proper psychoanalysis should persist at least for seven, eight or nine years'; he did not question the statement, as he might have, but replied irreverently—perhaps irrelevantly—that it takes the British longer to see a joke.

Many writers have compared the few available statistics of the outcome of psychoanalytical treatment with the results reported for other forms of psychotherapy, and for treatment solely by drugs, or by drugs reinforced with advice and attentive listening: they have even compared them with the natural course of untreated illness. Most of the inquirers find little to choose between the respective results—except that the method the inquirer habitually employs appears to yield better results than the others. It must be conceded, however, that collective findings are misleading if applied without qualification to individual cases: there can be no reasonable doubt that some patients derive great benefit from psychoanalytic treatment, as indeed from other forms of treatment, but they are apt to be overshadowed in group data by the unfavourable results obtained in ill-chosen or inherently unresponsive patients.

Since Freud and those coming after him have insisted that no one is competent to carry out psychoanalytical treatment unless he has himself been psychoanalysed, some of the present unease among psychoanalysts centres on the conformity with his analyst's views and suggestions which is commonly required of the aspirant before his training analysis and his supervised analysis of two patients can be judged complete. It is the familiar story of orthodoxy on guard, rigid, institutionalized and exigent. Dr. Edward Glover has drawn attention to this danger, and in America psychoanalysts who are not content with the present state of psychoanalytic practice and theory question the need for such prolonged and expensive training as is now customary. In the American Psychoanalytic Association there were, in 1963, 1,300 members: their psychoanalytic training occupied approximately 4,000 hours for each individual, spread over several years and costing about £9,000. The membership of the British Psychoanalytical Society in 1964 was 273, and the length of training was seldom less than four years.

Another feature of psychoanalytical training which causes disquiet is the widespread assumption that the analyst must remain neutral; he is to be as impersonal as a looking glass, reflecting in such a way that the patient sees himself and his behaviour most plainly. But the looking-glass might turn out to be like Alice's. Many now hold that carefully maintained detachment by the analyst works against its intended purpose, since it leaves the patient feeling that he is unsupported in his struggles. To him it must seem that, like the metaphysical poets, such analysts behave

rather as beholders than partakers of human nature; as beings looking upon good and evil, impassive and at leisure; as Epicurean deities, making remarks on the actions of man and the vicissitudes of life, without interest and without emotion.

Psychoanalysis as a form of treatment has provided the livelihood of those who studied psychoanalysis as a field of psychological inquiry, but it has never rivalled the latter in interest and output. Papers on therapeutic technique have been few, in contrast to the Niagara of books and articles on 'metapsychology', the substance of things looked for, the evidence of things not seen.

'Without metapsychological speculation and theorizing—I had almost said fantasy—we shall not get a step further', wrote Freud apropos of the 'taming' of instinctual demands so that they harmonize with the activities of the ego. But before he had published the speculations which resulted in the ego, id, superego topography of the mind, Freud had laid down in 1922 his four articles of belief, 'the cornerstones of psychoanalytic theory'—recognition of the theory of resistance and repression, the importance of sexuality and the Oedipus complex. How far he regarded the detailed instinctual hypotheses as metaphorical statements or as scientific constructs is hard to tell. He raised the point with Einstein: 'It may perhaps seem to you as though our theories are a kind of mythology . . . but does not every science come in the end to a kind of mythology like this?' It seems probable that Freud accepted his elaborate metapsychological structure as a real mental apparatus, not an explanatory fiction. However, he modified his views continuously, in the light of facts observed during the course of psychoanalytic treatment. It is notoriously difficult to express the theory in terms of an empirical system which can be checked by experiment. It has been urged that this is an inevitable stage in the development of a science—the phlogiston phase, as it might be called—when hypothetical entities, forces and analogues are made to do duty for unrefuted facts and experimentally confirmed relations. To such an argument it can be replied, as it was ten years ago by B. F. Skinner, that we have learnt, or should have learnt, enough about the nature of scientific thinking to avoid some of the mistakes made in the history of older sciences; the Freudian language of libido and cathexis, psychic energy, processes, tensions, systems and forces differs from the seemingly analogous conceptual languages of physics and biology in that it does not, like them, concern itself at all with things that have spatial relations and can be related to one another in the real world. Of course this objection has no force if the methods of thought appropriate to the physical sciences, and for the most part to the biological sciences, are held to be essentially inappropriate for the *Geisteswissenschaften*, or at any rate for psychoanalysis and its 'meta-psychology'.

The interplay between philosophy and psychoanalysis has been changeable and inconclusive. Lancelot Law Whyte and Siegfried Bernfeld have shown how much Freud owed to earlier and contemporary philosophers. Though partly aware of the debt, he expressed distaste and incapacity for philosophy. 'Even when I have moved away from observation, I have carefully avoided any contact with philosophy proper. This avoidance has been greatly facilitated by constitutional incapacity'—though in 1896 he wrote that his original ambition had been to attain understanding of human nature through philosophy. In due course his theory has been examined by philosophers, in some cases (by Ernest Nagel, for example) with destructive intent or effect, in others with partial acceptance (e.g., by J. O. Wisdom). The most recent and elaborate, but not by any means the most pellucid, philosophical study comes from Professor Paul Ricoeur of Paris. As a pupil of Roland Dalbiez, he begins with an avowal of cardinal disagreement with his master. Dalbiez concluded his notable study of psychoanalysis with the barbed tribute 'l'oeuvre de Freud est l'analyse la plus profonde que l'histoire ait connue de ce qui, dans l'homme, n'est pas le plus humain'. But my enterprise, says M. Ricoeur, was born of the opposite conviction: 'c'est parce que la psychanalyse est de droit une interprétation de la culture qu'elle entre en conflit avec toute autre interprétation globale du phénomène humain'. For him it explores the most distinctively human of our characteristics, the creation of a culuture, and the instrument of this exploration is linguistic analysis. In *De l'interprétation* he engages in a subtle hermeneutic exercise, a study of symbols and the nature of interpretation. Taking up the problem from the point where he had left it in his last book *Le Symbolique du Mal*, he insists that interpretation is the intermediary between the symbol, with its double meaning, and the act of reflection, consciously performed—the *cogito* of the famous phrase. After restating some epistemological difficulties—and giving Freud's Draft Project for a Scientific Psychology rather more significance than it warrants in this context—M. Ricoeur examines the validity of the psychoanalytical interpretation of culture, particularly as expressed in Freud's writings on art, morality and religion; everything that psychoanalysis can say about these, he maintains, is determined by the space-energy model of 'meta-psychology' and by the paradigm set in the interpretation of dreams, which have become the first term in an endless series of analogues, reaching from the oneiroid to the sublime. The archaeological metaphors and analogies which played so large a part in Freud's thinking are given central importance by M. Ricoeur. He stresses the temporal factor inherent in this genetic approach, and discerns in the theory of narcissism the most advanced point of 'archaeological' thinking at the instinctual level. Narcissism is the reservoir of libido, the original form of desire to which one always returns, 'il est ainsi la condition de tous nos dégagements affectifs et de toute sublimation'. But there is also in M. Ricoeur's view an implicit teleology, to be set alongside the predominant determinist theme: the arguments for it, which require Hegelian dialectic to be brought to bear on the issue, are murky and unconvincing. It is improbable that psychoanalysts will find much that consorts with their lines of thought in Professor Ricoeur's book, though such respectful treatment of metapsychology by an unanalysed philosopher of distinction will surprise and please them.

The influence of psychoanalysis upon the outlook and assumptions of contemporary society is sometimes compared with that of Marxism. In both cases it is difficult to go beyond a comprehensive impression and a plausible guess. Experts sometimes venture farther. Thus Professor E. H. Gombrich declared in *Encounter* (January, 1966) that Freud's influence on the practice and criticism of art in the twentieth century is all-pervasive, and that it is his teachings which were largely instrumental in undermining and destroying the rich cultural tradition in which he had been nurtured. Many professional observers of social change have credited or blamed psychoanalysis for its contribution to the loosening of sexual mores. Moscovici, a French social psychologist, has reviewed the steps by which psychoanalytical concepts are restructured as they penetrate society, and given body and objective 'entity' as collective categories; the technical language becomes a common dialect (using 'complexes', 'transference', 'acting out', the 'depressive position', 'libido' and all the rest), it pervades judgment, and may affect behaviour. On the other hand, there are also alert onlookers who dispute the tenets and methods of psychoanalysis when applied outside the medical sphere and by their forceful criticism lessen the degree of its acceptance or nearly strangle its extension to fields of human activity towards which it has stretched out tentative pseudopods. Professor Morris Ginsberg, for example, contemplated the claims Freud made to illuminate 'the nature of human groups, the foundations of morals and religion, and indeed of all the elements of culture'; he decided that the claims were 'so far-reaching that it was the plain duty of sociologists to come to terms with them', and in the process of doing so he made it hard for anyone who had read his critique thereafter to take as well-authenticated the applications of psychoanalytical theory to problems of war, morality, and crime.

Whether psychoanalysis is a science has been debated so long and with such sterile results that it is safe to conclude the question is falsely posed. Certainly the methods of psychoanalysis are not those of the natural sciences, its findings are scarcely open to replication and possible refutation by experiment, and it leans heavily on explanatory intermediate concepts which are of great range and imprecision. If we accept Professor R. B. Braithwaite's view that a scientific theory is one in which high-level theoretical statements are linked through rules of interpretation to low-level observational statements, then psycho-analysis qualifies for inclusion unless the elasticity of its rules of inter-pretation and the distance between high level and low level put it out of court. Kenneth Colby, the Research Chairman of the San Francisco Psychoanalytic Institute, writing an Introduction to Psychoanalytic Research, makes an epigrammatic concession: 'Psychology has been precise about things that do not matter much, whereas psychoanalysis has been sloppy about things that matter a great deal'. It is more important that the contrast between the two subjects should lose its point than that a scientific accolade should be conferred on either.

The unkindest charge that can be made against psychoanalysis is that it shows too many of the characteristics of a religion. Disciples gathered round the Master; defections, schisms and heresy; scriptures reproduced with Masoretic devotion; faith in reified abstractions; and a prolonged ritual preparation of oblates—all of these have their close parallels in the history of sects and cults. Suspension of doubt and a mind cleansed of disbelief are common characteristics of the adherents to a new faith. *Addictus jurare in verba magistri*, the average psycho-analyst or analytically inclined physician subscribes to the basic tenets and the metapsychology of analysis so compliantly that his common sense comes under suspicion of having been lulled into torpor. Masserman, himself a prominent American psychoanalyst, put this to the test. Invited to address a group of physicians, he solemnly presented them with a ludicrous, sustained parody of dynamic formulations centred on the ingrowing toenail. He employed, as many analysts do, imprecise terms and formulas which could not be tested as to their validity or meaning; consequently his exposition reads like a grossly far-fetched exercise in freewheeling interpretation, in terms of libido, cathexis, regression and sexual symbolism. To Masserman's extreme surprise, members of his audience later congratulated him on the 'analytic perspicacity with which I had derived the specific dynamic formula for the etiology and possible therapy of that hitherto unexplored psychosomatic disorder—ingrown toenail'.

65

It would be unjust and absurd to take such credulity as a common attribute of psychoanalysts, or of those who expect psychiatrists to spin out improbable fantasies in lieu of psychopathology. The mature psychoanalyst knows how to communicate, and to adjust his language and his interpretations to the measure of his correspondent or interlocutor, and he has adequate ways of judging whether a colleague is running off the psychopathological rails. It is not among such men that one discovers that Simple Simon fervour which recalls the extremes of intellectual capitulation and shallowness characteristic of some cults.

Although the accessions to psychoanalytic theory since Freud's death have been of little weight in comparison with the colossal edifice of ideas and hypotheses that he reared, there are significant respects in which orthodoxy has shifted its ground. Some of the deviations and amendments enjoy only a local vogue and limited acceptance. Melanie Klein's views, for example, might be included in the canon in this country now, but in the United States few would call her theories orthodox, especially those concerning the very early fantasy life of babies, their alleged capacity to experience anxiety and institute defences, and the conflict in them between life and death instincts. In almost all countries, however, ego-psychology has acquired a more central position in psychoanalysis, the notion of psychic energy is less confidently used, more attention is paid to the patient's present life situation than formerly, and the part played by transference and counter-transference in the therapeutic relation is being reshaped.

Psychoanalysis has had its chief efflorescence in the United States, and it is the Americans who have been showing the greatest vigour lately in re-examining the whole structure. Walking to some extent on the same road as the schismatics Karen Horney, H. S. Sullivan, and Erich Fromm, psychoanalysts of the standing of Franz Alexander, S. Rado, Roy Grinker and Jules Masserman have ventured on some radical departures from the Freudian body of theory. Less drastic shifts of emphasis, giving much attention to the relation between the real environment and the developing child which is involved in the process of 'internalizing' the world, have been put forward by recognized leaders of psychoanalysis such as David Rapaport, Heinz Hartmann, and Erik Erikson. Parallel though not identical changes of standpoint have taken place in this country; but there has been less demand here than in America for clearer statement of hypotheses and stricter methods of test and verification.

It is impossible to think or write about psychoanalysis without reverting to the extraordinary qualities of its creator. Ernest Jones has set them out as fully as he could, but the copious flow of Freud's correspondence published since Jones's biography helps us to see aspects of his complex personality through non-apostolic eyes. His stature is not diminished, but some of the contradictions and surprising elements mentioned by Jones are intensified. There are traits and avowals that seem out of character, like his blunt admission to Pfister that 'I have not found much good in the average human being. Most of them are in my experience riff-raff, whether they proclaim this or that ethical doctrine or none at all', and 'In private life I have no patience at all with lunatics. I only see the harm they can do . . .' But in the latest volume of letters (exchanged with Karl Abraham, his Berlin disciple and wise counsellor) the surprise lies in their busy attention to mundane detail. Freud seems immersed in personal imbroglios and practical matters. The bulk of his correspondence with this gifted recruit turns on the domestic politics of the growing movement, its sometimes petty, sometimes bitter internal struggles, its piecemeal successes, and its remarkable capacity for attracting to it difficult, clever, unreliable, ambitious men, as well as men of outstanding firmness and integrity, like Abraham. The violence of the opprobrium Freud cast on those major defectors, the heresiarchs Jung and Adler, and on outspoken opponents like Alfred Hoche and A. A. Friedlaender, is understandable; but it conflicts with the ideal picture of a dispassionate psychologist, averse from moral judgments and tolerant of human weaknesses. Not without reason Percival Bailey calls Freud unserene. Another unexpected feature of his personality was evident in his unmeasured esteem for the psychoanalytic insight and lofty character of that strangely many-sided woman Lou Andreas-Salomé. Though the kind of philosophizing she loved was obnoxious to him, and her way of life the antithesis of his, he was able to write that:

her intimates had the strongest impression of the genuineness and harmony of her being, and discovered that all feminine weaknesses, perhaps most of the human weaknesses, were alien to her nature or had been overcome in the course of her life.

Her assessment of him in turn had less of the superlative about it, but attributed to him genius and nobility. When she first met Freud at the beginning of her sixth decade, she described it as a turning point in her life, and she wrote later of her

respect for the simple heroism of the man. To be sure the heroic and the all-too-human elements lie close together, especially for the psychoanalyst. . . . Confronted by a human being who impresses us as great, should we not be moved, rather than chilled, by the thought that he perhaps attained his greatness only through his weaknesses?

A Psycho-Analytic Dialogue. The letters of Sigmund Freud and Karl Abraham. 1907–1926. Edited by Hilda C. Abraham and Ernst L. Freud. Translated by Bernard Marsh and Hilda C. Abraham. 406pp. Hogarth Press and the Institute of Psycho-Analysis.

SIGMUND FREUD/KARL ABRAHAM: *Briefe, 1907–1926.* 375pp. Frankfurt: S. Fischer.

The Freud Journal of Lou Andreas-Salomé. Translated and with an Introduction by Stanley A. Leavy. 211pp. Hogarth Press and the Institute of Psycho-Analysis.

LOU ANDREAS-SALOMÉ: *In der Schule bei Freud.* Tagebuch eines Jahres 1912–1913. 214pp. Munich: Kindler Taschenbücher.

NORMAN S. GREENFIELD and WILLIAM C. LEWIS (Editors): *Psychoanalysis and Current Biological Thought.* 380pp. Madison: University of Wisconsin Press.

DAVID STAFFORD-CLARK: *What Freud Really Said.* 264pp. Macdonald.

PERCIVAL BAILEY: *Sigmund the Unserene.* A Tragedy in Three Acts. With foreword by Roy R. Grinker. 127pp. Springfield, Illinois: Thomas.

PAUL RICOEUR: *De l'interprétation.* Essai sur Freud. 534pp. Paris: Éditions du Seuil.

6

PSYCHIATRIC DICTA

Aubrey Lewis

Psychiatry does not welcome dogmas, but it has its quota of 'received Tenets and commonly presumed Truths' in which 'our reviewing judgments do find no satisfaction'. Some of these are opinions held about psychiatrists, others are the opinions of psychiatrists about their subject. Here are a few of the latter, casually assembled:

Mental hospitals were custodial in purpose, now they are therapeutic.
Philosophically, psychiatrists must be monists.
The essence of psychiatry is to be found in personal relations.
Medical students will not take psychiatry seriously unless they know that questions in it will be part of their final examination.
There has lately been a revolution in psychiatry.

There are fairly obvious reasons why these opinions are widely held: they have some elements of familiar truth, and are, like many other generalizations, too loose to be open to direct examination and refutation. They invite comment rather than argument.

Mental hospitals were custodial in purpose, now they are therapeutic.—The first of the quoted dicta is expressed more fully in the following passage from an admirably progressive and enlightened book on administrative therapy:

During the last twenty years institutional psychiatry has undergone numerous and profound changes. From being the medical officers of custodial institutions, concerned with security, with preventing escapes, and protecting society from their charges, psychiatrists have become the medical members of therapeutic communities, attempting to help and understand those placed in their care and to build a way of life that will help them soon to emerge as whole people.

The contrast is dramatic, and gratifying to everyone who wants the mentally ill to be brought from darkness into light. But is it overstated? Many of the modern virtues were in evidence in the past; and the modern virtues are lacking in some of our modern institutions. The virtues are indeed not so modern, as good witnesses testify. Adolf

Meyer, for example, visited the mental hospitals of Scotland in 1893 and praised unstintedly the freedom and respect which the patients enjoyed in all of them, and the very individual attention which the nurses paid to their feelings and needs. Bror Gadelius, the professor of psychiatry in Stockholm, described the social opportunities and freedom of activity available to patients in the early 'nineties. Many other authors could be cited, from the beginning of the last century onwards, who recorded the far from custodial attitude adopted in many hospitals where therapeutic effort was conspicuous. Of course the conceptual framework was expressed in a different idiom: it is sometimes pointed out that these men worked in the main on empirical lines which derived from humane conviction rather than from detailed psychological theory. That is so, but theories shift, and derivation from them is not always a virtue. Indeed the current model of the therapeutic community has developed in our time less as a deliberate application of psychological theory than as a product of gradual change in the climate of opinion, favouring a freer, more permissive attitude to deviants and a more egalitarian relation between patients and those who care for them.

Psychiatrists are monists.—As a recent textbook put it, 'bodily functions and mental functions are best regarded as aspects of different levels of intergration of the biological functioning of the individual as a whole'. A more emotional assertion to the same effect was Stanley Cobb's: 'I solve the mind-body problem, therefore, by stating that there is no such problem. The dichotomy is an artefact, there is no truth in it, and the discussion has no place in science. . . . Metaphysicians can argue the problem ad nauseam, and their nausea will be proof of their futility.' This robust attitude is strangely in contrast with the dualist language of psychiatrists writing on psychosomatic topics and with the widespread adoption by psychiatrists of the concepts and assumptions of Freud, an emphatic dualist. For the most part they like to believe that 'pluralism and pragmatism were liberating factors in throwing off dogmatic dualism', but there is a strong Cartesian flavour in most of their statements about mental happenings. Operationally, at any rate, they are dualists.

Essential psychiatry is about personal relations.—Psychiatry is a branch of medicine: it is concerned with all the functions of human beings—physiological, psychological, and social. None is more essential than the other for psychiatric understanding. It is true that in psychiatry the presenting phenomena are often conspicuously in the psychological and social field, but undue emphasis on these can have as damaging an effect on clinical judgment as their neglect. Some question this. There are medically qualified psychotherapists, for example, who agree with Freud's conclusion that for the practice of psychoanalysis a medical training is not necessary. Accordingly somatic and social measures of treatment are handed over to others by psychoanalysts and by psychotherapists who take this view. The patient, it may be thought, is in danger of falling between two stools. It is no comfort that one of the stools is marked 'essential'.

Medical students need an examination paper in psychiatry.—The argument runs on familiar lines: unless the student knows that he will be examined separately in a subject, he will suppose that his teachers and examiners do not think it of much importance, and he will feel safe to concentrate his energies on other, weightier subjects. This view is not in keeping with the often expressed desire of medical students to have fuller teaching of psychiatry than they get in some schools. Moreover, it rates too low the intrinsic interest of the subject when competently taught; and it implies that the kind of knowledge which can be tested by questions in a written paper is worth cultivating in a subject which, at this stage of a doctor's training, should be pre-eminently clinical. Happily, in many schools the student may encounter a psychiatric problem in his clinical examinations: he will then do well or ill according to his education and capacity, but he can hardly prepare himself for such a clinical test by hard reading. Supervised clinical clerking in psychiatry is more valuable than lectures and mastery of a textbook, and it does not require the goad of an imminent ordeal to excite interest in it.

There has been a recent revolution in psychiatry.—But a revolution implies the overthrow of what was established, and the aftermath of a revolution often derides the aims of the revolutionaries. The changes in psychiatry have not been like that, and do not deserve the sounding name given them by enthusiasts. The enthusiasts differ about the nature of the revolution they acclaim, some seeing it in community care, others in the advent of the tranquillizing drugs, or in behaviour therapy. It has been a common and invigorating habit of psychiatrists to rejoice that they live in an age of rapid and impressive advance: 'bliss was it in that dawn to be alive'. The advances are there, but they have enough of the perishable and uncertain about them to make 'revolution' too confident a word.

Sir Thomas Browne offered wise counsel about hasty appraisal. 'In this Encyclopædia and round of Knowledge, like the great and exemplary wheel of Heaven, we must observe two Circles; that, while we are daily carried about, and whirled on by the swing and rapt of the one, we may maintain a natural and proper course in the slow and sober wheel of the other. And this we shall more readily perform, if we timely survey our knowledge.'

Problems Presented by the Ambiguous Word "Anxiety" as used in Psychopathology

AUBREY LEWIS

London

The number of articles on anxiety listed in Psychological Abstracts in 1927 was three. By 1931 it had risen to fourteen, and by 1950 to thirty-seven. In 1960 it was two hundred and twenty-two, and in 1966 it was still over two hundred. It may be concluded that the subject to which the term refers rapidly increased in importance or in vogue in the last decade, and that it would be as well to define what the word means. This is an awkward undertaking because different meanings are rampant. It is best to examine first the ordinary or vernacular meaning in various languages, and then to review its more precise meaning in the technical language of psychiatry and psychology.

The hypothetical Indogermanic root is *Angh*. In Greek this appears in αγχω to press tight, to strangle. In the Thesaurus Latinae Linguae αχθυμαι, to be weighed down with griefs and αχθυς, a load, a burden, trouble, are also related to *anxietas*.

The relevant Latin words contain the *Angh* root. They are *angustus, ango, angor, anxius, anxietas, angina*. In all these the notion of narrowness and constriction is present, literally or metaphorically, and there is usually discomfort or deficiency, too, as in English 'straits'. *Ango*, to throttle, follows the Greek closely but with more emphasis on the figurative meaning, to cause pain, to vex. Between *angor* and *anxietas* Cicero states a firm distinction: *angor* is transitory, an outburst; *anxietas* is an abiding predisposition: "anxium proprie dici qui pronus est ad aegritudinem animi, neque enim omnes anxii, qui anguntur aliquando; nec qui anxii, semper anguntur". The idea of pressure he says, is in *angor* — "angor est aegritudo premens". Other writers did not adhere to these distinctions: thus in the glossarium *anxius* is equivalent to "*tristis, cruciatus, angore affectus*", *angor* to "*dolor, metus, timor*". It is however Cicero's differentiation of *angor* from *anxietas* that prepares the way for corresponding usages later e.g. *anxiété* and *angoisse*: *anxiété* would be the lasting constitutional attribute, *angoisse* the transitory attack. It is noteworthy that although *angor* and *anxietas*, like the corresponding Greek words, denote distress, they scarcely include the idea of uncertainty and fear which has become an important feature, but they tend to stress sadness and disquiet — "anxius qui animi inquietudine et dolore angitur; nimis sollicitus tristis".

French usage may be considered next. *Angoisse* is defined by Littré (1863) as a feeling of constriction in the epigastric region with difficulty in breathing and great sadness, and as "grande affliction avec inquiétude", while *anxiété* is "angoisse de l'esprit", and "état de trouble et d'agitation, avec sentiment de gêne et de reserrement à la région précordiale". The two terms were therefore practically synonymous in 1863: at that time the word *anxieux* had not been admitted to the Dictionary of the Academy. Littré laid it down that *inquiétude anxiété*, and *angoisse* are three degrees of the same condition; just as Kant had established the gradation in German — Bangigkeit, Angst, Grauen, Entsetzen, Furcht.

A dictionary definition, even in Littré, may be questioned. In 1890 Littré's definition of *anxiété* and *angoisse* was rejected by Brissaud who was not prepared to regard *anxiété* and *angoise* as almost interchangeable terms differing only in the relative severity of the condition they denoted. Brissaud maintained that for the acute condition with feelings of imminent death, the proper term is *anxiété*; whereas *angoisse* — or more specifically *angoisse physique* — refers to the feelings of constriction in the chest and being stifled. Brissaud however complicated the issue by calling *anxiété* '*angoisse intellectuelle*'; he said that morbid *anxiété* is indefinable and that its indefinability is its most characteristic feature. From that time there have been lively disputes in France about the proper use of these two words. Littré was again objected to, on account of his statement that in ordinary usage *anxiété* is a mental state of trouble and agitation, whereas *angoisse* is associated with a mental state of extreme sadness. Niceties of language were battled over. Thus Pitres and Régis in 1902 insisted that *angoisse* is compounded of fear and doubt; Boven in 1935 said that graded in the scale of severity restlessness (*inquiétude*) is the mild form, then comes *anxiété*, and the worst is *angoisse*. Boutonier in 1945 agrees, while also holding (like Cicero) that *angoisse* is a more transitory emotion than anxiety. She adds, however, with rather less lucidity, that "there is something ambiguous in *angoisse* and also in *anxiété*".

In German the idea of narrowness and onstriction is traceable in the words *eng* and *bange*, as well as in *Angst*. The Deutsches Wörterbuch of the Brothers Grimm states that "Angst ist nicht bloss Mutlosigkeit sondern quälende Sorge, zweifelnder beengender Zustand überhaupt" and give an informative quotation from Luther: "Angst im ebraischen lautet als das Enge, und ich achte das in Deudschen auch Angst daher komme, das Enge sei, darin einem bange und wehe wird und gleich beklemmet gedruckt und gepresset wird, wie denn die Anfechtungen und Unglück thun, nach dem Sprichwort'es war mir die weite Welt zu enge' " In Luther's translation of the Bible he uses Angst where the Authorised Version usually has 'distress', 'straits' or 'anguish of soul'.

The word was extended to cover a state of needless fear (aus unnötiger Furcht) and the element of dread was strongly incorporated in it. (e.g., "war von Furcht und Ängsten gepeinigt": Goethe). In the seventeenth century Angst could also mean 'longing'.

The Italian *ansia* similarly contains the idea of longing — desiderio ardente e con principio di dolore — but it can be a shorter form of *ansieta*. *Ansieta* denotes "a state of the body or the mind in which pain, doubt or desire make us waver between longing (*ansia*) and a feeling of constriction or anguish (ondeggiare tra l'ansia e un principio d'affanne o d'angoscia)". (Tommaseo and Bellini 1895).

In the Dictionary of the Spanish Academy *angustia* means distress, anguish (aflicción, congoja) while *ansiedad* is a state of restlessness or depression (inquietud o zozobra de ánimo). Lopez Ibor comments that the word *ansiedad* has a morbid note that is not found in the word *angustia*, and that the differentiation must have occurred after the sixteenth century as, in Covarubbia's Dictionary (1611) *angustia* and *ansia* were both stated to mean oppression of the heart, feeling of mental constriction; corporis vel animae cruciatus; *ansiedad* was not mentioned in it.

In English we have in this cluster anxiety, anxious, anguish, and anger: formerly there was also ange. Concisely, the relevant items from the Oxford English Dictionary are:

'ange' meant trouble, affliction: in plural, straits.

'anger' had, as a now obsolete meaning, trouble, sorrow.

'anguish' means excruciating or oppressive bodily pain; or severe mental suffering.

'anxious' means 1. troubled in mind about some uncertain event; being in painful or disturbing suspense.

2. full of desire and endeavour; solicitous, earnestly desirous (e.g. 'anxious to please')

'anxiety' means 1. uneasiness about some uncertain event.

2. solicitous desire to effect some purpose.

3. (at least since 1661) a condition of agitation and depression, with a sensation of tightness and distress in the precordial region.

There are, it is clear, in various languages some common features of this group of words, but there are also differences that make translation dubious or deceptive. Literal and figurative feelings of constriction and distress, sadness or pain, are usually implicit in the usage of the languages considered above — and in others, of which Hebrew is an outstanding example. Nowhere is the association of tightness and distress more plainly given linguistic expression than in the literal and figurative meanings of צר.

In some European languages, including English, 'anxiety' may denote only desire, without distress (e.g., Nelson's dispatch "The General seems as anxious as any of us to expedite the fall of the place"). This is found also in Latin (cf. "quaerendi, judicaudi, comparandi anxietas"), and in Italian, but not in modern German, French or Spanish.

The German word '*Angst*' is not flanked by other derivatives of the root, as is the case in the rest of the languages reviewed. It is the most influential word of them all, from the psychiatric standpoint; yet it signifies a degree of fear that is far from inherent in the English word 'anxiety' or some of the other terms considered. Muret Sanders gives as German equivalents of anxiety, Schreck, Furcht, Bestürzung, and as English equivalents of Angst, besides anxiety and anguish, "agony, dread, fear, fright, terror, consternation, alarm, apprehension". These are terms appropriate for a far more shattering emotion than our 'anxiety' which may be scarcely more than 'concern', (as in Darwin's "few persons feel any anxiety from the impossibility of determining at what precise period in the development of the individual, man became an immortal being"). It is clear that, in the commonly used meaning of the word, it would be misleading to translate '*Angst*' as 'anxiety'.

This incomparability of seemingly similar or identical words has harassed a number of readers and translators. Since the line of demarcation between the literary or vernacular and the technical psychiatric usage of the word 'anxiety' is indistinct, the complaints of translators need to be recorded here before the technical term is more closely examined. Lowrie, the translator of Kierkegaard's "The Concept of Dread", says "the very title of this book reveals a serious lack in our language: we have no word which adequately translates *Angst*. In the first translation of fragments of Kierkegaard published by Professor Hollander in 1924 he used the word 'dread' and everyone has agreed to continue it — after a desperate search for something better. The Spanish translation uses *angustia*. . . both the French translators use *angoisse*. These words rightly indicate the distress of the moment but do not suggest what is essential to the experience Kierkegaard deals with, that it is an anticipation of the future."

Edouard Pichon deals with the problem as French translators encounter it. He distinguishes between the words concerned with fear — *peur, crainte, terreur, frousse, frayeur, effroi* — and *anxiété* and *angoisse*. He exclaims, rather petulantly that "it is time to make an end of the perpetual confusion occasioned by translation of the equivocal German term "*Angst*". He illustrates the confusion by citing Kastrationsangst and Todesangst.

Wandruszka likewise stigmatised *Angst* and *Furcht* as deceptive words: to try and assign to them separate content "is like making a stroke of the pen in turbulent water". James Strachey, the translator of Freud's complete works into English, wrote a special note on his difficulties with *Angst*. Recalling that Freud did not consistently observe the distinction he himself drew about the use of the word, Strachey asserted that *Angst* may on occssion "be translated by any one of half a dozen similarly common English words — fear, fright, alarm and so on — and it is therefore quite unpractical to fix on some simple English term as its sole translation". He deplored the universal adoption of 'anxiety' as the equivalent for *Angst* when used as a technical term: the remoteness of 'anxiety' from any of the uses of the German *Angst* made it unsuitable, but it is too late to rectify the error. Finally Strachey objected strongly to the translation of *Angst* simply as "morbid anxiety": it is, he wrote, ill-judged because there is the theoretical problem, discussed by Freud, of whether and why *Angst* can be sometimes pathological and sometimes normal.

Loosli-Usteri, with Swiss impartiality, indicated German and French usage alike: "the situation is anarchical", she declared, "*angoisse* and *anxiété* are loosely interchangeable in meaning and so are *Angst* and *Furcht*". A short polyglot table which she drew up showed the inexactitude prevailing in this area.

Lopez Ibor believes the linguistic situation has influenced thinking, "the fact that there is only the one word *Angst* has relieved the Germans of any necessity to separate and distinguish between *angustia* and *ansiedad* . . ." The great influence of the German psychiatrists has led many other authors to forget such distinctions, even outside the German tongue . . . . In Spanish *angustia* and *anciedad* are now used indifferently; because of the influence of foreign languages".

There can be little doubt that the attention paid to anxiety in the last ten years or more has been largely due to the adoption of Freudian concepts and to some extent of Freudian metapsychology. But some writers go rather too far in this direction; they believe that psychiatrists only lately woke up to the prominence of fear states in mental disorder. Thus Sarbin recently wrote "The word anxiety was hardly used in standard medical and psychiatrical textbooks until the late 1930's. It was a result of Freud's writing about *Angst*, translated anxiety, that the term now has wide currency." Such a statement is only justified if it is tacitly assumed that non-English writings do not count. Kraepelin in the second edition of his textbook, which appeared in 1887, devoted

considerable space to *Angst*, differentiating if from *Aengstlichkeit*. Aschaffenburg,in the volume of the Handbuch dealing with symptomatology (1915),
likewise gave much space to *Angst*, as did the majority of German authors
of psychiatric textbooks from the beginning of the century. Wernicke's description of *Angstpsychose* occurring in the involutional period had a particularly
powerful effect, from the publication of his Grundriss onwards. French textbooks (such as Régis's Précis 1914) deealt fully with *angoisse* and *anxiété*,
recalling the debates, in the nineties and subsequently, in which Brissaud,
Lalanne, Féré and Souques were prominent. Devaux and Logre published
their monograph *Les Anxieux* in 1917, and F. Heckel's "*La Névrose d'Angoisse*"
came out in 1927, the year after Janet's classical study "*De l'angoisse à l'extase*".
It is therefore only a parochial restriction to Anglo-Saxon writings that can
lead to such an assertion as Professor Sarbin made. In the psychiatric textbooks of England and America in the first quarter of the century, it is true,
the word anxiety does not occur prominently, but fear and agitation do, and
would be the equivalents of *Angst*.

It is possible that the concept of anxiety has been made familiar to many
because of its prominence in existential philosophy, which began with Søren
Kierkegaard and was given wider currency by theologians like Tillich and
philosophers like Heidegger, Jaspers and Sartre. Influential though
Kierkegaard's writings have been they are arcane for the uninstructed reader.
"Dread is different" wrote Kierkegaard, "from fear and similar concepts
which refer to something definite, whereas dread (*Angst*) is the reality of freedom
as possibility anterior to possibility;" "he who through *Angst* becomes guilty
is innocent, for it was not he himself but *Angst*, an alien power, which laid
hold of him... there is nothing in the world more ambiguous (than *Angst*)".
"Angst is the dizziness of freedom which occurs when the spirit would posit
the synthesis, and freedom then gazes down at its own possibility." These
quotations from the standard translation of Kierkegaard's book "The Concept
of Dread" sufficiently indicate the abstruseness of his theory, and the obstacles
in the way of equating *Angst* as he and his successors understood it with *Angst*
the psychological concept used in psychopathology. Some have however
essayed the task, linking anxiety, as Kierkegaard did, to freedom and self-
consciousness, but paying less regard to his insistence that *Angst* lays bare
all finite aims, and discovers that they are deceptive: "no Grand Inquisitor
has in readiness such terrible tortures as has *Angst* and no spy knows how to
attack more artfully the man he suspects". Dr. Boutonier, in her sympathetic
review, points out that Kierkegaard's intuitions are close neighbours to ambivalence: "dans l'ambivalence primitive, instincts destructifs et instincts con-
structifs ont la même force et les mêmes droits." To pursue this further would

77

be to engage in study of the psychopathology and the metaphysics of fear, which is not within the intended scope of this paper.

Anxiety as a technical word in psychiatry has passed through two main phases: first as a qualifying term for the agitated depression of melancholia, secondly as a qualifying term for a neurosis in which subjective feelings of alarm are associated with visceral disturbances. The first had its title — anxiety psychosis — conferred by Wernicke; the second, *Angstneurose*, was christened by Freud. The former has never had much currency outside Germany, and is now little used. The Freudian usage calls for detailed consideration in view of its central role in dynamic psychopathology. So does the parallel French, for a different reason: it was more critically examined and more discriminatingly used than the German term, on which British and American psychiatrists have relied, accepting its deceptively close translation as anxiety.

The French psychiatrists have made manful efforts to define the two terms of art — *angoisse* and *anxiété*. As already indicated in this paper ordinary language as defined in Littré was not precise enough for clear thinking and exact classification. The most distinguished guide through the corresponding maze is Janet. In 1903 he proposed to regard as *angoisse* a diffuse emotional perturbation of the whole individual, "sans rapport avec une pensée deter-minée"; following Ribot — and Cicero — he considered *anxiété* to be a vague but permanent state: "où l'anxiété au lieu d'être rivée à un objet toujours le même, flotte comme dans un rêve et ne se fixe que pour un instant au hazard des circonstances. M. Freud, " Janet adds " a beaucoup insisté sur cet état constituant ce qu'il appelle la 'névrose d'angoisse' ". He goes on to emphasise that *angoisse* may be mental (possibly accompanied by headache and feeling of depresonalisation) or 'visceral' (e.g. respiratory and cardiac disturbance). A quarter of a century later he links *anxiété* closely to depression, as the ancients did: "la tristesse peut prendre la forme de mélancolie, d'anxiété, d'angoisse morale"; and he summed up the relation of *anxiété* and *angoisse*: "l'anxiété n'est qu'une angoisse répétée à propos d'un grand nombre d'actions et étendue à toute la vie." He added that there is a constitutional predisposition to *anxiété*.

Edouard Pichon followed Janet's lead, with more stringent definition. For him *angoisse* is a process in which intense and acute mental suffering synchronises with a subjective sense of constriction of the throat, tachycardia and other visceral disturbances; *anxiété* is chronic mental state, in which there is sub-jective discomfort of neuro-vegetative origin, and a characteristic facies.

There were, however, slightly dissonant voices. Déjérine and Gauckler in 1911 wrote that *angoisse* is "une impression physique qui s'oppose a l'anxiété, impression physique (tightness of epigastrium, feeling of suffocation) . . . , c'est une diffusion physique d'une émotion psychique qui s'amplifie progressivement dans la conscience et qui crée psychiquement l'anxiété a laquelle l'angoisse est souvent liée."

Baruk in his Traité (1959) elaborates the varieties of *anxiété*, which he clearly regards as a comprehensive term, *angoisse* being much less important: "on distingue en général, l'anxiété, malaise essentiellement moral, comme la crainte d'un malheur, et l'angoisse qui est un malaise beaucoup plus physique, comme par exemple la sensation du coeur serré, la gêne respiratoire, la peur de se trouver mal." He describes an *"anxiété purement metaphvsique"* in the early stages of schizophrenia without any *angoisse physique*, and maintains that many organic diseases have *angoisse* without any anxiety. Like many writers, he says that the difference between *anxiété* and fear (*peur*) is that the latter is occasioned by some evident and verifiable danger, and disappears when the danger disappears; whereas the danger which brings on anxiety is psychological, consisting of images and recollection of past dangers, evocation of future dangers, or awareness of insidious or impending disorders, of the body or the mind. Baruk is one of the few authorities who dwell on the advantages of anxiety and the calamities that can be brought about by its absence e.g. after leucotomy. Baruk uses the term "anxieux constitutionel" (introduced by Lévy-Valensi) to denote the patient with *anxiété* as Pierre Janet used the word.

Henri Ey has written a lengthy and well informed study of pathological anxiety. He begins by acknowledging the distinction implicit in the terms: *angoisse*, he says, is, in medical psychology, an emotional disturbance experienced in the face of imminent danger, and characterised by bodily phenomena, whereas *anxiété* is a more general affective state. But in a footnote he says he will use *angoisse* and *anxiété* indifferently, and the succeeding pages bear out this threat or apology, in which he follows Dr. Favez Boutonier. It is therefore not difficult to bring his subsequent use of these terms into line with English usage, on purely etymological grounds, but perplexing statements follow, regarding crises of anxiety. As Ey sees it, these crises of morbid anxiety can occur in melancholia (in the form of stupor, agitation, confusional oneiroid state, or perplexity) in schizophrenia, in dementia, in manic-depressive psychosis and in epilepsy; it can alternatively appear as a neurotic disorder *"névrose d'angoisse"* or as *"anxiété constitutionelle"* of which there are three clinical types: cyclothymia, neurasthenia and hypochondria. In spite of the erudition and occasional subtlety displayed in Dr. Ey's review of the different aspects of anxiety, it cannot be said that his effort to bring together French views and those of Freud and some German psychologists and philosophers have brought clarity into the scene. He could not subscribe to the deceptively simple medical usage stated succinctly by Brissaud: *angoisse* and *anxiété* are necessary terms for two distinct phenomena "un phenomène physique d'angoisse et un phenomène purement psychique, l'anxiété". No doubt Dr. Ey rejected this over-sharp distinction because a purely psychological distinction without bodily accompaniments is as elusive and uncommon as physical expressions of anxiety without any subjective accompaniment. The disjunction can occur, but rarely and in very special circumstances.

Because of his influence on the language of psychopathology, Freud's use of the term *Angst* is of special importance. Significantly he wrote in the 25th of the Introductory Lectures that *Angst* itself needs no description: "everyone has presumably experienced this sensation, or, to speak more correctly, this affective conditions, at sometime or other"; and he added that the problem of *Angst* is a "nodal point ... a riddle of which the solution must cast a flood of light upon our whole mental life." He was, evidently, at a much earlier period of life, indifferent to the problems of translation inherent in the word *Angst*, since in an article he wrote in French in 1895 he used the two words *angoisse* and *anxiété* as though they were synonymous: "in the group of phobias, this emotional state is always one of *angoisse*, while in true obsessions other emotional states ... may occur just as well as *anxiété*."

The main article bearing on his technical use of the term appeared in 1895, when he made the case for delimiting *Angstneurose*. In this article he quoted Hecker who had in 1893 written about "*Angstzustand bei Neurasthenie*". Freud described the syndrome in terms of ten prominent features: 1. general irritability, 2. anxious expectation, 3. acute dread (*Angst*); fear of death, for example, 4. varying combination of these with accompaniments, which he lists, 5. night terrors, 6. vertigo, 7. phobias, 8. digestive tract disturbances, 9. paraesthesias like those of hysteria, 10. the symptoms may be chronic and accompanied by little anxiety. This was an elaborated version of the views stated in drafts which Freud had sent to Fliess. In the second draft, (1893), Freud had written that *Angstneurose* appears in two forms — as a chronic state and as an attack of anxiety. He then considered that "periodic depression must be regarded as a third form of anxiety neurosis, an attack of anxiety which may last for weeks or months." In the fifth draft (1894) he wrote that "anxiety is the sensation of an accumulation of another endogenous stimulus — the stimulus towards breathing—which cannot be worked over psychically in any way." The actiology of anxiety neurosis was at the centre of Freud's preoccupation at this time, and his conception of the term 'anxiety' in the syndrome "anxiety neurosis" (which he called the somatic counterpart of hysteria) has to be inferred. He was convinced that frustrated sexual discharge and the resulting accumulated tension accounted for the generation of anxiety. Later he construed anxiety as a repetition of the experience of birth — "which involves just such a concentration of painful feelings, of discharges of excitation, and of bodily sensations, as to have become a prototype for all occasions on which life is endangered, ever after to be reproduced again in us as the dread or 'anxiety' condition".

The chief variation in Freud's views on the aetiology of anxiety was experienced in his "Hemmung, Symptom and Angst" in 1926. Essentially this consisted in his abandonment of the conception of anxiety as transformed libido, and recognition of it as a reaction to situations of danger. Consequently he distinguished between realistic and neurotic anxiety. *Angst*, he now held, has an unmistakable relation to expectation. It is indefinite and lacks an object: "in precise speech we use the word *Furcht* rather than *Angst* if it has found an object. Real danger is a danger that is known, and realistic anxiety (*Realangst*) is anxiety about a known danger ... neurotic anxiety is anxiety about an unknown danger. By bringing this danger which is not known to the ego into consciousness, the analyst makes neurotic anxiety no different from realistic anxiety". "A danger situation is a recognized, remembered, expected situation of helplessness. Anxiety is the original reaction to helplessness in the trauma and is reproduced later on in the danger situation as a signal for help." There is some looseness in the expression of these views, and in the interchange of the use of terms *Angst* and *Unlust*: "anxiety is characterized by a specific character of unpleasure, (*Unlust*) acts of discharge (through visceral innervations) and perception of these acts."

In 1929 Ernest Jones sought to clarify the matter. He drew attention to the allied concepts anxiety, fear, dread, fright, panic, and apprehensiveness, and stated that "in psychopathology the term 'morbid anxiety', or 'anxiety' for short, is widely employed to designate a particular collection of phenomena, one which can be distinguished from those grouped round the name of fear". The distinction rests on two features: the disproportion between the external stimulus and the response to it, and the disproportion between bodily and mental manifestations. Since, however, Jones and Freud himself recognise that 'realistic anxiety' and 'morbid anxiety' may coexist in the same person, to distinguish between fear (which can be taken as a normal phenomenon) and anxiety (taken to be morbid) it would be necessary to have some standard of proportion and some quantitative measure for recognising disproportion. This, as Jones admitted, is hardly practicable: "I do not think, however, that sufficiently accurate observations have yet been made for us to establish with any sureness a direct correlation between the disharmony in question and the extent to which the response is pathological". There has been a good deal written about the 'normality' of anxiety, but it is unprofitable to pursue it:

it rests partly on looseness of terminology and partly on opinions about the psychopathology of anxiety which go beyond the purview of this note. Many of the difficulties of definition have been accentuated by uncertainty in the use made of such words as 'danger' and 'expedient'. Thus Freud wrote: "an increase in unpleasure which is expected and foreseen is met by a signal of anxiety; the occasion of this increase, whenever it threatens from without or from within, is called a danger," and he says it is the business of the ego to protect itself from danger by means of anxiety. Yet elsewhere he wrote that "the development of anxiety (is) the inexpedient element in what we call anxiety or dread ... In my opinion anxiety relates to the condition and ignores the object, whereas in the word 'fear' attention is directed to the object; fright ... relates specifically to the condition induced when danger is unexpectedly encountered without previous anxious readiness. It might be said then that anxiety is a protection against fright." Not without reason Freud adds, in the following sentence "it will not have escaped you that a certain ambiguity and indefiniteness exists in the use of the word 'anxiety' ".

The psychoanalytical usage of the word *Angst* cannot be entirely divorced from the general psychiatric usage in German-speaking countries. In the late part of the nineteenth century the concept which Angst was meant to convey had more to do with involutional melancholia than with what came to be called anxiety neurosis. Wernicke gave currency to the term 'anxiety psychosis', covering what was later called 'agitated depression' or 'anxiety melancholia'. Through Wernicke's pupil and faithful intellectual heir Kleist, the condition was further studied and made to include the "degenerative psychoses". Leonhard, inheritor of Kleist's views, has fused the *Angstpsychosen* with the *Glüeckspsychosen*, much as mania and depression were fused into one bipolar cycloid disease. Leonhard has urged that in extremes of unpleasure anxiety is always experienced, but in the *Angst-Glückspsychose* it is associated with suspicion, ideas of reference, terrifying hallucinations and hypochronidrcal ideas: there may be also self-reproach. Leonard makes some distinction between "pure anxiety psychosis" in which there are always paranoid features, and "*Angst-glückspsychose*"; in the former there may be little agitation: the patients are 'petrified' with fear. Kleist was disposed to make this a point of relevance to the further division of the *Angstpsychose*, according to whether there was excessive agitated movement or stupor. It is necessary to bear this usage of *Angst* in mind, though it has not been adopted in most countries, because it may become a part of the generally accepted classificatory system of East Germany.

A better known strand of psychiatric opinion may be derived from Kraepelin though he picked it up and developed, rather than originated, it. Thus Roller in 1880 had written "Wenn aber in der grossen Klasse von Seelenstörungen, die wir unter dem Namen der Melancholie zusammenzufassen pflegen, etwas typisch ist, so ist es die Angst, sei es dass sie als solche, sei es dass sie in allerlei Transformationen und Verkleidungen auftritt ... Die präcordiale Angst ist bekanntlich eines der kostantesten Symptome." He emphasised that *Angst* had for a long time attracted the close attention of psychiatrists. Kraepelin, seven years later, in the second edition of his textbook, devoted considerable space to *Angst*, especially as an accompaniment of melancholia. The tension state of anxiety often, he stated, provided the background of mood in mental disorder in either restlessness, excitement and discharge of emoton or in inhibition of all voluntary movement; such general states of extreme *Angst* are especially to be seen in certain forms of melancholia and paranoia as well as in rabies and the physical diseases affecting respiration and the circulation. Passing from these *Angstpsychosen* to milder forms he described *Aengstlichkeit* (a condition corresponding closely to French *anxiété*) in which there is a persistent sense of helplessness in the face of some threat; it may be recognised passing by gradual steps either into the constant terror of some impending danger or, in the other, direction, into the accepted range of normal behaviour.

By 1909, in the eighth edition of the textbook, Kraepelin again described *Angst* as a combination of unpleasure with inner tension which involved the whole bodily and mental state. He enumerated the many manifestations in posture and expression, in groaning, screaming, and running away, vertigo, feelings of weakness, palpitations and precordial pressure, falling, dyspepsia, tremor, sweating, urgency or incontinence and diarrhoea; in the beginning the *Angst* occurs without any stimulus of which the sufferer is aware, but gradually the feelings of discomfort settle into more or less definite fears. *Angst* may be oftenest met with in the severe depression of manic-depressive disorder but it occurs also in delirium and in the extensive clinical group of phobias. The description of the varieties of anxiety is fuller than in other similar works, but much of it concerns the phobias, whose relation to obsessional disorders is a common theme in other detailed considerations of anxiety states.

A contemporary German writer, (Panse) in a monograph on *Angst* und *Schreck* assumes that *Angst* and *Furcht* (fear) are practically indistinguishable in subjective feelings and bodily disturbances; he agrees however with Hoche that *Angst* is distinct from *Schreck* (fright, consternation) in that the latter need not be unpleasant, and he stresses the suddenness with which the individual is overwhelmed in *Schreck*, as against *Angst*, (e.g. by an earthquake). Another prominent contemporary writer however, groups together *Traurigkeit* (sadness), *Schreck* and *Angst* as important causes of breakdown. Many German psychiatrists regard *Angst* — and *Schreck* — as 'vital' feelings, (in the sense in which

Schneider and Lopez Ibor have used this elusive term) though *Angst* is considered by them to be more elemental and instinctive, whereas fear (*Frucht*) is rather a rational affair. However, "die körperlichen Begleit — und Folge — erscheinungen jeder Art Angst sind die gleichen wie beim Schreckerlebnis".

Italian psychiatrists define anxiety as "sentimento di attesa penosa" and *angoscia* as "ansia grave senza contenuto ideativo". Many of them (e.g. Disertori, Bini, Rubino) distinguish between free-floating *angoscia* which they equate with Freud's *Angstneurose*, and the *angoscia* which is intimately and irrationally fixed on some definite idea, as in phobias. The former occurs in crises coming out of a clear sky, with a feeling of imminent catastrophe and with intense bodily manifestations, Somewhat confusingly Italian writers describe also a "*nevrose d'ansia*" which occurs in episodes of primary, non-reactive anxiety and is of varying intensity. Bini and Bazzi have a further category of 'psychogenic' *ansia* which is a reaction to some calamity or exceptional stress.

The Spanish view, most fully presented by Lopez Ibor, is close to the French: in *angustia* (*angoisse*) the physical side of the affective disturbances is predominant, in *ansiedad* (*anxiété*) the psychological; the former is more static, the latter has movement, a feeling of unquiet expectation; *angustia* is more deeply 'vital', more visceral. Delgado, of Lima, defines anxiety neurosis (*anjustia*) as a 'vital' affective state which disturbs and hampers activity and occurs spontaneously or under some stress to which the reaction is disproportionate and continues independently of the cessation of the stress; it is also characterised by the intensity and variety of its bodily symptoms. He disagrees with Lopez Ibor's view of a nuclear, non-psychogenic, "anxious thymopathy" which can be grouped, as an endogenous affective state, with the manic depressive group. Another Spanish authority (Mira) emphasised the necessity to demonstrate that the syndrome is mostly psychogenic before diagnosing anxiety neurosis: he recognised *angustia* as severe *ansia* lacking any ideational content.

Amid this welter it might be hoped rather than expected, that psychiatric usage of the term 'anxiety' in the English speaking countries would be more consistent, or more exact, or more uniform. In a standard work, Allbutt's System of Medicine (1899), the term 'anxiety' is not used technically, and 'anxiety neurosis' is described but not delimited, the disorder being grouped with obsessions and other forms of 'neurasthenia': "peculiar dreads and oppressions which do not tincture the whole being as insanity does... these dreads or 'obsessions' are besetting thoughts, impulses or anxieties which have their origins within... such are false apprehensions of evil, fears of fears, recurring impulses, or, again, peculiar bodily oppressions or disturbances — cardiac, respiratory, pelvic... a dread of formless evil." It took about a quarter of a century before the French or the German usage of 'anxiety' became general in Great Britain or the United States. Thus in England a text-book appeared in 1928 which had no reference to 'anxiety' in the Index, and this conditon was mentioned only fleetingly under the heading of Psychasthenia. Another author of a textbook (Stoddart) reported in the Preface to his third edition, which appeared in 1919, that he had become "convinced of the truth of Freud's doctrines" and had therefore added a new chapter, on the Anxiety Neurosis. The American psychiatrist, William A. White, in the eighth edition of his textbook (1921) wrote that he wished to carry the student further into the realm of the newer, more dynamic interpretative psychiatry: he devoted half a page (in a book of 355 pages) to the 'anxiety neurosis of Freud' and three or four lines to stating that in involutional melancholia depression "often gives rise to a state of anxiety with marked precordial distress, difficulty of breathing, and some motor agitation". T. A. Ross, contributing an extensive section on 'the Anxiety Reactions' to the Anglo-American Oxford Loose-Leaf Medicine (1936) stated at the outset that he included in the word 'anxiety' "such emotional states as doubt, mental conflict, boredom, disappointment, that is to say depressive emotional states . . . The mental symptoms (of anxiety reactions) are insomnia, fears, phobias and apprehensions, depression, failure of concentration, poor memory, shyness in company, bashfulness, sense of inferiority, various disagreeable ideas, the sense of unreality."

Since these far from subtle or precise uses of the term were prevalent, there has been considerable change in the Anglo-American approach to anxiety. This can best be conveyed by some quotations from more or less contemporary American psychiatrists, Norman Cameron wrote in 1947 that "we designate as anxiety the predominantly covert skeletal and viceral reaction which, for an unhampered and uninhibited person, constitutes the normal preliminary phase of emotional flight, but which for some reason is prevented from going on into its consummatory phase." . . . In a monograph on 'Anxiety and Stress' by a Chicago group (1954) anxiety is defined as "the conscious and reportable experience of intense dread and foreboding, conceptualized as internally derived and unrelated to external threat." The authors go on, however, to say that it is not always possible to differentiate the fear response to actual real danger from the objectless anxiety response. To a trivial danger the organism may react as though it were a matter of life and death; anxiety tends to be chronic, fear to be transient and preparatory to appropriate behaviour. Anxiety is always accompanied by weakening of ego boundaries; the person may be unable to distinguish self from object. Because of the many meanings of the word 'anxiety', in both common and scientific parlance, Grinker and his colleagues restrict the term to 'free anxiety', meaning the conscious emotional experience and ignoring the accompanying somatic and psychological changes. In this conception of anxiety, 'unconscious anxiety' becomes a contradiction in terms.

An English investigator recently stated (1961) that a legitimate and potentially useful definition of anxiety was the "conditioned form of the pain-fear response" involving automatic arousal and skeletal motor discharge. She was taking this definition from a suggestion by two American investigators and was criticised by another American writer for thus accepting an electro-physiological explanation and calling it a definition.

Many psychologists define anxiety in terms of the subject's score on certain items in the Taylor Manifest Anxiety Scale or the Minnesota Multiple Personality Inventory — an operational definition, (buttressed potentially with measures of eye blink conditioning etc.). Critics emphasise that the scale measures and defines only manifest anxiety. Other workers stress the need to recognise 'unconscious anxiety' but do not define it.

A special issue affecting definition, in regard to which there is much written but little clearly established, is anxiety in children (including night-terrors). The problems in childhood are dealt with mostly by educational psychologists such as Claparède and his pupil Dr. Loosli Usteri: it would require a separate paper to give a comprehensive account of views about the differentiation of normal from pathological anxiety in children, and the consequences for delimitation. Dr. Loosli Usteri offers as a definition "anxiety is that state of inner unrest and insecurity which arises from imbalance between the forces making for development and those making for permanence and fixity:" nothing operational about that! She adds that she realises her definition goes beyond the bounds of empirical science. She defends her definition on the ground that in childhood the forces of development are, of course, more powerful than in the adult, and the tensions appearing as imbalance therefore more severe.

CONCLUSIONS

Enough evidence has been drawn from the usages and writings of a few countries to give a conspectus of the situation. It is obviously far from complete — the literatature of Russia, Scandinavia, Japan, Holland and many other countries has not been searched. But, as it stands, it provides a sufficiently disturbing picture. Evidently while many voices proclaim that anxiety is the alpha and the omega of psychopathology, and that it permeates every sort of mental disorder, there are even more voices insisting that anxiety means what they choose it to mean.

Leaving aside the existential use of the word and concept, we can try, as others have, to provide an acceptable distillate from current and past definitions. A list of the characteristics of anxiety, in its technical sense, could be:

1. *It is an emotional state, with the subjectively experienced quality of fear or a closely related emotion* (terror, horror, alarm, fright, panic, trepidation, dread, scare). It should, for example, be different in its specific quality from anger, and indubitably recognised as being like fear. It may be harder to tell it from depression, subjectively experienced.

2. *The emotion is unpleasant.* It may be a feeling of impending death or collapse.

3. *It is directed towards the future.* This is implicit in the feeling that there is a threat of some kind, an impending danger. Hence anguish, which combines the ideas of present pain and present agony of mind is inappropriate for anxiety although the etymologically equivalent terms such as *angoisse, angustia* are widely and perhaps legitimately pressed into service in other languages.

4. *There is either no recognisable threat, or the threat is, by reasonable standards, quite out of proportion to the emotion it seemingly evokes.* The threat, if there is one, will almost always come from outside but can be from within: e.g. a man who coughs up a trace of blood may conclude that his life is threatened from within.

5. *There are subjective bodily discomforts during the period of the anxiety.* The sense of constriction in the chest, tightness in the throat, difficulty in breathing, and weakness in the legs are conspicuous; there are others mostly representing the subjective side of what is also objectively manifest.

6. *There are manifest bodily disturbances.* Some of these are of functions normally under voluntary control (e.g. running in panic, agitation, screaming, sudden defaecation); other are of functions not wholly or at all under voluntary control. Of these phenomena there are many varieties e.g. dryness of mouth, sweating, horripilation, tremor, vomiting, palpitation, giddiness, abdominal pain: and others physiological and biochemical, that can be detected with appropriate methods of investigation.

The first, second, third and fifth of these characteristics of anxiety may be inferred from the patient's demeanour and conduct even though he says nothing about what he is feeling, but for the most part the psychiatrist will need to be told by the patient about them, if he is to assess them satisfactorily. The others (fourth and sixth) in the list, can be objectively determined. It will sometimes be necessary and proper to conclude that there is anxiety (especially in the chronic neurotic patient) even though there is no certainty that the patient is experiencing appropriate emotion, but before this conclusion is reached

(e.g. in 'effort syndrome') the relevant objective features of somatic disturbance should be indisputable and characteristic.

It is necessary to list also those attributes which at some time or place have
been included in the criteria of anxiety, but can now be dispensed with:

Anxiety may be

1. normal (student taking an examination) or pathological. An 'anxiety
neurosis' or 'anxiety' state is, ex vi termini, pathological.

2. mild or severe.

3. mainly detrimental to thought and action, or in some respects advantageous.

4. episodic or persistent (chronic).

5. due to physical disease (e.g. delirium tremens) or psychogenic.

6. accompanying other features of mental disorder (e.g. in melancholia) or
alone.

7. may for the duration of the attack affect perception and memory or may
leave them intact.

These characteristics are therefore not criteria for the recognition of anxiety.
When anxiety is, however, pathological and severe, it will usually be detrimental
to thought and action, will be accompanied by other features of mental disorder
(especially depression) and will affect perception, memory, judgement and other
cognitive abilities.

After this disturbing review of the varied meanings attached to the word
'anxiety', the question arises "should we do away with it?" It has had a short
life as far as psychiatry in the English speaking countries goes, and has not
endeared itself to French and German authorities on psychiatric terminology.
In 1950 Rado wrote, "In current psychiatric usage anxiety denotes fear with
some qualification which differs from school to school, if not from writer to
writer", and he proposed very firmly to drop the word altogether. Similarly
Sarbin, in 1964 launched an attack on "Anxiety: Reification of a Metaphor"
on the grounds that it has had confusing referents and is postulated to be a
mental state: "the mentalistic and multi-referenced term anxiety has outlived
its usefulness. Unless a convention is called to decide or more precise existing
referents for the term it would be better to discontinue employing it in scientific
discourse". The prospect of killing the term is slender, as is the prospect of
a successful convention devoted to making the concept and word scientifically
respectable. It would, however, be a step in the right direction to get agreement
on either substituting the term 'fear' for it, with adjectival qualification, or
stating necessary criteria, as has been suggested in the conclusions of this paper.

88

EMPIRICAL OR RATIONAL ?
THE NATURE AND BASIS OF PSYCHIATRY*

AUBREY LEWIS

Kt, M.D. Adelaide, F.R.C.P., Hon. LL.D. Toronto

EMERITUS PROFESSOR OF PSYCHIATRY IN THE UNIVERSITY OF LONDON
AT THE INSTITUTE OF PSYCHIATRY, LONDON S.E.5

I AM sure that everyone who has been honoured by being chosen to give the Linacre Lecture has made it his first duty to acquaint himself as fully as he can with the character and achievements of Thomas Linacre. The known facts about this great humanist and physician are on the whole meagre, and they have been so often rehearsed by previous Linacre lecturers that it would be repetitive and probably superfluous for me to remind you in detail again of the rich friendships Linacre had with men like Erasmus, Budé, and Colet; of his contributions to philology; or of that most magnificent and far-sighted of his major actions, the foundation of the College of Physicians.

Linacre as a Translator

To his contemporaries it was the translations he made of some of Galen's writings that constituted his chief service to medical learning. Scholars vied with each other in praising the elegance and fidelity of the translations: Erasmus and others declared that Galen spoke better Latin, through the mouth of Linacre, than he had spoken Greek in his own person. In the first of these translations to be dedicated to the King, Linacre made plain his admiration for Galen, whom he set very close to Hippocrates; and he ridiculed the moderns who tried to relieve their envy by finding fault with some trivial niceties and carping at a few passages in Galen's innumerable writings. His profound veneration for Galen is attested not only by his explicit praise but still more by his willingness to devote his time and effort to the translation of so much of Galen's writings. It is true that in the sixteenth century Galen reigned supreme among medical authorities, and that

---

* The Linacre Lecture, delivered in Cambridge on May 6.

many others besides Linacre set about turning Galen's voluminous works into Latin, as earlier they had been turned into Arabic, but Linacre stood out in this industrious band because of the concision and easy mastery of Latin which he displayed.

The Linacre lecturer has his attention specially directed to Galen by the injunction that he should devote his lecture to expounding and illustrating three of Galen's treatises—the *De Sanitate Tuenda*, the *Methodus Medendi*, and the *De Elementis et Simplicibus*. Although this was not laid down in the Letters Patent made public in October, 1524, eight days before Linacre's death, but was stipulated in the Statutes drawn up under Elizabeth in 1570, it is obviously incumbent on the lecturer to consider whether in these three works there are matters still meriting our regard. I have gone a little way towards meeting this obligation in that I have read the *De Sanitate Tuenda* and, sadly, confirmed the statement of its most recent translator that " to the impatient modern reader . . . a great deal of Galen's Hygiene seems prolix, repetitious, tedious, and needlessly controversial and dialectic ". The *Methodus Medendi*, consisting of fourteen books, is a still more formidable undertaking to read—to translate it must have been a work of supererogation. The biographer of Linacre, Dr. Noble Johnson, described it as " not less formidable in its length than incomprehensible in many of the theories contained in it " and said the meaning of its doctrines was intelligible only to God and Galen. I have not attempted to read it.

It seems at first sight strange that Linacre, a man who was one of the foremost scholars of his time, who had great responsibilities as domestic physician to Henry VII and Henry VIII and as tutor to the Prince of Wales, who was a penetrating judge of excellence, vir severi judicii, a grammarian who had " mastered learning's crabbed text ", a travelled man who had lived within the family of Lorenzo the Magnificent, it was strange that such a man should have devoted a large part of his life and scholarship to translating medical works open to such objections as succeeding ages have made to Galen. The answer is, of course, that Galen is not to be judged piecemeal, that he would never have attained to so unquestionable a primacy as he enjoyed until the seventeenth century, if he had not provided a coherent theoretical scheme of pathology based partly on anatomical and clinical observations, and a digest of all the medical knowledge—or what passed for medical knowledge—in the period between Hippocrates and Imperial Rome of the second century. Professor Scott Buchanan has stated it forcibly and disrespectfully. " It is difficult even for the inquiring reader to follow Galen's diffuse, verbose, meandering style with anything like a sympathetic comprehension . . . There is so much rhetoric in his works that one is tempted to use the scissors ruthlessly in order to amputate and eliminate

90

his sentimental ravings. But . . . this would be a fatal mistake . . . Galen was heir to almost a thousand years of Greek thought and culture, and he was bringing it all to bear on the professional problems of medicine . . . Galen's writings are a medical interpretation of Greek life and thought, and have a great deal to do with the tradition of humanism in all subsequent European thought."

Bearing this in mind and still anxious, if I could, to pay regard to Linacre's avowed respect for Galen, I looked for his contributions to psychiatry, turning first to works with such hopeful titles as *On the Passions and Errors of the Soul* or the sections on melancholia in *De Locis Affectis*; but these turned out to treat either of ethics or of the supposed pathology with which the reader of Galen soon becomes uneasily familiar. As Sarton bluntly put it, it is a waste of time to discuss this pathology embodying the connection between the elementary qualities or the humours as Galen conceived them; he rendered a disservice to the progress of medicine—as others have done since—by postulating forces to meet every need; a spurious and irrefutable schema is made to satisfy the multitude of those who are content with a set of reified abstractions and who are fond of words without observable referents.

Although Galen had a shrewd insight into psychological situations—he was evidently quick to spot a covert emotional upset, as several anecdotes record—he nowhere puts forward an orderly statement about mental illness, but often proffers instead a subtle, pedantic disquisition on what other writers have said, for example, about melancholia. Or, having set forth the Hippocratic hypothesis of the four main humours, he deduces how too much or too little of these could affect the brain and cause disorder in the primary qualities of dryness, moisture, warmth, and cold, which would lead to mental illness.

It would not be profitable on this occasion to go further into Galen's psychiatry. He does, however, open another door which leads into the very centre of current psychiatric thinking.

Empirics and Rationalists in Galen's time . . .

Galen was not only a great anatomist and a successful clinician, he was also a philosopher, and body-physician to a philosopher-emperor, Marcus Aurelius. In several of his writings this is stressed. There is his essay on the proposition that a good doctor must be a philosopher: in it he says " a true physician must be well versed in the rational method of thought so that he can tell the classes and varieties of disease and the indications for particular remedies in the individual disorders ". This is a subject to which he returns more than once. It arises from the divisions then prevailing between doctors on the ground of their professed method. There were, as Galen puts it, three main sects in Greco-Roman medicine: the empirical, the rational, and the methodist. The methodist, though important, has less relevance for us than the other two. The rational and the empirical are clearly contrasted in the essay which Galen addressed to students, to enlighten them about the sects. " Those who rely exclusively on experience are called ' empirics ', those for whom reason is their point of departure are ' rationalists '. These are the two most prominent sects in medicine . . . The first are also called ' observers ' or ' memorisers ', the second are ' dogmatists ' or ' analogists ' . . . The empirics make observations, collect the observations of others, and use the method of inferring like from like. The rationalists study all the possible causes—water, climate, air, food, habits, way of life, and diathesis, because they believe that only by studying all these factors can they arrive at the proper therapeutic indications." And then, rather startlingly, he declares that the therapeutic measures taken by the empirics are the same as those used by the rationalist, but the method of arriving at them is different.

Where Galen himself stood is not immediately clear. In the book which is now known only in its Arabic version, as in some other articles, he says " Do not think these are my own views: I give each side of the argument and I leave it to the reader to decide which is more correct." But there is ground for thinking that he inclined to the rationalist side, though well enough aware of the strong points in the empirical argument, and ready to incorporate it in his practice. In the *Ad Pisonem*—a work which is usually attributed to him—he comes out more plainly. He declares that Hippocrates, whom he reveres, was the author and head of the rationalist sect. " We do not practise medicine like the people who call themselves empirics working only from experience, who declare that they fix on some medicaments from study of dreams and in fact may cure a patient haphazard; we search out with every possible care everything that reason can alone discover and examine it with the utmost thoroughness." And in another passage he says: " The rational sect looks for the causes of disease, and their treatment proceeds by the principle of contraries . . . Four characteristics denote the rational sect: the inspection of nature, the logic of causes, the estimation of signs, and treatment in accordance with the causes. The empiric sect does not diagnose the disease nor look for the cause; they are content to observe the phenomena."

What divided the two sects is clear, but it is easy to forget that the empirics had a particular virtue: they made experiments—not, it is true, controlled laboratory experiments—but still experiments. Thus of Serapion we are told that he was the first to declare that the rationalist doctrine was of no value in medicine: only practice and experiments counted. But Galen made experiments too. It may fairly be concluded that he took the best from both sects. In the analogy which Bacon drew in the *Novum Organum*, Galen can be regarded as figured by the bee. " Those who have treated of the sciences," wrote Bacon, " have been either empirical or dogmatical. The former like ants only heap up and use their store; the latter like spiders spin out their own webs. The bee, a mean between both, extracts matter from the flowers of the garden and the field, but works and fashions it by her own efforts. The true labour of Philosophy resembles hers, for it neither relies altogether or principally on the powers of the Mind, nor yet lays up in the memory the matter afforded by experiments of natural history or mechanics in its raw state, but changes and works it in the Understanding."

To the picture of medicine in Alexandria and Rome in Galen's time with its rival schools there are some analogies in our own day, immensely different though the two worlds are. In contemporary psychiatry, which is the theme of this lecture, there are cleavages of opinion and practice. Some psychiatrists rely mainly on drugs and other physical methods of treating the body, in order to relieve mental illness, others concentrate on psychological treatment addressed to the underground drives and the emotions which influence behaviour. Some adhere closely to the freudian pattern of psychoanalysis: others to the jungian doctrine or discipline, or to behaviour therapy. There are expansionists who want fresh worlds to conquer, and astringent sceptics who maintain that mental illness is a myth, fostered in the interests of a group of medical psychotherapists. The contrasts can be dramatic and as explicit as that of the rationalist and the empirical sects in the second century. The word " sect " applied to contending psychiatrists is likely to be rejected and resented because it nowadays implies a religious devotion or an unquestioning faith: but it seems still apposite for those who have strongly held convictions about matters of theory and practice which are by no means well attested, though fervently and powerfully urged. There is, of course, a large central group who deplore the divisions and want a synthesis. These are the majority.

The shibboleth which distinguishes the extreme psychiatric rationalist is " descriptive psychiatry "—a pejorative term which he pronounces with evident distaste—whereas the contemporary sign of the extreme empiricist is his fond hope that for every mental disorder specific curative drugs will be found or specific physical procedures, and that social and psychological influences will prove to be wholly understandable by the light of common sense and worldly wisdom.

... and Today

It is a pity that the word " empiric " has had a bad meaning as well as a good one for the past four hundred

93

years: it has been as likely to denote a quack as to be applied to a close and dispassionate observer of phenomena, like Bunsen or Sydenham. The word " rational " has acquired no such taint in the course of the centuries: certainly not in a medical context. Nevertheless it seems the right word for that undue proliferation of ideas into all-explaining systems which prevailed in Greco-Roman medicine and which we still have with us in modern versions.

In Galen's essay insisting that the doctor should be a philosopher we might now substitute scientist for " philosopher ". Many and acrimonious, however, have been the disputes about the scientific status of the psychiatrist and his proper field of study. The contention has not been profitable. The difficulty lies in defining the concept " scientific ", especially now that it carries with it a built-in letter of credit. Professor Blackett recently cited two definitions: one is brief, " scientific method consists of a systematic method of learning by experience "—a definition that would have fitted the Greek empirics (if there had been agreement about what is systematic). The other, veering towards tautology, runs: " scientific method may be defined as that combination of observation, experiment and reasoning (both deductive and inductive) which scientists are in the habit of using in their scientific investigations ": this requires a consensus about who are scientists and what their habits are, which can more surely be arrived at in regard to the physical and biological sciences than when the social sciences are in question. The most difficult case to examine is psychoanalysis, considered as a method of investigation linked to a theory. On this there has been much high debate.

The nature of psychiatry, scientific or not, could be expressed with some confidence when it was almost entirely concerned with the forms of insanity and defect to be met with in the special institutions variously known then as madhouses, asylums, or retreats. The neuroses were the province of the general physician or the neurologist; psychological anomalies in children were the pædiatrician's concern. As specialisation has increased, and the confidence of the psychiatrist (as well as other people's confidence in him) has grown, the field of action has become larger, the experience much wider, the responsibilities more heavy. Thus, in a current rather conservative textbook there is a lengthy chapter on The Psycho-somatic Diseases, another on Behaviour Disorders

94

in Childhood and Adolescence, followed by one on Behaviour Disorders in Old Age, and other chapters deal with The Drug Addictions, Psychiatry and the Law, Psychiatry and the Practice of Medicine and Surgery, and, finally, Psychiatry and Society. There would be general consent that these are all, or nearly all, topics in which the psychiatrist has a legitimate concern, as much as in the more traditional areas such as the psychoses, subnormality and the psychoneuroses.

The common feature in these diverse themes is abnormality of behaviour, irrespective of whether it arises wholly or partly from physical disease, environmental stress, disturbed upbringing, inherited abnormality, or cultural circumstance. The so-called psychosomatic disorders are an exception to this general statement: there may be no manifest abnormality of behaviour in the patient with one of these conditions such as asthma, or peptic ulcer, or ulcerative colitis. It might be surmised that they come within the psychiatrist's range because he can treat them more effectively than other physicians can, but this is not so either. His participant role depends on two assumptions, or observations; namely, that emotional factors play an important part in determining the occurrence, persistence, and severity of the conditions in question, and that psychiatrists know a great deal about emotional disturbances and how to cope with them. This, which may be considered the rationalist approach, is disputed by the empirical critic who reports that in the treatment of " psychosomatic " disorders the psychiatrist's record is not one of steady triumph. At this point the rationalist may well point out that every illness is psychosomatic, in so far as it is accepted that human beings are biological organisms, in whom body and mind are different aspects of their unity; it is in the prominence of the mental component that one disease may differ from another and be called, for convenience, psychosomatic. This is true, but it does not follow, in logic or in fact, that because the mental component is conspicuous, the somatic component will respond to the therapeutic efforts of the psychiatrist doing his best for the whole man.

At various times and places it has been the lot of the psychiatrist to offer advice and explanation of social phenomena which would not' in preceding generations have seemed in any sense his professional business. Sometimes he has claimed expert competence in order to justify his intervention, sometimes he has had the role

95

thrust upon him. A section of society has invoked his aid and treated him as a social engineer; or, other measures having failed to alleviate or stave off some catastrophe attributable to human folly and perversity, statesmen, governments, or other architects of policy have turned to him—usually covertly—in desperation. Their action has been dependent on rationalist thinking. The line of thought starts from the principle I have just referred to, namely that psychiatrists know about the springs of human conduct and the aberrations they can produce, which may become manifest as mental disorder of one sort or another: they know this about individuals and about groups, therefore (the argument runs), they may be assumed to know it about larger aggregations, such as nations. The achievements of psychiatrists entrusted with such extended social responsibility have not been commensurate with what was hoped for from them, or by them. However disappointing the results so far, the effort continues; not, I think, to any considerable extent in this country, but in the United States, where the Group for the Advancement of Psychiatry, a progressive section of the specialty, has in a recently published series of reports extended their professional concern to such matters as international relations, the psychodynamics of desegregation, forceful indoctrination, and the threat of nuclear war. These are matters in which every citizen, no matter what occupational group he belongs to, has an abiding interest and involvement, in one way or another: but when it is postulated that the psychiatrist can provide expert guidance, it must be objected that alone he can accomplish relatively little either in studying the phenomena, elucidating the causes, or suggesting preventive measures and remedies. In conjunction with people from other disciplines he can through research throw light on certain elements in problems of this public or political type, but when he essays to proffer advice motu proprio about the prevention of adolescent crime, or how to deal with a psychopathic dictator, he is not on terra firma. In such situations psychiatrists do well to brood on the dictum of Charles Darwin, that "ignorance begets confidence more frequently than does knowledge".

A recent instance of the feeling which this issue arouses was provided by a gathering of French psychiatrists. One of the most distinguished and authoritative of them, Dr. Henri Ey, expressed his strongly felt doubts about the psychiatry of childhood and the way in which "vague concepts of anomalies of infantile

96

character or development result in thousands of francs being wasted ":

"Voyez vous tout le problème de l'extension de la psychiatrie en général est un problème tres considérable . . . Si nous nous presentons comme l'opinion publique se represente la psychiatrie, c'est à dire comme un homme qui doit venir en aide à tous les conflits, à toutes les situations malheureuses de l'humanité, à tous les debats de conscience de l'humanité, à tous les problèmes politiques mêmes (disent certains) . . . nois risquons de nous présenter devant les Pouvoirs Publics c'est à dire devant ceux qui payent, dans une position totalement indéfensable."

Another prominent psychiatrist said that this extension of the scope of psychiatry was the subject of an old and passionate dispute, but that:

". . . il s'est dégagé dans notre groupe une très belle unanimité pour demander à nos assemblées de prendre une position ferme de condamnation des tendances psychocratiques: nous demandons que cette position ferme soit prise fondamentale-ment au nom de notre science, au nom de notre technique, au nom de la connaissance que nous avons des dimensions fondamentales qui fondent notre action devant les problèmes humains."

Psychiatry, then, is the study of abnormal behaviour from the medical standpoint: it is therefore concerned with diagnosis, prognosis, prevention, and treatment. Knowledge acquired by it, and the methods it has developed, may well be applied to the study of non-medical problems, but to facilitate that is not a primary function of psychiatry and psychiatrists today, however much they welcome such a fruitful borrowing from them, as they in turn borrow from other branches of medicine and from still wider stores of method and knowledge. This view I am putting forward of the medical nature of psychiatry may be contested from several directions—wrongly, I think. There are those who maintain that there is nothing properly medical about mental disorders which do not spring from recognisable physical disease. Others, less committed to a root-and-branch upheaval, would bring in larger battalions to supplement the medical contribution. Thus Lawrence Kubie, a much respected American psychia-trist, has said that " psychopathology as a discipline, as a theoretical system, as a field of understanding and as a technique of exploration must escape the confines of the medical clinic and merge with human culture ". This is an aspiration rather than a programme.

The extension of psychiatric services into the community which has followed the 1957 report of the Royal Commission and the ensuing Act, inevitably quickened the concern of psychiatrists with social conditions, as they impinge on the causation and the treatment of mental illness. Psychiatrists' interest in social aspects led to an efflorescence of sociomedical investigations, usually conducted in association with sociologists, statisticians, and kindred workers. These have added, and seem likely to add further, to our understanding of the social factors and consequences of mental disorder, defect, and such abnormalities of behaviour as drug-dependence and suicide. They have not so far materially extended the frontiers of psychiatric practice, but well may, in time to come.

It is the common fate of new and vigorous fields of knowledge to be at first unsteady in their aims and scope, especially if their advance rests less on progress in new instruments and techniques than on bold innovating ideas and the invasion of hitherto virgin territory. Sociology, for example, as Professor Ginsberg has pointed out, suffered from claiming to be a kind of scientia scientiarum purporting to give a complete explanation of human life and even to supply a whole phiiosophy. Specialisation acts fissiparously, setting at a further distance the establishment of valid general principles. On the other hand the barriers set up between sciences become hindrances to development: these are themes dealt with by Sir Harold Himsworth in the Linacre lecture of 1955. I refer to them now only to justify my reluctance to assert with any confidence that the borders and purview of psychiatry have the fixity which attaches to the scope, say, of newtonian mechanics.

The Foundations of Psychiatry

This being, very briefly, the present nature and business of psychiatry, on what foundations does it rest? In discussions of medical education there is much reference to the basic sciences. In the Pickering Committee's report on the new medical school at Nottingham, for example, it is laid down that:

" The older scientific disciplines are based upon experiment, measurement and hypotheses that are refutable. This is the hard core of exact science, around which a modern curriculum must be developed. In our present context, the basic disciplines are chemistry, physics and mathematics . . . On them are based several biological disciplines which are becoming

98

almost as rigorous, including physiology, biochemistry, genetics and biometry; the more general and experimental aspects of pharmacology, pathology and morphology may be regarded as extensions of physiology. From an educational point of view these should be the main ingredients of the preclinical curriculum. Newer, and as yet much less susceptible to accurate measurement and precisely formulated hypotheses, are the behavioural and social sciences. So are the clinical sciences, except in so far as they are extensions of physiology, genetics and biometry into the field of disease."

It is a convenient usage to talk of the bases of psychiatry but it would be juster, perhaps, to change the metaphor, and to speak of the sources from which it draws information and the models which it has been happy to copy. We cannot appraise these unless we have considered what are the problems which they have served to clarify or solve. The phenomena of mental illness offer many such problems presented by the symptoms and the course of illness: in other words, its " natural history "—a familiar but not a happy term, since a disease is only a fiction and we make a false analogy in picturing it as having a life of its own, with changes as time passes. But it can be agreed that the disturbed behaviour and the course that characterise any mental illness set out the crucial medical problems— i.e., what will happen, which is prognosis, and what will relieve or end the illness, which is therapy.

For a long time there has been, as I said earlier, a perceptible cleavage in psychiatry between, on the one hand, those who made it their business to observe, with the utmost fullness, all the relevant morbid phenomena and to classify them, and, on the other hand, those who wanted to go behind the phenomena, to make out the pathology, without being delayed or misled by surface appearances. The former, empirics to a man, fell into the pit of overconcern with classification, degenerated into labelling and sorting: the latter, rationalists of undoubted lineage, devised systems and hypostatised forces, sometimes without appreciating how easily closer observation could stultify their misconceived explanations of imperfectly studied behaviour.

Undoubtedly foremost among the empirics was Kraepelin. If the name " empiric " carries even a slight flavour of spuriousness and dishonesty, it is inappropriate to use it of Kraepelin, a man of scrupulous intellectual integrity. It is customary in some psychiatric circles to belittle the contribution he made to psychiatry, on the ground that he only described and labelled, and has been superseded by more penetrating, dynamically minded psychiatrists attuned to underlying forces and deep therapeutic needs. Nevertheless the diagnostic categories he worked out are still in general use, and his descriptions are valid and exemplary. The justification of his empirical approach may be seen in our present research efforts in epidemiology. One of the most promising methods now being employed on a large scale is to ascertain the frequency with which a particular variety of mental disorder occurs in some given populations, to compare these, and seek to relate disparities in their incidence to disparities between the respective populations in other respects which may be relevant. There are, for example, striking differences in the frequency with which schizophrenia appears in different social groups. These differences prompt some hypotheses which it would be very desirable to explore—hypotheses bearing on the social causes and effects of schizophrenia. But the whole project has its point of departure, its raison d'être, in a measurement of the proportion of schizophrenic persons in a given population: if the diagnosis was mistaken and based on divergent criteria of schizophrenia, or on different ways of examining the mental state, the case for further inquiry is much weakened. Psychiatrists know that the criteria of schizophrenia applied in different countries, or by different groups and sects, are not uniform: and that some psychiatrists examine the mental state of their patients cursorily, or with a strong bias, while others are systematic and relatively detached or rigid. The more closely the diagnosing psychiatrists approximate to one method and share common diagnostic criteria, the less disparity may there be in the apparent incidence of schizophrenia in various populations. Those who have been trained on the lines which Kraepelin exemplified will show high diagnostic reliability and concordance with colleagues. But Kraepelin, after all, has been dead for forty years and there are divergent schools of thought in the psychiatric world. Those who are pursuing epidemiological inquiries, especially those who are comparing the incidence in different countries, are hampered and at times nonplussed by the fact that diagnostic procedure and the details of clinical examination are not safely comparable; it has therefore been found necessary to go back to the foundations; that is, to inquire closely into methods of examination and diagnosis and to ensure, if possible, that the same condition in a single patient will not be diversely investigated

100

by different clinicians and diversely diagnosed. So important is this matter and so fundamental that a large part of the resources of the Mental Health Division of the World Health Organisation is now deployed on its study in a number of countries; and it is given a high place in the research supported by the United States National Institute of Mental Health. The research harks back to Kraepelinian empiricism.

Epidemiology, applied now to the study of such diseases as schizophrenia, is not usually thought of as a basic science; it has too much of the clinical in it, I suppose. But the clinical sciences can properly be directed at such fundamental questions as the method of medical or medicopsychological examination. This is all the more necessary when the phenomena to be observed and classified are mutable, complex, wide-ranging, exceptionally difficult to measure, and wayward. Human behaviour deserves these adjectives.

Turning now to the traditional basic sciences in medicine, there is none of them which can be considered wholly irrelevant to psychiatry, though of course the significance of, say, anatomy is muted. But even in that case, if anatomy is what anatomists now study, it merges at many points into physiology, anthropology, and other sciences: and it is highly germane to psychiatry. A fairly simple instance is the investigation and measurement of constitutional types, and a complex instance is the part played by the reticular system in consciousness. This is, of course, the situation that has developed in very many areas of scientific inquiry: old fences have been broken down, and embargos lifted. It would be difficult to point to any single science that has not changed its shape, and so far as the sciences most obviously converging on psychiatry are concerned, this has been conspicuously the case.

To illustrate what has been happening, a biological science may be taken—genetics. After the pre-scientific speculations about degeneration, and blastophthoria, anticipation, and other supposed hereditary influences on the occurrence of mental disorder and defect, there was a long initial phase in which the chief methods of investigation were pedigree analysis and twin studies. These valuable methods added materially to our knowledge, but were restricted by their dependence on available statistics as well as by the diagnostic uncertainties in psychiatry, and by the discovery that mendelian ratios could not be found in the major psychoses, so that various additional explanations had to be pressed into service. The forms of mental defect which could not be laid at the door of gross physical disease such as myxœdema or birth injury were attributed to polygenic inheritance, without much hope of precision in expanding this vague statement.

But technical and other advances in biochemistry made it possible to enucleate a number of varieties of inborn metabolic errors which were accompanied by mental defect. In most such cases the abnormality was found to be genetically determined, a single gene substitution. A specific enzyme defect could thus be used as the means of identifying a hereditary form of mental disorder, which might be treatable when recognised early. Phenylketonuria was the first of these to be recognised: the number is growing. The basic science is neither genetics nor biochemistry alone, but the two in conjunction, defining a more or less treatable abnormality. Mongolism tells a rather dissimilar story, inasmuch as the condition was recognised by clinical observation, without the aid of laboratory or other technical procedures, but its causes were a matter of speculation until the development of chromosomal studies. These disclosed that trisomy of the 21 autosome is responsible for the intellectual and bodily peculiarities of these people. If the clinical characteristics of the phenotype were not so readily identified, it is questionable whether this condition would have been distinguished from other forms of retardation before the cytological observation had been made. The search for distinctive biochemical features is energetically made, not to delineate a morbid entity—that has been done—nor primarily in the hope of remedying or preventing the disorder, but in the hope that genes may be located on the trisomic chromosome.

It is noteworthy that all the quantitative changes in autosomes so far recorded have been associated with mental retardation in the affected person. There is an inseparable connection between genetics, biochemistry, and clinical and psychological abnormality here, and advances brought about by invoking one of the basic sciences may, and indeed usually do, result in advances in the other aspects too. Whereas some forms of mental retardation have in this way been much illuminated, the genetic study of schizophrenia has been virtually at a standstill. It is highly probable, however, that if a particular group from among the schizophrenic multitudes could be found to have a specific biochemical disturbance— periodic catatonia comes nearest to it—detailed genetic features of that condition would be intensively—perhaps successfully— looked for: conversely a genetic means of isolating a special group of schizophrenics would set the stage for more concentrated biochemical inquiries.

How promising these lines of inquiry can be is shown by current interest in the genetic constitution of another heterogeneous collection of people whose undesirable behaviour may raise psychiatric problems—the criminals. Here the biochemical line of approach has not seemed appropriate, but genetic investigation has demonstrated that certain abnormal sex-chromosome complements—chiefly an additional X or an additional Y chromosome—could be found in unusual numbers in men under care in the special security hospitals for mentally

102

abnormal persons who have dangerous or criminal propensities. The men with an additional Y chromosome are taller than average: it is not unreasonable to suspect a biochemical anomaly, but at all events, as Court Brown has surmised, " the finding of the XYY male in his setting in these criminal groups may be the most important discovery yet made in human cytogenetics, and it may provide a powerful lever to open up the study of human behavioural genetics. The four abnormal sex chromosome complements (XXY; XY/XXY; XXYY; and XYY) may, in varying degrees, influence intelligence and behaviour ... Cytogenic studies of criminal groups are likely to be rewarding in helping to further our understanding of the nature of criminal behaviour."

The aspiration is bold, perhaps over-bold: but when advance has been rapid in any field of knowledge, hopes rise fast and fresh ground is ploughed. The dramatic advances in genetics have had this effect, and it is certain that among the basic sciences of psychiatry genetics occupies an assured place.

The Medical Curriculum

It would obviously not be feasible to review here the grounds on which biochemistry, physiology, and pharmacology are basic to the study and practice of psychiatry. The pressing question at the moment is not whether they are essential, but whether the essential elements in them which the psychiatrist should learn can be adequately taught within a crowded curriculum. The educational problem is dealt with in many ways in different schools, and it would be presumptuous at this time to say that an ideal solution had been found. But whereas working methods have been developed over many years for teaching these traditionally recognised basic sciences, the path is incomparably more rocky where another equally important group of basic sciences is concerned. I mean the social services. They have been neglected in medical education until very lately. Under the general heading " behavioural sciences "— which I take to be practically synonymous with " social sciences "—may be included sociology, psychology, anthropology, and, I should think, demography, education, and criminology. The *Index Medicus* includes statistics also under this head. Some of these may be thought tangential rather than basic. But however this is decided in respect of, say, education and criminology, there can hardly be any dispute that in principle psychology, sociology, and anthropology are sciences basic to psychiatry.

Systematic teaching of these sciences in medical schools has been until recently for the most part per-

103

functory or negligible. The reasons lie partly in distrust
of these sciences, and partly in tradition and complacency.
Complacency says that doctors have always paid regard
to social and psychological factors, and that the art of
medicine has consisted in the intuitive understanding
and deployment of such factors. Tradition says that it is
only anatomy and physiology, flanked by biochemistry,
pathology, and pharmacology, that are the true preclinical sciences in which every medical student should
have a thorough grounding. This tradition is being
eroded, however, and complacency has become less
whole-hearted of late. Powerful voices acknowledge a
wider need; the draft recommendations of the General
Medical Council stated that " in the Council's view the
study of human structure and function should be
combined with the study of human behaviour. The
Council considers that instruction should be given in
those aspects of the behavioural sciences which are
relevant to the study of man as an organism adapting to
his social and psychological, no less than to his physical,
environment. Instruction in the biological and sociological bases of human behaviour, normal emotional and
intellectual growth, and the principles of learning theory
should also be included." This is explicit, and puts the
behavioural sciences squarely in their place among the
Institutes of Medicine. It contrasts with what was the
enlightened standpoint of fifty years ago, when these
subjects were silently excluded from the " laboratory
sciences basic to medicine " by men as far-sighted as
Flexner and William H. Welch.

But although there is now, and has been for some
time, unequivocal acceptance of the necessity to include
them in the medical curriculum, not only in the preclinical period, but again in the postgraduate period, and
although some schools have tackled the problem
energetically, it is on the whole through half-hearted
and tentative espousal that the accepted policy is being
gradually brought into effect. To account for this
hesitation there are the familiar obstacles to the addition
of anything further to the curriculum, and, more particularly, as I have said, distrust of the social sciences—
distrust of their relevance, at any rate in the form in
which they are pursued in university departments;
distrust of their scientific status; and distrust of their
language.

The distrust is not an expression of irrational hostility,
I think, but a surviving prejudice which had some

104

justification a few decades ago. Much of what was then studied in psychological laboratories seemed arid and remote to medical educators and medical students; much of what was studied in departments of sociology seemed wordy philosophising; anthropologists seemed to be chiefly interested in the behaviour of preliterate peoples with curious beliefs and outlandish customs. In short, there was misunderstanding and uncertainty about common ground, which kept social scientists and doctors at some distance from each other. These barriers are being broken down. The extension of epidemiological research into the field of chronic diseases and particularly into mental disorders has led to collaboration between social scientist and clinician; their joint studies have made clear to the psychiatrist how dependent he is on the methods and concepts of the sociologist, for example, for elucidating the environmental factors in the causation and treatment of disease. To understand the effect upon mental health of rapid cultural change and admixture, such as is happening in so many societies now, he has to turn to the social anthropologist, who can throw light also on the behaviour of large groups (going much beyond the lively speculations of Wilfred Trotter).

Dependence on these sciences—sociology and anthropology—is clear, but there is still, apparently, not enough solid development and common ground between them and medicine generally, according to medical educators, to warrant their inclusion on other than an experimental footing, among the basic sciences taught in the preclinical periods. That they should be an intrinsic part of the education of the pyschiatrist, to be acquired or amplified after graduation, is, however, undisputed: they undoubtedly should be, if the teachers are available. The intricacy of the relation between individual and society is a further reason for concentrating this instruction on the postgraduate period. Social and cultural conditions that lead to widespread mental abnormality are fostered and perpetuated through the very symptoms they have generated: it is, as Leighton pointed out, a circular or spiral relation, making the interpretation of findings a complex matter, too difficult perhaps for the tiro to unravel . . .

The Role of Psychology

As to psychology there can be no doubt: it is as much a basic science of psychiatry as physiology is a basic science of physical disease (if the familiar dichotomy is to be sustained); and since the psychological aspect of all disease is in principle significant, psychology is a proper component of the preclinical scientific training of all medical students. It is true that there are branches of psychology which have little evident bearing on medicine, and the efforts to teach them may fall on stony soil, but that is the common problem of teaching all the basic sciences—what to include, what to omit. In the University of Cambridge there could be no great problem in this regard, since the psychological studies pursued here during the past forty years have had an obvious relevance to medical issues. This was recognised by the Council of the Senate when they suggested to the Goodenough Committee a quarter of a century ago that a research and training unit in psychiatry might be established in Cambridge which would be based on association between the hospital and the department of experimental psychology so strongly established here. Of many examples which might be adduced to illustrate the force of this suggestion—some day, no doubt, to be realised—the most telling and cogent is afforded by the psychology of remembering, as it occurs normally and in disease.

But, despite such arguments and proposals, in most medical schools it has been only with laggard steps that psychology has been worked into the curriculum. When the British Psychological Society made an inquiry, eight years ago, they found that out of 22 medical schools, 15 had more or less serious doubts of the value of the instruction they provided in psychology: " frequent changes in syllabus and method of approach seemed to reflect this dissatisfaction. The attitude to psychology among teachers and clinicians was often unsympathetic, and students not infrequently came to regard psychology as a non-factual study of little importance. Thus, although there was agreement that some psychology ought to be taught, in practice it was being taught on a small scale, half-heartedly, and with somewhat doubtful success." Things have improved since then, but there is still a long way to go.

If it were not for psychology, a great deal of psychiatric practice would be empirical, in the less admirable sense of the term. Psychology has provided methods, concepts, experimental findings, generalisations, and systematic knowledge about an impressive array of functions and phenomena—perception, learning, speech and communication, development, group dynamics, attitudes and opinions, and much else. The parallel I drew between physiology and organic medicine, on the one hand, and psychology and psychiatry on the other, is, however, admittedly less close than might be wished, because of the very different stage of development reached respectively by psychology and physiology, and because of the rarity with which the psychiatrist has had as thorough a training in psychology as physicians commonly have in physiology. The psychiatrist, alive to this uncomfortable situation, has too often been disposed either to depreciate what the fundamental science of psychology can offer, or at the other extreme to accept uncritically every test and finding put forward by psychologists, eager to illuminate the abnormal.

Many psychiatrists who have little pleasure in the painstaking procedures and cautiously guarded conclusions of the experimental psychologist, find their psychological haven in psychoanalysis. Ernest Jones, addressing the American Psychiatric Association in 1944, said: " by medical psychology I chiefly mean psychoanalysis, because there does not seem to be much medical psychology nowadays outside of psychoanalysis and its imitations ". This hardy assumption is not likely to be so plainly stated now, but it is implicit in a good deal that psychoanalysts write. No one conversant with the history of psychiatry could deny that psychoanalysis has profoundly influenced it, and still does so. Whether it is to be properly regarded as one of the basic sciences or, as Ernest Jones and other psychoanalysts would say, as the basic science of psychiatry, is a question endlessly debated—for the most part unprofitably. The most penetrating and subtle of recent reviews, that of Prof. Paul Ricoeur, rejects the claims of psychoanalysis to be a science at all: its propositions do not permit of empirical validation; " Enfin nous serons ramenés à la critique la plus radicale, celle de la logique des sciences. Nous lui ferons l'aveu qu'elle demande: que la psychoanalyse n'est pas une science d'observation." From which it would follow that psychoanalysts are of the rationalist, not of the empirical sect. This is indeed the verdict of historians (like Shryock), as it is of philosophers (like Popper). Shryock would range psychoanalysis alongside those 18th-century systems which were characterised by use of unduly selected data, loose reasoning, unchecked speculation and the careless use of analogy and reified forces " to bridge gaps ". This is an adverse judgment which takes no account of the powerful influence psychoanalysis has had on thought and practice, nor of the modifications and reformulations by which psychoanalysts, well aware of weaknesses and uncertainties in their discipline, have tried to make it more conformable to recognised scientific requirements. At this juncture it is more seemly to wait for better evidence of the acceptability or refutation of psychoanalytic theory than to engage in repetitive examination of its claims to being scientific in some sense of the word. During this period of suspended judgment it would be legitimate to regard it as poised midway between the humanities and the behavioural sciences.

The humanities cannot, by definition, be classed as sciences, but history and ethics, and, in the long run, philosophy are branches of knowledge from which medicine draws sustenance. For Galen they were inseparably one. The distinction between rationalist and empiricist was for him a philosophical one, with ethical and historical overtones. It would be straining words unduly to maintain that the humanities are basic to medicine today, but that does not mean they are remote and irrelevant. This is particularly true of their relation to psychiatry. Concerned as he must be with the multi-farious aspects of human behaviour, the psychiatrist is inescapably caught up in problems that cannot be fully dealt with by scientific inquiry. This I take to have been the argument put forward by a recent Linacre lecturer, Robert Platt: " the first trend of clinical science which I regret is that which tends to divorce its teaching from the appreciation of human values in the practice of medicine; and we must not forget that in the practice of medicine, ethical judgments, about which science has nothing to say, decide upon action to be taken." But in amplifying this theme Lord Platt went a good deal further: " the psychological factors in illness may be far more important than the disordered functions which science can measure . . . there is a side to human behaviour in health and disease which is not a thing of the intellect, which is irrational and emotional but important. It is the main-spring of most of what we do and a great deal of what we think. It is being explored by psychiatry but is in danger of being neglected by clinical science." That is, of course, good doctrine but it asserts by implication that the irrational and emotional elements in human behaviour cannot be the subject of scientific study and measure-ment. This, I think, is unjustified; it ignores the extensive contributions to scientific knowledge of these matters made by psychologists and psychiatrists. The data of human behaviour can be profitably quantified and studied by experiment, without postulating conflict between interior, immeasurable forces, " superb in their indefiniteness " as Freud put it. What we loosely call the irrational in human motives and conduct can be inquired into scientifically by psychologists, in a way distinct from the approach of the theologian, the moralist, the existentialist, the psychoanalyst, or the historian.

The basic sciences of medicine are so-called because they provide the essential foundation on which medicine has been, and is being built, by the use of their methods, and by the deductive application of laws and relationships which have been established in them. If I am right in supposing this is what the term " basic science " means, it is closely akin to the term " pure science ". The distinction between pure and applied science is under a cloud because it so often is taken to imply a kind of snobbery, a spurious rank-order of intellectual merit. This hierarchical notion is, by common consent, unwise, if only because, in the long run, unless the pure sciences have evident application to useful ends, like those of medicine, they are unlikely to receive from society enough support to permit their full progress. " The true and lawful end of the sciences is that human life be enriched by new discoveries and powers " (Bacon). Kapitsa recently put the current standpoint clearly. " When I think over the developments in science I am most amazed at the general change in attitude towards it. In my youth they spoke of a ' pure science ', science for the sake of science. This is no longer said. Science is judged as a necessary part of the social order—as its very useful and urgent component . . . We may speak of the division of science into fundamental and applied, but we must stress that this division is artificial, and it is difficult to designate the point where fundamental science ends and applied begins."

Few would dispute this, I suppose, though they might still see the " basic sciences " as more exact, more assured, more abstract, richer in well-supported explanatory generalisations. If the position of medicine in this matter is closely regarded, the growth of clinical science adds force to the contention that the distinction between " basic " and " applied " science is an arbitrary and shifting affair, depending as much on the intention or motive of the scientist and the vantage-ground from which he works as on the nature of his research. In the narrower field of psychiatry, however, recognition of this has led regrettably to some overweening claims. Ives

Hendrick, for example, of the Harvard Teaching Unit, recently wrote: " dynamic psychiatry today should be considered, together with anatomy, pathology, physiology and chemistry, as one of the basic sciences of medicine . . . Dynamic psychiatry is basic in the same sense as the other medical sciences: it originates in an area of observation which other basic sciences do not study . . . Like other basic sciences, dynamic psychiatry is therefore rooted in its own specific areas of empirical investigation, and depends primarily on its own techniques." Professor Bond of Western Reserve University, in a slightly more restricted formulation, spoke recently of the " body of observation and construct which is the ' basic science ' of analysis. This body of material is woven into a theory that is true theory ".

Extravagant or premature attempts to glorify psychiatry by putting it among the basic sciences of medicine are as little likely to further its growth as are attempts to enthrone it among the social sciences. Its place in medicine has become secure without such advocacy, and its dependence on other disciplines (to which it has in turn made valuable contributions) does not detract from that station within medicine but rather makes it firmer.

Which is it to be?

It is time to come back to Galen and to recall the sects which divided doctors into contesting camps—the rationalists, as Galen's predecessor, Celsus, described them—" who profess a reasoned theory of medicine [and] propound as requisite, first, a knowledge of hidden causes involving disease, next of evident causes, then of natural actions [physiology] and lastly of the internal parts [through autopsy]. And the empirics who " do indeed accept evident causes as necessary, but they contend that inquiry about obscure causes and natural action is superfluous . . . even philosophers (they say) would have become the greatest of medical practitioners, if reasoning from theory could have made them so." And Celsus went on, with prescient wisdom, to weigh up the whole matter: " Since all these questions have been discussed often, in many volumes and in large and contentious disputations, and the discussion continues, it remains to add such views as seem nearest the truth. These are neither wholly in accord with one opinion or another, but hold a sort of intermediate place between divers sentiments . . . Nothing adds more to a really rational treatment than experience." This intermediate

110

position was that taken up not only by Celsus but, as we saw earlier, also by Galen a hundred years later: and it is, I believe, the judicious position likely to be taken up by prudent, " discreet, groundedly learned " men of today as they contemplate those twentieth-century psychiatric disputations which reflect the ancient contention between tough-minded and tender-minded men, the empirics and the rationalists.

I do not doubt that the contemporary scene offers instances of this contentious division in other fields besides psychiatry; instances also of how the division is being closed and the contention allayed, as is happening in psychiatry. Even outside medicine altogether, it seems that empiricism and rationalism, in transfigured guise, now often walk hand in hand. Whom can I cite better than Sir Karl Popper? He maintains that the differences between classical empiricism and rationalism are much smaller than their similarities, and that both standpoints are mistaken. He avows himself " both an empiricist and a rationalist of sorts " but he cannot ascribe either to empiricism or rationalism its classical role as a source of knowledge. There are, in his view, no ultimate sources of knowledge; knowledge comes from critical examination apolied to assertions derived from any source whatever, including of course observation and experience. What makes science in some sense both rational and empirical is the way it grows, through the overthrow and replacement of theories, so that it progresses deeper and deeper into the problems.

So long as rationalism is relentlessly critical, and not a cartesian intellectualism, Professor Popper gives it his blessing: and he says, not inconsistently, that empiricism in some form or other, although perhaps in a modest and modified form, is the only interpretation of scientific method which can be taken seriously in our day. These views certainly fit the present state of knowledge and study in psychiatry. If, in the words I quoted from Henry VIII's charter to the Royal College of Physicians, the subject is to be furthered by men who are " profound, discreet, groundedly learned, and deeply studied in physic ", it is by way of enlightened empiricism and critical rationalism that they will achieve that aim. Psychiatry is working in that direction, not without success.

I would like to have been able to finish by recalling that Thomas Linacre approached the problems of medicine—and particularly of psychiatry—in this spirit of critical rationalism. But it would not be true, nor in keeping with the spirit of his time. Authority prevailed then over inquiry, and refutation of accepted doctrine was no virtue. Nevertheless Linacre was steeped in the Greek learning, and he was, as his friend Erasmus said, a man of most acute and refined judgment. I hope it is not too far-fetched to suppose that if he had not been deflected into translating Galen, he would have encountered and pondered that aspect of Greek thought on which Prof. E. R. Dodds has enlightened us, and would have appreciated the necessity for studying the irrational factors in behaviour if we are to reach a realistic understanding of human nature and the means to mental health.

112

Periodicity

Aubrey LEWIS

London

Most of what has been written about the periodic course of mental illness has been directed at the affective disorders, in which recurrence and alternation can strikingly occur. The ancient writer most frequently quoted in this context is Aretaeus. The relevant passages are: " There is a lowness of spirits, from a single fantasy, without fever; and it appears to me that melancholy is the commencement and a part of mania ... The bile passes upwards and downwards in cases of melancholy, but it also affects the head from sympathy, and the abnormal irritability of temper changes to laughter and joy ". And again (in Moffatt's translation): " The melancholic cases tend towards depression and anxiety only ... if, however, respite from this condition of anxiety occurs, gaiety and hilarity in the majority of cases follows, and this finally ends in mania. Summer and autumn are the periods of the year most favourable for the production of this disorder, but it may occur in spring."

Here, then, are two cardinal features: regular seasonal recurrence, and the switch from one emotional extreme—melancholy—to its polar opposite—manic gaiety. It has often been pointed out that the terms ' mania ' and ' melancholia ' comprehended many conditions which, neither in the time of Aretaeus nor in the succeeding eighteen centuries, would have been what we now understand by these diagnostic terms. But it is clear that the contrasted emotional disturbances were in the forefront of what Aretaeus was emphasising in the passages quoted. It is a little less evident in the related assertion of Alexander of Tralles, in the sixth century, who said that there is a cyclical swing from melancholia to mania, but added that mania is nothing but melancholia in a more intense form. The general idea of a cyclical alternation, imprecisely formulated, persisted into the nineteenth century.

In the seventeenth century we find Willis stating the long-accepted observation in vivid terms " Saepe haec duo (melancholia et mania) quasi fumus et flamma se mutuo excipiunt ceduntque ". More soberly he stated " Post melancholiam sequitur agendum de mania quae isti in tantum affinus est, ut hi affectus saepe vices commutent et alter uter in alterum transeat; nam diathesis melancholica in pejus evecta furorem accersit; atque furor defervens non raro in diathesin atrabiliariam desinit ". As a practical gloss on this Morgagni added " quin saepius dubitantes medicos videas, hinc taciturnitate et metu, hinc loquacitate et audacia in eodem aegro subinde alternatis, melancholicum an maniacum pronuntient." Obviously, from this passage, we can infer that circularity was a widely known and accepted phenomenon in mental disorder. It was not only in respect of melancholia and mania, but also in what was then understood to be hysteria: Robert Whytt, for example, was keenly interested in the periodicity of some forms of nervous affection called hysterical: he set them alongside migraine and epilepsy, which he likewise observed in regularly recurring form.

By the nineteenth century, and indeed at the end of the eighteenth, the details are sharper, the semantic confusion more explicit. Pinel describes what he calls " degeneration into mania ": a patient who has been for years a slow, isolated, deluded, self-absorbed melancholic, may pass into a manic state: " ils éprouvent, après plusieurs années, une sorte de révolution intérieure par des causes inconnues, et leur délire change d'objet ou prend une forme nouvelle ". The factor of periodicity and the factor of affective disturbance have become remote and negligible.

It was not until the eighteen-fifties that the modern view was asserted by Baillarger and J. P. Falret. Falret proposed the name ' folie circulaire ' for " une certaine catégorie d'aliénés chez lesquels cette succession de la manie et de la mélancolie se manifeste avec continuité et d'une manière presque régulière ". He rejected the common assumption that the alternation occurred by chance. Baillarger proposed the name " folie à double forme " for the same condition, characterised " par la succession de deux périodes régulières, l'une d'excitation, l'autre de dépression ". He did not, like Falret, include a lucid interval in his concise description of the essentials but he agreed with Esquirol that the succession of phases is very regular.

So far as France was concerned that was the decisive step. Although Morel, Dagonet and Régis criticised the new concept, for the bulk of French psychiatrists henceforward the periodic sequence excitement-depression, or the converse, recurring in the same individual, was indicative of one disease. Magnan put stress on the periodic and unitary nature of the disorder. Putting forward the term ' folie intermittente ', he admitted within its scope alternating, circular and other forms " mais on s'assure aisément par l'histoire clinique des malades que ces distinctions reposent sur des caractères assurément très apparents, très saillants, mais néanmoins secondaires et limités à une phase épisodique de la maladie ".

For Germany it was, of course, Kraepelin who adopted and established the unitary conception of this disorder. In the second edition of his textbook, published in 1887, he characteristically took somatic recurring conditions such as malaria as his point of reference for intermittent disorders, and defined the ' periodic psychoses ' as those in which there is a fairly regular alternation of a morbid with a relatively normal state. He dealt separately with the circular cases: " ein in mehrfacher Beziehung abweichendes Bild bieten die sogenannten circulären oder cyklischen Psychosen: ... der Eintritt dieser Stadien selber ist völlig unabhängig von äusseren Anlässen; er vollzieht sich mit der grössten Sicherheit und Regelmässigkeit ". This insistence on the regularity of the periodic attacks is surprising: he declares roundly that the regular variation of phases is the characteristic feature of the whole morbid process. He enumerates separately three sorts of periodic psychosis—mania, melancholia, and periodic delusional insanity—and one sort of circular insanity.

By 1899, however, in his sixth edition he threw these distinctions overboard, and committed himself to the one fundamental and comprehensive disorder—manic-depressive psychosis. While admitting the changes of clinical form which make the term ' circular psychosis ' dubiously applicable for many patients, Kraepelin maintained that clinical similarities and similar course are so much more characteristic of the major affective disorder than its very irregular periodicity that the designation for it should not, as in the French terms, draw attention to the time relations and sequence but should refer to the clinical picture.

On this question of regular periodicity, Kraepelin expressed himself forcefully. It is rare, he said, for the recurring attacks of manic-depressive illness to show even approximate regularity: there is in the overwhelming majority of cases enormous variability in the length of the interval between attacks, and it is of little consequence to distinguish between simple and periodic forms of mania or melancholia, especially since similar imperfect periodicity is met with in epilepsy and in some forms of dementia praecox as well as in dementia paralytica; in other words, periodicity is not the decisive feature peculiar to any mental disorder.

At one time much emphasis was laid on the calendar-like precision of timing in some mental disorders. Rayner, for example, in 1899 wrote that in ' manie à double forme ' " the circuits in a given case usually occupy a wonderfully uniform period ". There is now, however, general agreement that exact periodicity is rare and Jaspers went so far as to say that, if strict mathematical periodicity is insisted on, there will be no periodic disorders left. The cases collected by Menninger-Lerchenthal and the cases of periodic catatonia observed in Gjessing's patients at Dikemark and in some other clinics contradict Jaspers's summary denial, but true instances of cyclic precision in time of occurrence are undoubtedly hard to find. This is due to the multiple factors which affect the manifestation of a recurring illness. Not so long ago the heavenly bodies, in their regular procession, were thought to influence the course of disease. Richard Mead, most respected of physicians, wrote in 1704 his famed treatise on " the influence of the sun and moon upon human bodies and the diseases thereby produced (e.g. the ' raving fits of mad people which keep lunar periods ')." Mesmer followed him, with his thesis ' De Planetarum Influxu '. As astrology and its offspring lost ground among educated people, the weather, the atmosphere, and other environmental forces were substituted as determinants of the course of illness, thus reverting to Hippocratic modes of thought. The atmosphere preoccupied Thomas Forster, who in 1817 published his ' Observations on the Phenomena of Insanity, being a Supplement to Observations on the Casual and Periodical Influence of Peculiar States of the Atmosphere on Illness '. Forster had had his attention drawn to the periodicity of mental disorders by J. G. Spurzheim.

I would not wish to imply that consideration of the influence of climatic conditions upon periodicity is as far fetched as astrological speculations are; climate is to be reckoned among the possible material and psychological influences in the environment which could prevent a biologically determined periodicity from being clearly manifest. In this context the speculations of Fliess spring to mind. He believed he had detected a twenty-three-day rhythm in a " nasal reflex neurosis " with a sexual aetiology. Freud was much interested in Fliess's hypothesis and in his letter to Fliess on December 6th, 1896, he wrote: " I cannot repress a suspicion that the distinction between neurasthenia and anxiety neurosis, which I detected clinically, is related to the existence of the two twenty-three-day and twenty-eight-day substances " and he refers to release of " the twenty-eight-day anxiety substance ". He did not pursue this line of thought, however, nor warm to Fliess's suggestion that periodicity, rather than treatment, might be responsible for recovery in neurotic illnesses.

Many psychiatrists have laboured the point that, although the affective psychosis is *facile princeps* in respect of periodicity, it is by no means unique in this regard. They point to the periodicity sometimes observed in obsessional disorders, in paranoid states, in hysteria, and in schizophrenia. Obviously the more powerful the environmental causes of a psychological illness, the less likely is it that any constitutional trend towards periodicity will be apparent in clear-cut form: nevertheless, many writers have observed such a sequence in patients with neuroses (Schultz, Kahn, Kehrer, Rouart, Lange, Abély, Soukhanoff, Carras). There is, however, so little known about the hereditary determinants of personality and predisposition, and the particular biological mechanisms governing or mediating mental variations which occur regularly, that it would be unprofitable at this time to put much weight on isolated cases, except the obsessionals (in whom the evidence of occasional periodicity is strong) and the schizophrenics.

Kraepelin, because of his principles of classification, could not be supposed to have any bias towards recognising periodicity in his patients with dementia praecox. Nevertheless he found that 2 % of his patients with that diagnosis had a periodic course: they were mostly women and had fairly short attacks; they eventually developed poverty of thought, impaired judgment, dullness and aboulia and he was satisfied that they were suffering from dementia praecox, and not from manic-depressive psychosis. There are grounds, often urged, for regarding these periodic forms of schizophrenia (including periodic catatonia) as mainly manic-depressive, or as a mixture of hereditarily determined schizophrenia with hereditarily determined manic-depressive psychosis. But, as Lange pointed out, there may be no evidence, either in the clinical picture, the habitus, or the family history, of a manic-depressive condition in these periodic schizophrenics. It is legitimate to adopt the standpoint, which Bumke so stoutly maintained, that biological rhythms appear in health and in disease, in the personality (whatever its form) and in the mental illness (whatever its form): but that some forms (types) of personality and some types of mental illness are particularly prone to show periodicity, whereas others, like schizophrenia, seldom do so. It is difficult, in writing and thought, to avoid the temptation to equate periodicity with ' cyclothymia ', i.e. with the affective or manic-depressive disorders. But this is not permissible while we remain ignorant of the neural and meta-bolic systems which respectively control particular rhythms and particular clinical patterns. Periodic catatonia illustrated the problem and occasioned the unceasing effort which Rolf Gjessing made to find its solution.

The strong tendency to regard ' periodic psychosis ' and ' manic-depressive psychosis' as synonymous is only one sort of semantic pitfall in this area. A number of adjectives are used loosely: periodic, rhythmic, recurrent, intermittent, remitting or relapsing, cyclical, cycloid, circular, alternating, episodic, phasic.

Jaspers defined two of the more important of these words: phase and period. ' Phases ', he ruled, are psychological changes, arising endo-genously or in response to inadequate stimulus, lasting weeks, months or years, and then disappearing with re-establishment of the *status quo ante*. ' Attacks ' are phases of very short duration. Phases are ' periodic ' when there is a regular time-interval between the individual phases, and a great similarity between these phases. Mugdan had earlier laid it down that " a system of events is periodic when at temporally equal intervals events occur that are logically related ".

There is a wide gap between these somewhat loose definitions, and the precision appropriate to the dimensions of cyclical behaviour. The confu-sion is exemplified by those clinicians, such as Falret and Rouart, who have tried to state a non-statistical criterion for distinguishing, say, between periodic and intermittent disorders: they have not been success-ful. Rouart quotes Falret to the effect that every mental disorder can be intermittent, with remissions and phases of aggravation, but that cir-cular insanity " varie d'intensité et de durée dans l'ensemble et dans chacune de ses périodes, soit chez les divers malades, soit aux divers accès chez le même malade ". How a remission is to be distinguished from a periodic variation is not made clear; unless it is by the persistence of some evidence of illness during the remittent phase of the intermittent psychoses. To complete the record of confusion, Rouart says that " ayant pris l'habitude de considérer tout ce qui était intermittent comme synonyme de psychose maniaque-dépressive . . . on s'étonnait de ce que des états intermittents évoluassent vers la démence précoce confirmée ". He rightly calls this a pitfall; but one has to bear in mind that Magnan called all the circular and alternating forms intermittent. Much contro-versy about the use of these terms has indicated that behind such words as ' remission ', ' periodic recurrence ' and ' relapse ' lurk assumptions about the nature of the disease process involved—that remissions, for example, occur in a chronic disease, intervals of health in an acute but recurring disease (manie et mélancolie par accès), and so forth. It is surprising that in Allbutt's System (1899) the well-informed article on Recurrent Insanity includes catatonia, on the same footing as mania and melancholia, and the author says, " as with other periodic insanities (in circular insanity) the influence of heredity . . . and the unfavourable prognosis are all strikingly exemplified". And again " although periodic insanity may begin at any age, it may be stated that if a patient, young in years, of hereditary tendencies to insanity, has a sharp attack of mental disease, and recovers speedily, the prognosis is unfavourable in this respect. Should there be signs of degeneracy on the first onset, dementia, or, more rarely, periodic insanity is to be feared ". This view is opposite to the prevailing opinion, then and now.

At this point it seems appropriate to consider a bold deviation from the accepted nosography—that propounded by Kleist and modified by Leonhard. It is difficult for anyone who has not been in the habit of using this classification to describe it. The chief interest, from the point of view of periodicity, lies in the cycloid psychoses, as Leonhard calls them, following Schröder. These are phasic disorders which run the same course as manic-depressive disorders, i.e. complete normality between attacks, but nevertheless show no affective symptom pattern. Kleist could not accept the customary explanation referred to earlier, viz. that they are mixed disorders in which there have been hereditary converging determinants of both manic-depressive and schizophrenic disorder. He considered that they are independent conditions. The cycloid disorders, in his classification, were of three kinds: the motility psychosis, the confusional (*Verwirrtheitspsychose*) and the anxiety psychosis (or, as Leonhard reformulated it, the anxiety-ecstasy psychosis). The derivation of this from Wernicke's conceptions is plain, but Wernicke did not stress the periodic nature of these conditions. Besides these three, the independence of which Leonhard considers he has confirmed by family studies, there are the atypical forms of schizophrenia: affective paraphrenia, schizophasia, and periodic catatonia. The last, made widely known through Gjessing's classical investigations, is not readily distinguishable from motility-psychosis: the chief difference consists in the observation that in the motility psychosis there is either hyperkinesis or akinesis (stupor), whereas in periodic catatonia both co-exist—the movements of an excited patient still show some akinetic characteristics, according to Leonhard; conversely he can discern hyperkinetic features in the grimaces and finger movements of an akinetic patient. It would be inappropriate to go into detail regarding the Kleist-Leonhard classification, its evidential support and its relation to the two great Kraepelinian groups, especially the manic-depressive. Kleist must be counted as the great heresiarch in the diagnostic church. The complications of his system have put it beyond the reach, and consequently outside the practice, of all but a small school of psychiatrists, even though some of his doctrine, e.g. regarding the monopolar nature of the ' phasophrenias ', is coming in by another route, through the work of Weitbrecht, Angst and others. Polonio's recent reports seem to be in line with the Leonhard standpoint.

Although it has often been pointed out that depressive or manic-depressive patients may not be phasic or recover, the tendency to regard periodicity as the interchangeable attribute of affective psychosis carries with it a corresponding tendency to assume that periodicity, coming as it does from within, so to speak, has a mainly hereditary cause. As Johannes Lange pointed out, in Morel's day and subsequently, the periodic psychoses were regarded as hereditary, and external causes were assumed for the simple non-periodic mental disorders: this was the fore-runner of the endogenous-psychogenic dichotomy of depressive states. The heredity of periodic manic-depressive disorders has of course been closely studied, and Leonhard has investigated the atypical forms from this standpoint: what emerges is strong evidence of genetic influence in periodic catatonia and cycloid conditions, but there is hardly enough unanimity in the findings to warrant rejection of the view that, when periodicity coincides with a non-affective clinical picture, a schizophrenic heredity can be detected or inferred. Gjessing reviewed the evidence and made an outspoken comment: agreeing with Tuczek, he affirmed that the dispute about whether combinations of schizophrenic and manic-depressive constitution produce the atypical pictures can be discussed endlessly, and " always with the same futile outcome: theoretical support can be found for every point of view ". Contributing to this inconclusive-ness is our ignorance of the effect of extraneous causes on persons pre-disposed to a particular psychosis: we are seldom sure, at any rate during the span of the first two or three attacks, how far the upset and recovery are ' autochthonous ', and how far a response to external stresses and stimuli. Even where the periodicity is of the most exact and predictable kind in a particular illness, we cannot, as Curt Richter has put it, be sure that we are dealing with a periodic disease, it may be only the periodic manifestation of a basic illness: periodicity may be abolished by medication (e.g. with thyroxin) but the basic catatonic features persist.

Inevitably the occurrence in women of oscillations in mental well-being has been related to menstruation. Though many supposed cases of this kind turn out, on close examination, to be randomly related to the phases of ovulation, such observations as those of Wakoh and Krasowska are instructive: acute episodic confusional states, atypical in form and of good prognosis, came on commonly in the second half of the cycle. But what the relation is and how mediated remains unknown.

I shall not attempt to re-examine the justification for the concept of one manic-depressive psychosis. Dr. Angst has dealt with this at length in his monograph, and he will doubtless be clarifying the matter in his address. Nor, of course, will I embark on an account of the meta-bolic studies which have been made with the purpose of correlating biochemical with clinical fluctuations: others here are dealing with it, and in any case these studies have not so far materially affected nosology.

On the whole, periodicity seems to have contributed in pretty equal proportions to the clarification, and the clouding, of psychiatric nosology.

References

Alexander, Trallianus: De Arte Medica. Lausanne, 1772.

Angst, J.: Zur Ätiologie und Nosologie endogener depressiver Psychosen. Berlin, Springer, 1966.

Aretaeus: The extant works. Edited and translated by F. Adams. London, Sydenham Society, 1856.

Baillarger, J.: Note sur un genre de folie. Bull. Acad. Med., 1854, *19*, 340.

Bumke, O.: Lehrbuch der Geisteskrankheiten. München, Bergmann, 1929.

Dagonet, H.: Traité élémentaire des maladies mentales. Paris, 1862.

Ey, H.: Etudes psychiatriques. Etude n⁰ 25. Paris, Desclée de Brouwer, 1954.

Falret, J. P.: Mémoire sur la folie circulaire. Bull. Acad. Med., 1854, *19*, 382.

Fliess, W.: Der Ablauf des Lebens. Wien, 1906.

Forster, T.: Observations on the phenomena of insanity. London, Underwood, 1817.

Freud, S.: The origins of psycho-analysis. London, Imago, 1954.

Gjessing, R.: Beiträge zur Somatologie der periodischen Katatonie: IX. Mitteilung. Arch. f. Psychiat., 1960, *200*, 350-365.

Jaspers, K.: Allgemeine Psychopathologie. Berlin, Springer, 1965.

Kleist, K.: Die Gliederung der neuro-psychischen Erkrankungen. M'schr. Psychiat. Neur., 1953, *125*, 526-554.

Kraepelin, E.: Psychiatrie. Leipzig, Abel, 1887.

Kraepelin, E.: Psychiatrie: sechste Auflage. Leipzig, 1899.

Lange, J.: Die endogenen und reaktiven Gemütserkrankungen. In Bumke's Handbuch der Geisteskrankheiten. Berlin, Springer, 1928.

Leonhard, K.: Die atypischen Psychosen. In Psychiatrie der Gegenwart, Bd. 2. Berlin, Springer, 1960.

Magnan, V.: Leçons cliniques sur les maladies mentales. Paris, 1897.

Mead, R.: A treatise concerning the influence of the sun and moon upon human bodies. Translated by T. Stack. London, 1748.

Menninger-Lerchenthal, E.: Periodizität in der Psycho-pathologie. Bonn, 1960.

Morel, B. A.: Traité des maladies mentales. Paris, 1859.

Morgagni, G. B.: De sedibus et causis morborum. Venice, 1761.

Mugdan, F.: Periodizität und periodische Geistesstörungen. Halle, 1911.

Pinel, P.: Traité philosophique sur l'aliénation mentale. Brosson, Paris, 1808.

Polonio, P.: Cycloid psychoses and reactions. M'schr. Psychiat. Neurol., 1954, *128*, 354-364.

Rayner, H.: Melancholia and hypochondriasis. In Allbutt's System of Medicine. London, Macmillan, 1899.

Régis, E.: Précis de psychiatrie: cinquième édition. Paris, Doin, 1914.

Urquhart, A. R.: Recurrent insanity. In Allbutt's System of Medicine. London, Macmillan, 1899.

Weitbrecht, H. J.: Offene Probleme bei affektiven Psychosen. Nervenarzt, 1953, *24*, 187-191.

Whytt, R.: Observations on the nature, causes and cure of those disorders which have been commonly called nervous. Edinburgh, Balfour, 1767.

Willis, T.: Opera omnia. Amsterdam, 1682.

MEDICINE AND CULTURE

by Sir Aubrey Lewis

THE INTERPLAY between medicine and culture is close and mutual –
nowhere more so than in the psychiatric branch of medicine.
Psychoanalysis illustrates this in the twentieth century, as psychic
epidemics and witchhunts did in the Middle Ages. In current
psychopathology the effort to distinguish between pathogenic
influences which determine disease and pathoplastic influences which
shape it and give it content bears witness to the causative role
assigned to culture as it impinges on the individual. The difficulty of
distinguishing between the biological and the cultural determinants
in a given case is reflected in the alternative forms of treatment and
prevention that may be deployed.

Culture influences, if it does not wholly determine, what will be
regarded as illness. The concepts of health and illness are ill-defined,
in whatever society they are inspected, but pain and disability are
commonly recognised as indicators of a threatening change. Some
mental disorders come readily into this category because their
symptoms mimic physical disease: hysteria is the outstanding
example. But those forms of mental disorder which are recognised
through abnormal behaviour alone are in varying degrees repudiated
as indicators of disease, or admitted with reservations. In our own
culture this is crudely obvious in the case of psychopaths who
infringe the social code: and less crudely in the divided opinions about
eccentric deviants, mystics, and 'maladjusted' adolescents. Some
would classify such people as ill because their functions are impaired,
in ways that are or can be the outcome of physical changes in the
body, while others would classify them as socially deviant but
healthy by strictly medical criteria (which they equate with the
criteria of physical disease). Religious and moral trends in the
subculture affect this standpoint: thus the views of Heinroth in the
Saxony of 1817 were widely supported, those of Szasz in the United
States of 1960 are not: Heinroth's views, though violently contested,
had cultural roots, Szasz's seem an individual vagary.

The expectations which a society has of the scope of medicine
and its powers in dealing with psychiatric problems, are correspondingly diverse. Is the doctor the right person to deal with the
behaviour of sexual perverts, or with drug addiction, or indeed

with any disorder of conduct in adults, adolescents, and children? Changes in the attitudes adopted by various sections of society towards such questions are now rapid: and these attitudes determine whether people with difficulties of conduct will go to the doctor, or be referred to him by a court, or will expect a particular kind of treatment (as by drugs, or by surgical intervention, or psychoanalysis).

In other cultures, mental disorders of an obvious kind, such as gross psychoses, are still dealt with by minatory and punitive methods, as they once were in our society, or by rituals manifestly expressive of the way of life and persisting ideas and value-systems of the society in question. These may, as was the case in temple incubation and the Asclepian cult, reflect a highly organised and integral part of the culture, or may be an empirically regulated suggestive procedure, carried out by a professional group, now often called 'native healers', who stand midway between the sorcerer and the psychotherapist.

Conversely the expectations current in a particular culture may generate and shape pathological phenomena, like those of 'grande hystérie' which made Charcot's clinics at the Salpetrière famous, or on another level like those of the great religious revivals (Kentucky 1800; Jansenist convulsionnaires; Flagellants). It has lately been suggested that duly viewed in their cultural setting, these phenomena, however bizarre and like those of familiar mental disorders, are not necessarily pathological, since they conform to modes of conduct accepted by a minority, at any rate, as appropriate in the circumstances, and can be regarded as social devices for generating the great effort needed to effect changes. The argument is not convincing, but it is plain that highly abnormal behaviour, like that of the Salem community in 1690, can be favoured and evoked by a given culture; the closer it conforms to the expected pattern, the more rapidly and widely will it spread among previously and subsequently normal people.

The culture will greatly influence prevailing notions about the causes of mental illness. In many societies, if not most, animistic ideas on this score have been the rule. Possession by spirits of one sort or another has been the simple or complex etiology which has justified a remarkable variety of treatments and cruelties. In advanced subcultures the current medical and scientific views on causation are generally held, though the large areas of ignorance and doubt in these leave room for much divergence of opinion in even the most sophisticated. But there are many gradations between such sophisticates and simple people who look to a supernatural cause.

Regrettably, the sophisticated views about etiology seem more often associated with unwarranted assumptions about the medical role than with due appraisal of medical limits: 'one of the most curious results of the twentieth century growth of the social and psychological sciences has been the tendency to reduce all the traditional defects in the texture of human life to the status of diseases treatable by physicians. Just about all the seven deadly sins can now be explained on the basis of physiological or psychological disturbances of genetic or environmental origin . . . [The doctor] should know the limits of his competence; he is not all things to all men; he is not some sort of God on whom all burdens can be laid.' Robert Morison's plain words were addressed to an American audience but they apply elsewhere too, in cultures that scarcely regard the doctor as 'some sort of God' but put upon him many of the responsibilities once thrown on the priest and expect from him some of the miracles worked by the saints. He is credited with having unravelled much of the mystery of the causes of behaviour. Hence their trust in his therapeutic powers.

The introduction of preventive and therapeutic measures to control infection may depend for its success on alteration of the prevailing notions of causation in the given culture. New Guinea provides a clear example. Great changes have been effected in their way of life and beliefs, they have given up their warlike expeditions, ceased to strangle widows, and generally effected a drastic readjustment. But they oppose or disregard the regulations designed to prevent the spread of infectious diseases because they remain convinced that sickness is the consequence of supernatural forces deployed by sorcerers or spirits, and requiring to be combated by ritual procedures rather than by care in disposal of corpses and the use of latrines. Similarly pathological examination of specimens of faeces and other bodily excreta or fluids may be greatly hampered because of fears concerning harmful magic that might be practised through them.

Since mental disorder may be the outcome of infection, psychiatric services are hampered by these cultural effects. The psychiatrist's therapeutic activities may, hoever, fit readily into the belief-system of an otherwise medically awkward society: thus electrical convulsive therapy may be construed as a piece of ritual counter-magic.

Ayurvedic medicine is close to some systems of psychopathology and psychotherapy current in Western Europe, and presents similar obstacles to any attempt to evaluate or refute it. It is likely to survive longer because it springs from an ancient and established culture, and is buttressed by national pride and policy. Similar considerations possibly apply to acupuncture.

It is an open question how far the psychopathological system put forward by Freud derives from the study of culturally determined behaviour which he mistakenly took to be the expression of unalterable biological trends. Freud assumed that the people he observed were typical specimens of universal human nature, and therefore the attitudes of Victorian (Viennese) Society were believed to characterize human nature in general. The neo-Freudian acceptance of this view has not been accompanied with a corresponding systematic dissection of the culturally determined from the universal psychological attributes, though isolated tenets like the Oedipus complex are shifted from the latter to the former, in the light of anthropological findings.

It has been urged that culture and personality are essentially two aspects of a single phenomenon, and 'basic personality types' have been postulated for different cultures. The faulty assumptions in this have been pointed out by Leighton and others. Prominent among them is the dogma that the cultural influences under which a child is brought up during his earliest years are the chief determinants of his personality and of any pathological traits and symptoms he may develop. It is, however, evident that at all stages of life the pressures of the culture can mould the manifestations of mental illness, e.g. the effects upon mental health of moral opprobrium and the sanctions it entails.

The attitudes to such conditions as venereal disease or leprosy hover between the medical and the moral. The same is true of some neurotic illness and psychopathic personality. It is emblematic that for a century 'moral insanity' was a legitimate diagnostic term, consonant with the culture of Victorian England though, as Maudsley put it, 'this is a form of mental alienation which has so much the look of vice or crime that many persons regard it as an unfounded medical invention'.

In past centuries in Western countries, and still in many Asiatic and African countries, the mentally ill are quartered in the same places of detention as criminals. Foucault has analysed the cultural attitudes which in France determined this association from the days when leprosaria were turned over to the housing of society's outcasts, until the ideas of the Enlightenment and the Revolution led to the emancipation of slaves, the more humane treatment of prisoners, and the classification of the mentally sick with the physically sick, as objects of compassion and medical effort. Pinel in France, Chiarugi in Italy, Tuke and later Gardiner Hill in England were the voices and agents of a changing cultural approach.

The rapidity of change in culture where sexual taboos are concerned has not been demonstrated as yet to have an effect for good or ill upon the frequency, types, or course of mental disorder, though pronouncements are often made about it. The legal and administrative measures taken in different countries, however, clearly attest the changing attitude towards restriction, and social betterment. In Great Britain the permissive Mental Health Act of 1959 followed the report of the Royal Commission of 1957 which declared that 'in our view, as in the view of almost all our witnesses, individual people who need care because of mental disorder should be able to receive it as far as possible with no more restriction of liberty or legal formality than is applied to people who need care because of other types of illness, disability, or social and economic difficulty' and 'the recommendations of our witnesses were generally in favour of a shift of emphasis from hospital care to community care . . . we believe that the increasing public sympathy towards mentally disordered patients will result in a higher degree of tolerance'. Subsequent experience has confirmed this, in essentials, and similar developments are occurring in U.S.A. and other countries.

The assimilation of mental health services into the National Health Service in Great Britain has partly sprung from, and partly intensified, the cultural attitudes just referred to. It has had an effect upon the quality and number of those doctors who embrace psychiatry as their specialty, and has particularly averted the division of the psychiatrists into those who are chiefly occupied with psychotherapy carried out in private practice, and those who staff the public hospitals and extramural services for the psychiatrically ill.

That section of the mental health services which is devoted to the disabilities of the elderly has likewise been given much more attention, now that the changing age structure of the population and socio-medical concern with chronic disorders has led to a different attitude on the part of those who carry out public policy. The number of those who engage in para-medical work – sometimes called 'the helping professions' – has rapidly increased, in keeping with the change in cultural attitudes; nevertheless they are fewer than the demand for them.

There is a shortage of doctors in the developing countries of Africa and Asia, which can be partly remedied by recruiting suitable men and women and sending them overseas for training until the country is able itself to afford the required academic and clinical facilities. In present circumstances, it is not uncommon for these postgraduate students to be given precisely the same training as the doctors of the host country receive. No adjustment in the educational curriculum is made to prepare them for the conditions peculiar to their own country which they will encounter on their return home. So far as this rests on an educational programme wide and deep enough to equip them for a variety of national and cultural settings, it is hardly to be decried. But in some instances it cannot be regarded as an ideal preparation for coping with the psychiatric needs of a population very different from that in which they are being trained. Their knowledge of its culture may be firsthand, but instruction in matters of health education, epidemiological inquiry, and adjustment to cultural change is requisite but difficult to provide, and seldom provided.

It is generally conceded that rapid cultural change, collision between cultures, racial discrimination, membership of a minority group, impersonal alienation, loneliness and other features of modern societies can act as stresses. There are grounds for concluding that the total amount of illness attributable to such stresses has not changed in the last century and a half (in spite of many impressions to the contrary); there are also grounds for speculating whether some forms of mental disorder that have changed in their incidence and phenomena, have done so because of fluctuation in the social stresses at work in a given community. Hysteria and general paralysis (neurosyphilis) are examples. It is impossible to relate the incidence of these, any more than, say, of coronary disease, to the stresses which each culture imposes over a period of time. Suicide offers a more cogent example of the variations in incidence in diverse cultures, and under varying stresses in the same culture.

Besides the effects of culture on disease discussed so far, there are the effects of disease upon culture. The composition, size and health of a population – especially its mental health – will affect its collective way of life. The eradication of diseases such as malaria, tuberculosis, smallpox, or malnutrition, can have a profound influence on the culture, with rapid urbanisation, industrial development and perhaps competitive affluence coming in the wake of the medical reforms. No similar triumphs or toxic side-effects can be demonstrated in the case of mental disease, except where it is symptomatic of a treatable or preventable physical condition like trypanosomiasis.

Medical opinion on psychiatric matters can, however, modify the general attitude towards such problems as contraception, the termination of pregnancy for psychiatric reasons, and the effectiveness of various sorts of psychological treatment. There is some evidence that psychoanalysis has had a broad cultural effect; the public attitude to homosexuality may be an example.

The most conspicuous instance of the impact of psychiatric opinion upon a cultural issue is afforded by criminal responsibility. The judges gave their view in the McNaghten rulings, and the general public had no quarrel with them. As time has gone on the lawyers have given some ground but always under strong medical pressure; and the force of public opinion which led to acceptance of the plea of 'limited responsibility' in England would seem to have been mobilized by the strength of psychiatric conviction on the matter.

Some ill-effects upon the culture can be laid at the door of psycho-pharmacologists (among whom psychiatrists may be numbered). The introduction of drugs with temporary but dramatic action on perception and identity, such as lysergic acid diethylamide, mescalin, psilocybin and amphetamine, was the work of pharmacologists and chemists, but their utilisation in treatment by psychiatrists familiarized their vogue, which in small sections of society has been apparently harmful. It is significant that mescalin and lysergic acid were used as cult drugs in Mexico by the indigenous population. The potential effect of drugs that powerfully affect behaviour is an alarming subject for speculation.

More conjectural is the effect of medical propaganda against obesity. There is evidence that anorexia nervosa (persistent disinclination to eat) is on the increase: many of the young women who suffer from it started 'slimming', allegedly in response to this propaganda, and then found they could not keep their abstinence within bounds or conquer the aversion for food that they had developed. It may be, however, that other than medical influences were at work in the widespread warnings against overweight.

If, as seems not improbable, we shall presently have drugs which greatly lessen the continuance and severity of schizophrenia and other mental disorders, or if biochemical advances were to enable us to scotch such disorders at their birth, the effect upon society might be considerable, since the inroads these illnesses now make upon our productive capacity, our skilled professions, and our collective happiness are monstrous. Scientific advances often follow on technological advances, and in turn make further technological advances possible; and so on in an unpredictable sequence. The process need not stop there. Psychiatric advances can follow on advances in other scientific fields; and it is not fanciful to picture cultural changes – for the better – following on psychiatric progress, as it would on other medical discoveries.

INTRODUCTION: DEFINITIONS AND PERSPECTIVES

AUBREY LEWIS

Institute of Psychiatry, Maudsley Hospital, London

SINCE this symposium is about drug dependence, it is perhaps useful to consider at the outset the meaning of the term and its recent historical background. Semantic niceties are often unwelcome in scientific discussion, but some weighty and authoritative committees have thought it very important to get the right words for this condition or, as one might call it, this form of servitude.

The term which it superseded was 'drug addiction', itself recent. The Departmental Committee on Morphine and Heroin addiction, which reported in 1926, defined an addict as "a person who, not requiring the continued use of a drug for the relief of the symptoms of organic disease, has acquired, as a result of repeated administration, an overpowering desire for its continuance, and in whom withdrawal of the drug leads to definite symptoms of mental or physical distress or disorder". Here, the person is defined, not the condition and, strictly interpreted, it would seem that those who develop an overmastering craving for, say, morphine which they are being given for the relief of pain due to organic disease, are excluded from among the addicts. A less narrow but more colourful definition, put forward in 1935, was that "addiction is a state of bondage to a masterful drug, usually, but not always, of the narcotic class, and is manifested by craving, tolerance, intense discomfort of a specialized type on withdrawal of the drug, and tendency to relapse".

When the World Health Organization tackled the problem

some fifteen years ago, they ruled that a distinction must be drawn between addiction and habituation, and that "only the expressions drug addiction and addiction-producing drugs should be used in documentation with respect to substances brought under, or to be brought under, international control". In a gloss on this, they boldly asserted that "there are some drugs, notably morphine . . . whose specific pharmacological action, under individual conditions of time and dose, will always produce compulsive craving, dependence and addiction in any individual . . . Sooner or later there must come a time when the use of the drug cannot be interrupted without significant disturbance, always psychic (psychological) and sometimes physical. Such drugs . . . must be rigidly controlled". They go on to declare that "there are other drugs which never produce compulsive craving, yet their pharmacological action is found desirable to some individuals to the point that they readily form a habit . . . They do not need rigid control. There are some drugs whose pharmacological action is intermediate in kind and degree between the two groups . . ." In that first pronouncement by the World Health Organization, dependence was referred to loosely in passing, without emphasis.

Five years later (1957), a World Health Organization report dealt with the matter more summarily. Declaring that there are many and widely divergent views on what constitutes an addiction; and that the point at which drug use becomes drug addiction depends to quite an extent on the orientation of the observer, they define an addict as "a person who habitually and compulsively uses any narcotic drug so as directly to endanger his own or others' health, safety, or welfare". In this definition, the emphasis had been shifted to underline a social implication—the harm an addict may do to others. As a rule this is not included among the characteristics of addiction, though it is the main reason for interfering with the addict's freedom of action.

In 1961 an Interdepartmental Committee, of which Lord

Brain was Chairman, defined drug addiction as a state of periodic or chronic intoxication produced by the repeated consumption of a drug and showing five specified characteristics, one of which was "a psychological and physical dependence on the effects of the drug"; whereas drug habituation included among its characteristics "some degree of psychological dependence on the effect of the drug, but absence of physical dependence and hence of an abstinence syndrome".

Meanwhile the World Health Organization Expert Committee had been having second thoughts. They noted that their effort to differentiate addiction from habituation had not proved workable; and they proposed, in 1964, to use only one term, 'drug dependence', which could be applied to drug abuse generally. This is the dispensation under which we now live and hold symposia.

The Expert Committee emphasized that the description of drug dependence as a state is a concept for clarification and not, in any sense, a specific definition. They recognized five types of dependence, respectively related to morphine, barbiturate, cocaine, amphetamine and cannabis. They added that "alcohol is outside the terms of reference of the Committee, but is nevertheless an agent that can admittedly cause psychic and physical dependence". Psychological dependence was characteristic of all of the five types enumerated, but physical dependence, they recognized, occurred only in the morphine-like and barbiturate-like types (and, of course, alcohol).

Physical dependence is more fully described in the report as "requiring the presence of the drug for maintenance of homeostasis and resulting in a definite, characteristic and self-limited abstinence syndrome when the drug is withdrawn". In psychic dependence (1965) "there is a feeling of satisfaction, and a psychic drive that require periodic or continuous administration of the drug to produce pleasure or to avoid discomfort".

The criterion, therefore, of physical dependence on a drug

130

was taken to be the development of a withdrawal syndrome—an objective criterion; and the criterion of psychological dependence was taken to be a desire or need to take the drug, together with subjective appreciation of its effects. The characteristics of psychological dependence can, therefore, only be inferred from the statements and behaviour of the affected person; they may be heavily influenced by his candour, veracity and general psychological state and by the prevailing social outlook.

Physical dependence, for a given individual and a given dose pattern, usually takes an invariable form. Psychological dependence can vary according to the internal state of the individual and his circumstances at the time. No doubt craving is a real experience, but it is very hard to measure and state its limits.

In 1965 four experts who have played a prominent part in the study of narcotic drugs, prepared a statement on behalf of the World Health Organization. They emphasized that physical and psychological dependence on a particular drug may both develop, but that psychological dependence "can and does develop, especially with stimulant-type drugs, without any evidence of physical dependence and, therefore, without an abstinence syndrome developing after drug withdrawal". They also pointed out, less convincingly, that "physical dependence too can be induced without notable psychic dependence". Psychic dependence, according to them, is related to pharmacological action but is more particularly a manifestation of the individual's reaction to the effects of the specific drug—a nice distinction, somewhat hard to sustain.

It seems reasonable to conclude that once the abstinence syndrome has been adequately described for a particular category of drugs, it can be confidently applied, and is serviceable: but that the stated indicators of psychological dependence are too woolly to enable the term to be used with precision and uniformity. A hypochondriac, for example, may regularly take large quantities of salicylate for the relief, say, of headache,

131

declaring that he has a desire and a need to take it and that he "has subjective appreciation of its effects". It therefore conforms to the requirement specified for a drug which can produce psychological dependence. If this be conceded, it can be extended to apply to any drug which a hysteric may habitually take, or an obsessional feel compelled to have recourse to in order to relieve tension. Indeed, it goes further, and must be applied in the case of, for example, psychogenic polydipsia—a disorder easily mistaken for diabetes insipidus—in which the hysterical or obsessional patient, though physically healthy, has to consume very large quantities of water—water which we must then, I suppose, regard as a drug of dependence.

However, as I said at the outset, semantic issues are not in high favour when scientific problems are under discussion and it is well to agree that, for the time being anyhow, the terms and definitions promulgated by the World Health Organization are reasonable working tools. The important thing, at this stage of our ignorance, is not precise definition but the study of detailed issues, such as this symposium is concerned with. At the same time, the needs of the epidemiologist must be recognized. Assessment and comparison of the amount of drug misuse in given countries or regions is hampered if there is confusion about the significance of the governing terms. This handicap has a damaging effect on psycho-social research in particular. Because psycho-social issues bulk so large in the study of drugs, an exact meaning of psychological dependence needs to be devised and agreed upon.

It is informative to compare the situation as it is today with the situation that prevailed at the beginning of the century. Now the drugs which are mainly causing concern are grouped in six types—according to their similarity to morphine, barbiturate, alcohol, cocaine, cannabis and amphetamine; some would add LSD and khat. Sixty or seventy years ago, the list embraced four of these, viz. morphia, alcohol, cannabis and cocaine, and, in addition, chloroform, ether, chloral, sulphonal, phenacetin,

132

tobacco (as a stimulant and intoxicant), and tea and coffee. Alcohol and morphine, then as now, were given major consideration.

At that time, the principle of classification was not dependence but toxic effect on the central nervous system. Hence the inclusion of tea and coffee, then credited with more severe damage than was justified. Tobacco was included because it produced, in some people, "a peculiar psychological state in which hallucinations of sight and hearing obtain, and in which the patient passes through psychical waves of excitation and depression". The results of excessive coffee are painted in alarming colours: "the sufferer is tremulous and loses his self-command; he is subject to fits of agitation and depression. He has a haggard appearance . . . As with other such agents, a renewed dose of the poison gives temporary relief, but at the cost of future misery". Tea is no better: "Tea has appeared to us to be especially efficient in producing nightmares with . . . hallucinations which may be alarming in their intensity. Another peculiar quality of tea is to produce a strange and extreme degree of physical depression. An hour or two after breakfast at which tea has been taken . . . a grievous sinking . . . may seize upon a sufferer, so that to speak is an effort . . . The speech may become weak and vague . . . By miseries such as these, the best years of life may be spoilt".

I quote these passages not to amuse you (though that would be a proper aim after the tedious disquisition on terminology), but to point to the likelihood that some of the statements now made about canabis and other drugs much in the public eye, may seem to our successors overwrought. These drugs are, in some cases, suffused with a certain glamour (LSD is a good example), and, in other cases, violently reprobated on emotional rather than objective grounds. This is a recurring feature of the drug landscape. The writers I have just been quoting about tea and coffee were among the most eminent of their day—Clifford Allbutt, the Regius Professor at Cambridge, and W. E. Dixon, whose standing as a pharmacologist is well known. They were the mouthpieces

133

of enlightened opinion, and the problems that troubled them have a bearing on some of our own uncertainties. Thus, while fully aware of the miseries and harm entailed by the misuse of opium, they looked abroad and then at home, and wrote "opium is used, rightly or wrongly, in many oriental countries, not as an idle or a vicious indulgence, but as a reasonable aid in the work of life. A patient of one of us took a grain of opium in a pill every morning and every evening of the last fifteen years of a long, laborious and distinguished career. A man of great force of character, concerned in affairs of weight and of national importance, and of stainless character, he persisted in this habit, as being one which gave him no conscious gratification or diversion, but which toned and strengthened him for his deliberations and engagements . . . The habit had arisen on the not improper advice of a physican who found him liable to intermittent . . . glycosuria. The opium was continued, however, not on this account but for its own sake."

So rare and atypical an observation has no place as a guide to policy or treatment. It does, however, serve as a reminder that although we classify the dependent drugs according to a small number of types, there is immense individual variation in their pharmacological, and even more in their psychological and social, effects: and perhaps also that we may sometimes be too ready to adopt the prevalent distinctions between what are thought to be very harmful and what are thought to be comparatively innocuous drugs. The gradations of danger between consuming tea and coffee at one end of the scale and injecting heroin intravenously at the other, may not be permanently those which we now assign to particular drugs, and on which legislative action may be based. Amphetamine, for instance, and barbiturate move up the scale; cannabis moves down: and although alcohol retains its high place as a potentially ruinous poison, its abuse is not visited with the dire legal penalties held over the head of less damaging substances.

Edward Mapother and the Making of the Maudsley Hospital

The First Mapother Lecture, delivered at the Institute of Psychiatry, 26 March 1969

By SIR AUBREY LEWIS

I am particularly grateful for the privilege of delivering the first Mapother Lecture. I believe it will be appropriate to devote it to a review of Professor Mapother's life and his work in shaping the Maudsley Hospital, with which he is inseparably connected. It is nearly thirty years since his death. The course of events since then has shown on what sure foundations he built. Those like myself who had daily contact with him during the later years of his life felt great respect and admiration, as well as warm affection, for him; but it is only in the perspective of recent history that the full measure of his achievement can be seen: perhaps not even yet. In preparing this Address I have been mindful of what Sir James Crichton-Browne said when delivering the first Maudsley Lecture in 1920—'the last thing the donor of this Lectureship, retiring and shy of publicity as he was, would have wished would be that its inaugural discourse should be devoted to any elaborate eulogy of himself.' It is an Éloge rather than a Eulogy that I would wish to put before you this evening; Condorcet, a master of the art of obituary appraisal, said that an academic Éloge should not be a panegyric but an effort to report the truth about a scholar and to do him full justice.

EARLY LIFE AND CAREER

Edward Mapother was born in Dublin on 12 July 1881. At the age of 27, in 1908 he was appointed an Assistant Medical Officer at Long Grove Asylum by the London County Council. It may safely be assumed that from this date he had resolved to make psychiatry his life's work. The decision is in many ways surprising. Psychiatry at that time did not hold out the prospect of an attractive career; as the *British Medical Journal* put it, 'mental hospital work has

undoubtedly not been in favour with newly qualified medical men in years past', the principal reasons being slow promotion, the obligation to remain single while an Assistant Medical Officer, and the routine nature of much of the work. These faults were set out in frank and damning detail in the Report of the Committee appointed by the Medico-Psychological Association to consider the Status of British Psychiatry and the Position of Medical Officers, which was presented in July 1914. In 1917 a similarly unattractive picture of English psychiatry was drawn by Eliot Smith and T. H. Pear: we were backward and inert, they said, the ignorance of up to date medical knowledge on the part of many asylum medical officers was deplorable; research was trifling, our text books were inadequate, our system of treatment not conducive to recovery: other countries had faced the problems of mental disease which we had shirked. In this indictment the failings were somewhat exaggerated, but the general derogatory judgement was well-founded. Why then should an able and ambitious young doctor have ventured into this gloomy backwater? Mapother had distinguished himself as a student at University College and University College Hospital. He had been awarded two scholarships, he obtained honours in anatomy and Materia Medica, and medals in Pathology and Medicine. His father was a prominent surgeon, and he was himself preparing for a higher surgical qualification (he obtained his Primary Fellowship in 1909 and his F.R.C.S. in 1910, having got his M.D. in 1908). He had held a locum appointment in three institutions of the Metropolitan Asylums Board or the L.C.C. soon after he qualified, so that he had seen for himself the unrewarding conditions that prevailed at that time. It is often difficult to account for people's choice of a profession, and for the particular branch of the profession to which they devote themselves; it might seem particularly obscure in this case, but there are two main considerations which could have influenced it. They may be summarily named as Long Grove and Edward Dillon Mapother.

In 1907 the London County Council opened a new mental hospital, Long Grove, which embodied the best plan and facilities that could then be devised. More important, however, than these material provisions were the staff: Hubert Bond was the ablest and most enlightened of the medical superintendents in the Council's service and he had gathered around him an exceptional group of young men: the most brilliant of them was Bernard Hart (who had been Mapother's senior by two years at University College Hospital), and others were Henry Devine, G. F. Barham and J. E. Martin. Mapother when he first came to Long Grove as locum tenens, found an intellectual climate which was more like that of a University than of a mental hospital: the atmosphere was surely congenial. He joined the regular staff in 1908, and traces of his contribution to the stimulating activity there may be discerned in the 1912 preface to Bernard Hart's little classic, *The Psychology of Insanity* in which Hart thanked Mapother for much valuable assistance.

Edward Dillon Mapother was Professor Mapother's father. The family had been settled in Ireland since 1583, when Elizabeth I granted land in County Roscommon to Richard Mapowder, younger son of Sir Thomas Mapowder. The name came from the Dorset village called Mapledre in Domesday Book and still on the map as Mappowder. The Roscommon property remained in the family's hands until 1934. Seven generations after Richard Mapowder came Edward Dillon Mapother, the son of an official of the Bank of Ireland. He was a man of note in his day, and has a two-column entry in the Dictionary of National Biography. He was Professor of Anatomy in Dublin, President of the Royal College of Surgeons of Ireland, Medical Officer of Health for Dublin, and President of the Statistical Society of Ireland. He moved to London in 1888 when his son

Edward was seven years old, and died in 1908. He was evidently a man of great energy and public spirit. He wrote a number of books on Public Health, was surgeon to two hospitals, and concerned himself particularly with medical education and the fitness of the Dublin hospitals to teach pathology and other branches of medicine. In 1868 he published a book on the Medical Profession and Medical Education which had won him the Carmichael Prize. It contained the following passage on mental hospitals: 'In the three kingdoms there are 261 of the profession directly concerned with the treatment of insanity, and it is surprising that so little attention is paid to the subject in the Schools. In Ireland no lectureship on the subject exists, but a few pupils attend one of the public asylums'. Later in the book he returns to this theme: 'The importance of the study of lunacy in asylums may be again dwelt on. In a School of Medicine there should be a Chair of Psychology, normal and abnormal. The profession is not gaining respect in this department, for a late Lord Chancellor and other legal authorities in England viewed as absurd the idea that medical men were better judges of the matter than other people.'

It does not seem far-fetched to suppose that both when he aimed at a surgical career and when he switched to psychiatry Edward Mapother was to some extent influenced by his public-spirited, tough-minded, progressive father. There were more than surface similarities between the two in their attitude to perennial medical topics. A few more quotations from the father's writings evoke memories of the son's pointed expression of uncompromising opinion. 'Instances of superstition and credulity in medical matter have afforded matter for volumes— in fact they have been rich carcasses on which the worms of quackery have fattened . . . Every hospital and dispensary attendant, still more readily every practitioner in fashionable life, can call to mind cases in which patients believed themselves cured by inert medicines'. 'People will believe in medical absurdities who will reason soundly on aught else in nature, and there seems no folly so ridiculous that it will not find minds ready to adopt it'. 'Public opinion, stimulated by the statements and addresses of

136

many famous medical men, is gradually tending to the belief that hospitals are injudicious and old-fashioned institutions, and that a well organized system of home treatment is more calculated to aid the sick and at a lesser expense . . . This problem should be set at rest by the collection of reliable statistics and other data on the subject'. In spite of being engaged in much medico-political controversy 'because', as he said, 'of the rebellious spirit that is within me', this upright, outspoken man won much respect, and set a pattern for his son.

Long Grove Asylum would not, at the time Mapother entered it, have fallen from grace in the eyes of a young doctor who had high standards. The Superintendent, Hubert Bond, was strongly in favour of classification according to behaviour; the minimum of locked doors; shrubberies instead of walls and fences; half way homes for convalescent patients; abandonment of 'seclusion'; and other salutary 'modern' methods. Alert critics were examining sceptically the older accepted views: thus Sir John Batty Tuke declared that it was 'an open question whether, in a certain number of cases, asylum treatment did not tend to aggravate the disease and render it chronic. That a certain number recovered in consequence of it, a certain number recovered in spite of it, and that a certain number became demented because of it were, he believed, each and all equally true statements.' In the open-minded and questioning company of his fellow Assistant Medical Officers, Mapother found what his own mental disposition and his father's example attracted him to. It was by no means a wholly critical approach: their chief line of interest was the relation of mental illness to philosophy and psychology, and especially to the novel findings and theories of the Frenchman, Janet, and the Viennese, Freud. Although the neuroses were still regarded as lying in the province of the neurologist, the Long Grove group of psychiatrists had acquired, through reading and un-tutored experiment, a familiarity with the problems of neurotic behaviour that equipped them to deal with the disorders of that nature brought to the surface in the 1914–19 War.

Mapother joined the Army in 1914. He was at first attached to the French Army, and then did some surgical work at Étaples and Millbank. He was with an advanced dressing station during the battle of Loos, and saw some wholesale panic of large units. From December 1915 to July 1916 he was in Mesopotamia, and then in India where he did surgical work though much handicapped by sciatica, the aftermath of dysentery. He was brought home in the spring of 1917 and sent to Maghull, the training centre for treatment of neurosis in soldiers. He was then put in charge of two hospitals which formed the 'neurological wing' of a large general hospital. For nearly a year he was responsible for equipping these two hospitals, organizing the daily routines, and maintaining discipline: 700 men passed through the hospitals. This experience stood him in good stead later on. He was demobilized in March 1919, and four months later was put in charge of the Maudsley Hospital, then occupied by the Ministry of Pensions.

This was a fateful appointment, and it is the appropriate point at which to consider the previous history of the Maudsley Hospital, as a concept and as a place.

INCEPTION OF THE MAUDSLEY HOSPITAL

Towards the end of the last century the serious deficiencies of psychiatry in this country were well recognized, and enlightened public authorities cast around for remedies that lay in their power. London was foremost in this. In 1889, a London County Council Committee was set up, with Brudenell Carter as Chairman, to consider 'the advantages from a hospital with a visiting medical staff for the study and curative treatment of insanity'. Evidence was submitted by the most noted neurologists and other physicians of the day—Gowers, Ferrier, Buzzard, Crichton-Browne, Horsley, Jonathan Hutchinson, Allbutt, Batty Tuke and Andrew Clark. The Committee duly submitted a unanimous report:

1. 'Knowledge about the nature, prevention and cure of the diseased changes which underlie and occasion insanity is not commensurate with that regarding other kinds of disease.

2. 'This is mainly due to the circumstances that the patients have been withdrawn from ordinary methods of investigation and treatment.

3. 'The establishment of a hospital for the study and treatment of insanity with a visiting medical and surgical staff, would produce increased knowledge of the subject, and consequently of increased means of prevention and cure.

4. 'The legal disabilities of the insane and the necessity of subjecting them to some degree of restraint render it impossible for the hospital to be established by private benevolence.'

The report was justly criticized for accepting the view that visiting physicians without special psychiatric experience could be depended on to diagnose and treat the mentally ill competently; no action was taken on it by the Council. A few years later, however, they decided, on the advice of a similar committee, to set up a Central Pathological Laboratory at Claybury Asylum and they appointed as Director Frederick Mott, a prominent neurologist and pathologist. After the laboratory had been running for ten years, during which Mott and his colleagues had won for it an international reputation, it was provided with a separate building. Mott, a man of great energy and self-confidence, tackled some of the most challenging problems of psychiatry. He stimulated, or himself carried out, research into the syphilitic nature of general paralysis, endocrine and metabolic abnormalities in dementia praecox, the heredity of mental disorders, and other important questions. However, it is not my purpose to consider his scientific contributions—a future Mapother Lecturer may do so—but to review his share in the founding of the Maudsley Hospital.

Mott had broad views about what should be done to further clinical psychiatry. 'We need', he wrote in 1903, 'means of intercepting for hospital treatment such cases of incipient and acute insanity as are not yet certifiable . . . A certain number of cases would thus come under observation willingly and in time to retard the progress of the disease.' It was an idea he had advocated to the London County Council shortly after his appointment to their service. In 1907 he returned to the charge, and extended the scope of his proposal: 'Another fruitful field of study in psychiatry would be those early cases of uncertifiable mental affection

termed neurasthenia, psychasthenia, obsession . . . hysteria and hypochondria, which in many instances are really the prodromal stages of a pronounced and permanent mental disorder. Such cases are often in the hopeful and curative stages, and these, if studied carefully by trained medico-psychologists, could not fail to yield valuable results . . . If suitable postgraduate training in medico-psychology and neuropathology were established, doubtless the University and licensing bodies might be induced to establish a diploma.'

Henry Maudsley, then in his early seventies, welcomed this pronouncement; he decided to call on Mott to further the matter in the most practical way. He had retired from practice four years previously with a sizeable competence, and he was childless. The two men met, and were of one mind. Mott had recently visited, not for the first time, Kraepelin's clinic at Munich. He could therefore clothe the general proposals he had put forward in well-informed detail, and he knew what obstacles might be met on the rugged path which could lead to L.C.C. adoption of the expensive child that Mott and Maudsley wanted to put in its lap. Maudsley left to Mott all the negotiations with the L.C.C.: his identity was not disclosed until the Council had agreed to accept his offer of £30,000 for the stipulated objects: early treatment, research and teaching.

The proposal had a relatively easy passage through the L.C.C. Committees, and in December 1907 the Chairman of the L.C.C., with five other of the Council's dignitaries, called on Maudsley at his home and there was a harmonious conclave, in which it was agreed there should be 75–100 in-patients in the projected hospital, an out-patient department, and due provision for research; the Laboratory should be transferred from Claybury to the new Hospital. The hospital and Laboratory should seek recognition as a School of the University of London: students might make a payment for clinical instruction. Besides the medical officers on the staff of the Hospital, there would be visiting physicians 'for purposes of consultation'. The Medical Superintendent should not engage in any sort of private practice —a decision later reversed.

138

In February 1908 Maudsley wrote a formal letter to the Chairman of the Council ratifying his offer. In it he emphasized the part the hospital would play in educating doctors so that they would be 'furnished with the necessary instruction, and imbued, one may hope, with the earnest spirit of scientific enquiry and observation'. He reiterated his belief that the proposed hospital would do much to break down the isolation of psychiatry from general medical knowledge and research. As a solatium to the Council's natural concern about the financial commitment he added that 'in the end it might save some of the prolonged expenses of chronic and incurable insanity'. In a codicil to his will he left the L.C.C. another £10,000, expressly for research at the Hospital and Laboratory.

Maudsley's patience was greatly tried by the delays that ensued after the Council's acceptance of the gift. He believed, no doubt rightly, that the political party then in power at County Hall wanted to cut back expenditure and therefore found excuses for putting the business off. At last, tired of the delays, he threatened to withdraw his offer in a public letter. This had the desired effect: a suitable site was found at Denmark Hill and an area of 4½ acres purchased for £10,000. It was calculated that the total cost, including the construction and equipment of the building, would be approximately £20,000 more than Maudsley's gift. In the summer of 1913 building began: it went forward quickly and was completed at the end of 1914. In 1916 Mott's laboratory moved from Claybury to Denmark Hill. From May 1915 to August 1919 the Hospital was in use, with Maudsley's consent, for the care of neurotic (or, as they were called, 'neurological') soldiers and pensioners. From August 1919 until October 1920 it was occupied by the Ministry of Pensions for similar patients.

The London County Council began in 1919 to consider the administrative questions of principle and detail which had to be settled in accordance with Maudsley's intention. The chief of these concerned the desirable staff and the kind of patient to be admitted. The staff question had in fact been looked into in 1911: on the assumption that there would be 108 beds the appropriate medical staff was judged to be a superintendent, a resident medical officer, and a house physician: the nursing staff was to number 40. This was revised in 1919 by Mott and Mapother who assumed that there would be 144 patients. For these they recommended an appreciably larger nursing staff—a matron and her deputy, 9 sisters and 65 others. At the same time Mott proposed that the staff for the Laboratory should consist of the Director, three assistants (two of them technicians), and a lab-boy. In 1921 Mapother put forward, and gained approval from the Council for, a staffing scheme which included five doctors. A special Maudsley Panel of the Council's General Purposes Committee in 1919 proposed that the Medical Superintendent should be appointed for a period 'not exceeding six years', and that he should submit a six-monthly report to the Council of the 'nature and extent of his consulting practice'. When in due course these proposals filtered through to the Finance Committee of the Council, the curmudgeons spoke up: would it not be more economical to appoint a resident Medical Superintendent without special qualifications, 'so that the work of a special character should be provided for by employing specialists or consultants, possibly without payment of a fee'. The Maudsley Hospital Sub-Committee rejoined with a somewhat illogical argument: 'it was because of the desire to have constantly the services of a keen, energetic, able man that they decided to recommend that the tenure of office should be restricted to a period of six years.' The Finance Committee, no doubt slightly bemused, gave way.

The Sub-Committee a little later gave its mind to the relationship of the Medical Superintendent to the Director of the Laboratory. They concluded that the Director should 'have supreme and sole charge and control of the Laboratory . . . no other person whatsoever shall be entitled to possession of the keys of the Laboratory and Museum without his permission. He shall, for the purposes of clinical study have access to the wards at the hospitals but . . . he shall conduct the work so that it shall in no way conflict with that of the Medical Superintendent's. Research should be 'into the patho-

139

logy of insanity in all its bearings'. The strong and absolute terms of this recommendation point to the friction there had been between pathologist and clinician in Mott's Claybury days. Mott was a man of choleric temper, and the subordinate footing on which he stood officially in relation to the Medical Superintendent (Sir R. Armstrong-Jones) must have been irksome to him. Moreover, the Laboratory had to be run on a shoestring. In 1923 Mott's successor as Director, Dr. Golla, appealed for a larger maintenance: he was getting £200 a year, which provided for the routine expenses of the Laboratory, and he asked for a further £400 for research: his request was granted, but the money had to be found out of the Maudsley bequest of £10,000.

The other outstanding issue was the type and status of the patients to be admitted. In 1914 the Council considered whether the Maudsley Hospital should be empowered to take in 'voluntary' boarders. Under the provisions of the Lunacy Act, 1890, County Asylums were debarred from doing so, though Registered Hospitals and Licensed Houses could, and in Scotland there was greater latitude. In accordance with prevailing opinion, the Council decided that it was necessary for the Maudsley to be able to receive patients who came in of their own free will. They therefore obtained Parliamentary approval in 1915 for accepting and treating at the Maudsley 'any person suffering from incipient insanity or mental infirmity who is desirous of voluntarily submitting himself to treatment therefor.'

After the War there was a general move towards liberalizing the legal provisions whereby certification was the requisite preliminary to psychiatric in-patient care; people also deplored the fact that in the mental hospitals patients with early recoverable conditions were living cheek by jowl with the chronic certified. Christopher Addison in 1920, when he was Minister of Health, introduced a Bill promoting closer regard for this distinction, by authorizing homes or hostels entirely separate from the 'asylums' (as had been advocated by Samuel Gaskell as far back as 1860), but the Bill was thrown out by the House of Lords.

The Council's Sub-Committee planning the Maudsley Hospital had therefore to decide whether they should restrict admission to voluntary patients only. At the end of 1921 they took the definite decision in no circumstances to receive certified patients or have any certified for retention there. 'Under such conditions many persons suffering from incipient mental disease would be induced to offer themselves for treatment who would otherwise not do so'. There was some fear that there would not be enough voluntary patients to keep the hospital full!—but Sir Frederick Mott solemnly allayed these fears. The results of adhering consistently to this policy were examined closely by the Royal (Macmillan) Commission of 1924–1926.

MAPOTHER AT THE MAUDSLEY

In the records I have been able to consult there is nothing to suggest that there was competition for the post of Medical Superintendent of the new Hospital. Mapother's merits were well-known to the L.C.C., to Mott, and, I suppose, to Henry Maudsley via Mott. He had been in charge of the Hospital during its difficult Ministry of Pensions days and had an unrivalled grasp of the crucial issues that awaited him. He had, like Maudsley, a distrust of galloping speculation and abstractions, a sharp critical faculty, tenacity of purpose, and a set of convictions based on clinical experience and a humanist morality, which served him well. There seems to have been no question but that he was the man for the job. Events proved it so.

He prepared himself by visiting early in 1922 many active European centres: Munich, Burghölzli, Cologne, Amsterdam, Utrecht and others. In consequence, when the Hospital was formally opened by the Minister of Health in January 1923, Mapother stressed, in what he told the Press, that 'it is the first institution of the kind to be founded in Great Britain on the lines of the neurological and psychiatric clinics of the Continent and America, designed for the combined treatment and investigation of organic nerve diseases, neuroses, and incipient psychoses'.

Mapother's energetic preparations, and especially his timely approach to general practitioners, ensured a lively start for the new Hospital: during the first year 452 persons were treated

140

as in-patients and 560 as out-patients. Besides four whole-time doctors on the staff, there were 11 unpaid clinical assistants, and in his first Annual Report Mapother made an interesting comment. He wrote that in psychotherapy as in physical treatment 'it is the function of such a hospital as the Maudsley to encourage an unprejudiced trial of every form of treatment offering a reasonable prospect of benefit rather than harm . . . I am extremely glad that among those who have acted as clinical assistants there was a considerable proportion of definite adherents of psycho-analysis. Though I find myself incapable of accepting all the alleged facts of any school of psycho-analysis, or the concepts proposed to resume them, yet there is no doubt of the great advance which the intensive methods introduced by these schools have made in our understanding of cases'. Although, as we shall see presently, his views about some features of psycho-analysis came to be expressed in later years with some acerbity, qualified and discriminating respect remained his lasting attitude.

The Maudsley was an L.C.C. responsibility, readily shouldered and generously discharged, all things considered. This might not have been the case if the Council had not had in Mapother a far-sighted, disinterested adviser whom they could trust unreservedly. But there came times when he told them in good round terms that they were wrong, and that he would not give way. An early occasion for such combative candour came along in 1924. The Chief Officer of the Mental Hospitals Department of the Council laid it down that it was part of the Medical Superintendent's duty to see anywhere in London any applicant for treatment at the Maudsley; and that the fee for any consultation during which the question of admission to the Maudsley arose was rightly the property of the L.C.C.: as Mapother tersely pointed out this would have made almost all his takings from 'private practice' payable to the L.C.C., while leaving him to pay the expenses. He protested, and the matter was referred to the Clerk of the Council. This official in an interview with Mapother remained impervious to all arguments. Mapother then wrote a remarkable letter, some 1,600 words long, reviewing

the ground of contention, marshalling the arguments against the Council's ruling, and indicating the troubles the Council might be laying up for itself if it persisted in its penurious and shabby demands. The letter is a masterly statement, in tone and temper. It had the inevitable effect: the matter was promptly dropped and a letter was sent to Mapother confirming his rights of private practice. Commenting on the incident years later, he said drily that it illustrated the fact that enlightened selfishness may be necessary to avert conditions that would destroy an institution such as the Hospital. Two hundred and fifty years ago another witty psychiatrist, Bernard Mandeville, made a stir by pronouncing much the same dictum, with a wider bearing; most benefits to society, he held, spring from behaviour pursued from selfish motives: private frailties make public benefits. The paradox is an old one: it had the backing of Thomas Aquinas.

In spite of such brushes—or perhaps even because of them—Mapother obtained the Council's approval for steady expansion of the Hospital's work. Tangible developments included provision for more patients (they numbered 200 by 1935 plus an extra 35 in a ward of King's College Hospital). New buildings were set up: a large Out-patient Department (1936); a Villa to house disturbing patients (1932); a Children's Block (1937); a Wing for Private Patients (1938). Most of the burden for planning these extensions rested on Mapother, in conjunction with the Council Architect. He had a very clear grasp of what he wanted and how it could be achieved.

By the time war was declared in 1939 the number of beds, apart from the ward in King's College Hospital, had risen to 290. The medical staff had increased to 15, and the nursing staff to 143. Out-patient services had been instituted by the Maudsley staff from 1932 at three of the Council's general hospitals in North London; fifteen hundred psychiatric patients were seen there per annum, in addition to those (over three thousand) seen at the Maudsley itself.

The extension of the Maudsley's activities into general hospitals was regarded by Mapother as experimental. Thus the ward at King's

College Hospital which was taken over and run by the Maudsley from 1932 led him to an adverse conclusion: 'all experience derived from this ward supports the view that it is only under the special conditions of association with a psychiatric clinic that a single ward in a general hospital can properly deal with truly recent cases of mental and even neurotic disorder.' He feared that propaganda for such wards would delay his ideal, viz. affiliation of completely organized psychiatric clinics to teaching hospitals. He was, of course, the psychiatrist to King's College Hospital, and knew that the local Medical Officer of Health had advised the House Governor of that hospital that in the neighbourhood of the hospital there was no need for more beds for general purposes, but that the best contribution they could make to the hospital needs of London was by putting a ward at the disposal of the Maudsley. In the same area there were the mental observation wards or Acute Reception Unit at Constance Road Institution (now called St. Francis Hospital) to which Mapother became the visiting consultant. He was indeed a pluralist of no mean order. He had a busy private practice in addition to these appointments, and he was psychiatrist to the Ex-Services Welfare Society. And all this was accomplished in the face of frequent bouts of ill-health.

One of his most cherished projects was the creation of a neurological or neuro-psychiatric unit at the Maudsley. From 1934 onwards he made unremitting efforts to turn it into a reality At first he saw it as forming a liaison between King's College Hospital and the Maudsley and as a corollary to his belief that the future of psychiatry in this country depended essentially on its development as a branch of neurological science (though not as the clinical province of the neurologist). He approached Dr. Alan Gregg to ask if the Rockefeller Foundation would provide the funds for the necessary premises; the response was discouraging. Undaunted, Mapother considered putting up the money himself, as an anonymous donor: 'I knew a man', he wrote in a memorandum to the Chief Officer, 'who was willing to leave about £30,000 to the furthering of psychiatry after the death of himself and his wife and to

take my advice as to the projects he would commend to his Trustees. Thus it seemed that eventually what I desired might come to pass, though perhaps only thirty years later.'

To secure an appropriate site the L.C.C. had to be persuaded to use their powers of compulsory puchase. Mapother therefore sounded Sir Frederick Menzies, the Chief Medical Officer of the L.C.C.; Menzies was attracted by the proposal, which fitted in with his larger plans for utilizing the clinical resources of the Council's hospitals for research and teaching. Schedules were prepared, and in 1937 the Council's architect put forward a scheme for the proposed Unit—a four storey building housing 100 patients, which would cost £80,000 to put up. In a series of cogent briefs Mapother presented the case for going ahead with the Unit. It was to be predominantly for teaching and research, and Mapother detailed the investigations which might be pursued with profit in such a centre; he expected it to work in close co-operation with the neuro-surgical unit which Menzies was planning in South London. In 1937 Mapother therefore broached the matter again with Alan Gregg. The response was more positive this time. He was told that the Rockefeller foundation might make a substantial endowment (say £200,000) for research and teaching at the Maudsley provided that a comparable sum was obtained from a British source. Mapother then asked whether if the L.C.C. provided £100,000 for the neuro-psychiatric building and £20,000 a year for its maintenance this would meet the stipulation of a matching grant. The reply was encouraging, though no promise was made on behalf of the Foundation. So back Mapother went to the Council. The Finance Committee was obviously the crucial power. They took their time over it, partly on principle, I suppose, and partly because of the international situation; it was by now 1938, and trenches were already being dug in the parks. The Finance Committee laid down five conditions, of which the first was that the Unit should be the last main feature to be added to the Maudsley Hospital, and the fifth that an attempt should be made to obtain a contribution to the cost from the Government or the University, on the ground

142

that the addition was for teaching and research. The first of these conditions presented no difficulty—the Villa, the Private Patients' Wing, the Children's Block, the Out-patients Department, had all been successfully brought into being, and Mapother was ready to rest on his building laurels, if only he could get his neuropsychiatric Unit. But the fifth condition presented a formidable obstacle. The Finance Committee in February 1939 said they doubted whether the proposal should be proceeded with unless there were a promise of Government assistance. That was its death-knell in that form.

The academic standing of the Maudsley meant a great deal to Mapother, as it had to Mott. Mott had had to put up with some frustration in getting the University of London to recognize his laboratory when it was located at Claybury. He was determined that the Maudsley should be recognized as one of its Schools, and a diploma instituted for post-graduates. The University demurred at recognition because the teaching staff were not represented on the Governing Body. However, in 1924 the Maudsley received this status, on the understanding that the Advisory Board should consist of representatives of the teachers as well as of the Hospital Sub-Committee, and that within a specified period some further assurances should be forthcoming: these concerned the University's authority in deciding who should be an Appointed Teacher. The Council having given the required assurances in 1934, the obvious next step was to ask the University to establish Chairs, of which the first incumbents would be Mapother and Golla. Negotiations ensued to clarify the consequences for the L.C.C., and to overcome a difficulty which was blandly intimated in the written reminder that 'the general policy of the University is to exclude from professorships medical practitioners who might possibly find in their professorial status a means of augmenting their private practices and the emoluments derived therefrom'. But all the hurdles were surmounted, and in November 1936 the title of Professor was conferred on the two men, and their duties, inter alia, were 'to organize a department of clinical research'.

Mapother characteristically seized the oppor-
tunity to advance his proposals for reorganizing the medical staff of the Maudsley on lines which combined, as he put it, 'features of the Post-Graduate Hospital, Hammersmith, with others found at Voluntary Hospitals which undertake teaching of a special branch of medicine (such as the National Hospital, Queen Square)'. When the question of a professorship had been put before the Clerk of the Council, Sir George Gater, he had asked what would be the ultimate probable effect of the proposals upon the staffing of the Hospital. This was a heaven-sent opening for Mapother, to put the case for enlargement.

It does not appear that Mapother took an active part in the affairs of the Faculty of Medicine, except when the Diploma of Psychological Medicine was being re-furbished. I think one can detect his hand in a minor battle between the Advisory Committee of the D.P.M. and the Board of Studies in Psychology. The Advisory Committee said they had 'reason to think that the practice of psychotherapy by persons with training in psychology but who are not medically qualified is already prevalent, and that they are strongly of the opinion that such practice should not be encouraged and fostered by the University'. The Board of Studies in Psychology countered with a well-aimed *tu quoque*: 'Members of the Board are aware that so-called psychologists have occasionally attempted to practise psychotherapy without medical knowledge and without medical supervision, but this has probably not been more prevalent than the diagnosis and treatment of educational disabilities and irregularities of behaviour by medical men with no special psychological training or knowledge.' Honours were even.

MAPOTHER AND PSYCHIATRIC RESEARCH

The furtherance of research had from the outset been a main purpose of the Hospital. Maudsley left an additional £10,000 in his will specifically to this end. For some years this was the only fund on which investigators could draw for apparatus and any other expenses. Clinical research had to be done in the scanty spare time of the hospital staff. Central funds were negligible. In 1914 the Government made a grant of £1,600 to cover psychiatric research for the whole country for that year;

143

five grants of £300 each were allocated. The War put a stop to this extravagant profusion, this cascade of money for research. The London County Council could not see why it should support research from its own resources. It is therefore remarkable how much was in fact accomplished in the Hospital and in the Laboratory during the first ten years after the opening of the Maudsley.

Mapother fully appreciated the effect of these financial trammels. He approached the Commonwealth Fund of America (to whom he had been helpful in launching child guidance and the Mental Health Courses for Psychiatric Social Workers), and in 1931 the Fund created two whole time research fellowships at the Hospital and the Laboratory. This grant was renewed for four years. The holder of one of the fellowships in 1934 was Mayer-Gross, who had had to leave Germany. The persecutions in that country led the Rockefeller Foundation to provide personal grants for evicted German scholars and in the years 1934–35 Mayer-Gross and Erich Guttmann were supported in this way. But this was a small instalment of what Mapother had long wanted. In 1930, when he spent two months in the United States, he had called on Dr. Pearce of the Rockefeller Foundation to ask about the possibility of their endowing research at the Maudsley and the Central Pathological Laboratory. The matter was referred to Alan Gregg, who came over here and discussed the general proposal, particularly Mapother's view that 'the great lack of the Maudsley is research by real specialists in a number of subjects contributory to psychiatry, e.g. biochemistry, psychology, genetics.' Mapother then formally submitted to the Foundation a considered appeal for endowment of an Institute. This was an ambitious, detailed statement persuasively argued in an extensive document—almost a book. In effect it requested funds to provide for a Clinical Director-Professor and six senior workers in the fields of genetics; endocrinology; morbid anatomy; experimental psychology; infection, e.g. encephalitis; and metabolism. Mapother made incidental pungent observations. Thus with endocrinology he bracketed sexual processes: 'however limited his taste for pornography, no

psychiatrist can doubt the vast influence of sexual processes in relation to "functional" nervous disorder. But the need seems to be for a study of recent and current rather than remote situations, and for the quest of physical and chemical findings rather than the cult of dubious reminiscence.'

The appeal to the Rockefeller Foundation was submitted in March 1931. It was an inauspicious time: the economic depression was doing its worst. The Foundation at first decided that they would prefer 'a less extensive and more gradual development of the research activities of the Maudsley'. Then after some months they had to postpone any action on it because of the continuing economic crisis. That was in December 1931. Mapother took the matter up again after a decent interval and in a warmer financial climate, with the result that for three years, from 1935 to 1938, the Foundation provided the salaries of five senior research workers, two of whom worked in the Hospital, and three in the Laboratory. In 1938 they undertook to provide £25,000 for the ensuing five years, and the grant holders were thus assured of continuous support during the War. If it had not been for the Rockefeller subvention important developments in psychology would not have been possible, and the research programme built up in previous years would have been in jeopardy.

It would be difficult to convey the stimulus and help afforded during the thirties by Alan Gregg and by his colleague in the European office, Daniel O'Brien. I received much personal kindness from Dr. O'Brien which I am glad to recall.

All this turns on Mapother's grasp and foresight in securing the right conditions for research. But he was not inert in research himself, so far as his multifarious responsibilities allowed. His first papers (1911–1914) had a strong neurological bent: they were concerned with such topics as mental symptoms in choreiform disorders, aphasia in general paralysis, and intrathecal treatment of this disease: they contained no original observations of any consequence. But in 1922 he published a paper of very different tenor. It was a study in psychopathology, reporting in detail how fantasies of

144

childhood and adolescence had later provided the content of a young woman's schizophrenic delusions. He drew attention to the 'wealth of meaning which, without any far-fetched interpretations or assumptions, lay behind the apparently disconnected symptoms'. And he added: 'In practically all properly investigated cases of insanity, it is found that it is the result of the summation of multiple causes, effective in combination, though inadequate singly. It is this that renders all controversy between extremists of the physiogenic and psychogenic schools so futile'. 'Remote events cannot be regarded as specific causes'. While expressing dissent from some psychoanalytic tenets, Mapother and his collaborator, J. E. Martin, asserted roundly that 'the time is past for crying that Freud's findings as to the contents of the neuroses and psychoses are horrid . . . and for substituting witticism for criticism'. Nevertheless he allowed himself in subsequent years to combine the two, on occasion.

He made some incisive contributions to the assessment and treatment of war neuroses, including his evidence to the War Office 'shell-shock' committee in 1922. He also analysed a large series of cases of head injury, associated with psychotic disturbances; he enquired into the incidence and prognosis of the mental changes, and used his own case-records of 123 such patients seen in private practice, and over 100 others seen at municipal and mental hospitals of the L.C.C. Another topic to which he applied his critical judgment was the assessment of alcoholic morbidity in a given population. In this valuable paper he exposed the fallacy in many of the accepted statistics: it is worth remembering that his father had been President of the Statistical Society in Dublin. His other papers dealt particularly with the principles underlying an enlightened Mental Health Service and with administrative and clinical aspects of psychiatry. There were also two main addresses (the Bradshaw lecture of the Royal College of Physicians, and the Presidential Address to the Section of Psychiatry of the Royal Society of Medicine). He took great pains over the preparation of these testimonies: they contain his confession of faith, and his commination of error. He also wrote articles on voluntary sterilization on eugenic grounds, and official reports on the psychiatric services in India and Ceylon.

THE STAFFING OF THE MAUDSLEY

When the Hospital had been open for ten years, Mapother reviewed its situation and needs in a powerful confidential memorandum for the Council, a document of some 15,000 words, skilfully presented, and realistic. The picture of achievement was compelling: a bold building programme was being carried through, extended services were being provided, and the Hospital had grown steadily in reputation and status. But it had been uphill work, sometimes carried out only by hand-to-mouth expedients. Mapother decided that it was now advisable to outline a considered policy for the next decade. It would not be practicable to summarize this comprehensive statement, and I must confine notice of it to the argument for reorganizing the medical staff—a matter which Mapother rightly saw as of over-riding importance. His aim was that the Hospital and Laboratory should 'become the central resort of all psychiatrists of the British Commonwealth, and of such other English-speaking psychiatrists as come to Europe for study. Jointly the Hospital and Laboratory should carry on such functions as are performed for German psychiatry by the Clinic and Forschungsanstalt in Munich'. He recognized that the staff of the Maudsley was not already equipped to teach at this level 'the point is that such teachers should be created.' To this end the functions hitherto exercised by the Medical Superintendent should be divided between a medical administrator and a clinical director: the latter should have University status as Professor. The staff structure in other respects should cease to conform to the pyramidal pattern familiar in mental hospitals and should be assimilated to that of the teaching hospitals 'in respect of their best features'. There was a simplicity about the mental hospitals model for the Maudsley 'which is bound to be fatal to the complexity of its functions'.

To illustrate the crying need to overhaul the medical staff arrangements he recalled dispassionately the circumstances of his own

145

appointment: he had been told in 1922 that his tenure of the post could last only six years, and within that period would be held 'during the pleasure of the Council' and at a lower salary than other Medical Superintendents, 'with various other somewhat humiliating limitations'. The conditions were indeed such, he recalled, 'that no man of the necessary status and experience, but without private means, could have risked applying, unless he had been devoid of responsibilities to children and married to a wife who was willing that he should chance a fresh start from scratch at about the age of 45.' Mapother had even been refused any assurance that he would be reabsorbed into the other mental hospitals of the L.C.C. on the expiry of his six-years tenure at the Maudsley.

After a corresponding resumé of the conditions under which the other doctors had to work at the Maudsley, their handicaps and hardships led on to a summary broadside: 'the conclusion to which opinion of the medical staff at the Maudsley is tending may be summed up by saying that service there—except in a deliberately temporary way for a couple of years—is a trap, baited with scientific interest, which must be avoided in one's own interest and still more in the interest of an actual or prospective wife'. On another count Mapother urged that the Council's policy meant that the Maudsley could not have an adequate staff unless its Medical Officers were prepared to accept conditions which denied them a future. The future he had in mind was private practice and an honorary appointment to the senior staff of a teaching hospital—then the ambition of aspiring clinicians in most branches of medicine. Mapother argued that psychiatric private practice must expand because 'within recent years there has been a very rapid extension in what is recognized as the province of the psychiatrist—a multitude of minor anomalies both in child and adult are now regarded as suitable for reference to him, concerning which his opinion would never have been sought before the War'.

Developing the case for splitting up the Medical Superintendent's duties (which he enumerated with relish, under nine heads), he declared that they implied for their efficient performance 'a combination of gifts which would be almost supernatural . . . The present Medical Superintendent waives all claim to be considered as performing the above duties efficiently, and considers this impossible.'

I have dwelt on the arguments he advanced to justify reorganization of staff; they received much more detailed attention than these few extracts suggest, and were the prelude to an establishment plan which laid much stress on the value of Visiting Physicians, who would spend half their time in private practice and half (six half days a week) at the Maudsley. There should be three of them, each specializing in some division of psychiatry, e.g. disorders of childhood. Their functions would be closely comparable to those of physicians in a teaching hospital, except that 'to be useful, the amount of time would have to be more than is the case at an ordinary Voluntary Hospital, and more continuous,' and the posts should be salaried. He did not contemplate having Visiting Physicians to the Maudsley who would also hold a consultant position at another teaching hospital, except in the case of the post at King's College Hospital, which strengthened the intimate relation between the two adjacent hospitals, and the corresponding post at the Hammersmith Hospital, which has been held from the beginning by a member of the Maudsley staff. As he saw it, whole time medical officers of the Maudsley might hold minor honorary posts at a teaching hospital in preparation for the time when they would leave the Maudsley to take up a consultant post elsewhere, with private practice. No one at that time could foresee the radical changes which the National Health Service would bring about in the conditions of medical practice.

In 1936 his essential proposals for reorganization were made public in the Medical Superintendent's Report covering the previous four years. After that they germinated for a couple of years. In the autumn of 1938 they were formally submitted to the L.C.C. Sub-committee, where discussion turned mainly on two matters: should the next Medical Superintendent be allowed to engage in private practice, and what should be the relationship of the Medical Superintendent to the Clinical Director-Professor. There was strong opposition to private practice, and hesitation about making the relation of Superintendent to Professor a dyarchy of equals, with defined spheres of duty and authority. Most of the other details of staff reorganization were accepted by the Sub-committee: they concerned some twenty doctors of varying seniority; six of them to be part-time psychotherapists.

There is no indication that the threat of impending war was allowed to interfere with the sturdy nurture of these plans. In August 1939, Mapother asked the doctors then on the staff to read carefully the memorandum he had drawn up for the Sub-Committee, which he circulated with minor modifications. 'It is obviously desirable that the views of the medical staff should be known and that steps should now be taken to ensure that as far as possible the re-organization conforms to their wishes.' He said he would hold a meeting with them the following week and added that 'if time permits he will take an opportunity at the same meeting of informing the medical staff of proposed arrangements to take effect in the event of war'.

It turned out that the doctors were not of one mind about the proposals, though the majority endorsed them with reservations. They were much exercised about the suggested Visiting Physicians, and wanted their tenure of appointment to be limited to ten years or less. They were unanimous in their opinion that 'the position of the Assistant Medical Officers under the proposed scheme of reorganization was scarcely tenable'. The comments of the doctors, expressed in individual memoranda, were a rather painful disappointment to Mapother in so far as they denied the need for radical reorganization and approximation to the staff structure of teaching hospitals ('Voluntary Hospitals'). One memorandum declared that 'the Medical Superintendent, the Deputy Medical Superintendent, and possibly the Clinical Director should, at least, do regular weekly rounds of the wards, since it is only by this means that they can adequately supervise the running of the hospital'. *Autre temps, autres moeurs.*

Greater events now impended, and Mapother was intensively occupied with plans for the two war-time hospitals of the Emergency Medical Service into which the Maudsley was to be split and transplanted.

MAPOTHER AND PSYCHOTHERAPY

Among the disputed staff appointments were those designed entirely for psychotherapy. Here was an apparent conflict between Mapother's actions and his beliefs. He made provision for psychotherapy, while doubting the theoretical basis on which it rested in its most developed form, i.e. psychoanalysis. A concise statement of his attitude was put forward in 1932. 'The Maudsley Hospital has always stood, as its founder did, for the conception which may be termed the "continuity" of all forms of mental disorder and for the compatibility of treatment within one building of all grades of it. In speaking of the "continuity" of mental disorder, one means that this is a collective term for a medley of different anomalous reactions, and that the ratio in which these various anomalies are inter-mixed even in a single case is infinitely variable and so is the possible intensity of each anomaly . . . The vogue of such artificial simplicities as classification into "neuroses" and "psychoses" is dying out; so is belief in the view that clinical pictures can be isolated and given a descriptive label to which one can relate with any useful constancy a general causation, treatment and course, without the balanced considerations of a multitude of individual factors . . . There is no doubt that mental stress is the commonest single factor that can be identified in "functional" cases. There is equally little doubt that in most of these psychotherapy, however empirical, is the chief active contribution to recovery which is possible. . . . Personally I feel that if psychopathology is to rise like other branches of biology from the anecdotal to the scientific level, and if psychotherapy is to become rational and to define its limitations, then uncontrolled clinical findings must clearly be supplemented by observations as to the effect of standard experiences under experimental conditions capable of repetition.' That is a temperate statement: contrast it with one made in the Maudsley Lecture of 1925 by Shaw Bolton, the Leeds Professor of Mental Diseases: 'the Rasputin-like philosophy of

147

Freud, with its cult of largely naked votaries, is another example of the extraordinary methods of thought of the present day.' Mapother's essential criticisms of psycho-analysis, it is well to recognize, were not based on ignorance and prejudice: they have been put forward by prominent psycho-analysts themselves at one time or another. He particularly rejected animistic explanations and ingenious constructs, 'pinnacled dim in the intense inane'.

The last paper Mapother wrote was an appreciation of Freud's work for the Memorial Meeting of the R.S.M. held shortly after Freud's death. In it he acclaimed Freud's genius for 'fertility in hypothesis and the penetration with which he discerned analogies and connotations where they had never before been explicitly noted . . . He brought to psychology and psychiatry more of the imagination of the great artist than of the stolid objectivity and rigid logic of the scientist' . . . Years before, addressing the same group (the members of the Section of Psychiatry of the Royal Society of Medicine) he had pronounced a harsher judgment on what he believed to be the animistic vagaries and fallacies of psychoanalysis.

In this connection it is appropriate, though perhaps hazardous, to refer to Mapother's attitude to the Tavistock Clinic. It is sometimes assumed that the Maudsley and the Tavistock were engaged in a struggle for ascendancy, and that each disparaged the other. The most recent reference to the Maudsley's attitude towards the Tavistock was in the 1967 Presidential Address to the Royal Medico-Psychological Association, where it was stated that to the Maudsley the Tavistock was 'beneath contempt'. How far this is from the facts can be recognized from correspondence which Mapother had with Crichton-Miller and J. R. Rees. In April 1930 Crichton-Miller invited Mapother to speak at the Tavistock's Annual Lunch, and Mapother replied in appreciative but frank terms 'I think my official job would make it very difficult for me to speak without a lot of explanations . . . There is, of course, no rivalry whatever between the Maudsley and the Tavistock Clinic, but . . . I gathered that the lunch was to be followed by a sort of drive on behalf of the Institute of Medical Psychology.

Here again I personally feel that there is room for both, but we have always had at the Maudsley a programme of development which corresponds to a large extent with your plans for the Institute; I think it might be taken amiss by people with whom I am associated if I seemed to be publicly advocating the schemes of the other show'. In a further friendly exchange Mapother wrote 'I wholly disbelieve in cases that are purely psychogenic or physiogenic, and in establishment of units professing to treat their cases preferably by one method rather than according to the needs of the case. Restricting applications to patients that need only one line of treatment is a practical impossibility. Therefore I should genuinely like to see the Tavistock Clinic going out for a development of its ability to investigate and treat on physical lines as well as psychological lines, and this almost necessarily means obtaining beds. It is far enough from the Maudsley for no overlapping to occur . . .'

A year later Mapother wrote to give up his membership of the Medical Advisory Board of the Tavistock, explaining his reasons (which concerned efforts he was making to persuade the L.C.C. to increase the provision for treating neurotic disorders by psychotherapy and otherwise), and he prefaced his letter with the assurance 'I should like you to believe that my action is not prompted by any illwill or even criticism'. He added 'neither of us is at all likely to make depreciatory remarks about the other's institution'. Rees's reply was on much the same 'live and let live' basis. Despite his generally friendly attitude, Mapother did not at that time or subsequently see any reason for encouraging the L.C.C. to give the Tavistock Clinic financial support: his comments on an approach with this as its object were lengthy and characteristically thorough. His sympathies were also somewhat alienated by the propaganda put out in connection with appeals for funds; as he put it in 1936, 'it seems that the need to raise the wind for private institutions is thought to require extravagant over-statement about their powers'. Probably the fairest assessment of the situation was that made by Rees in one of his letters to Mapother (a propos of an excessive claim to which Mapother took exception): 'You no doubt see our mistakes and our failures and are no doubt critical of us, we should be short-sighted if we were not at times critical also of other people's work, including the Maudsley, but surely these criticisms are the sort of things we want to have given us . . .'

MAPOTHER AS TEACHER AND ADMINISTRATOR

Postgraduate teaching at the Maudsley had been organized first by Mott in 1920, and the pattern he established—a six months compressed course—was adhered to. The purpose was explicitly to prepare people for the Diploma in Psychological Medicine, and it met a national need. Mapother had the lion's share of the teaching of clinical psychiatry in this course. He also gave lectures and demonstrations every year to the medical students of King's College Hospital and the Middlesex Hospital and took part in more sporadic teaching at various postgraduate levels. He tended to be over the heads of his audience, not because of his diction, which was always clear, but because of the relatively abstruse neuro-physiological basis of his theoretical position. His most detailed statement of this was presented in his Bradshaw Lecture. This is not the occasion to attempt to summarize it; it was highly speculative, but it represented a bold effort to repudiate the charge of a purely destructive approach to fundamental psychopathology.

As a clinician Mapother was at his teaching best in the ward conferences he held three times a week. He insisted on precision regarding dates and the order of events; he expected biographical detail to be given in sensible perspective, in contrast to the notion that 'nothing is too banal to be important provided it is sufficiently remote', and he always called a spade a spade. He relied a great deal on his case-memory, and it was sometimes easy to predict which of the patients whom he had seen at Long Grove or in his military experience he would cite to illustrate his opinion of the patient being presented to him. It was often clear that he held, with William James, that 'large acquaintance with particulars often makes us wiser than the possession of abstract formulas, however deep'.

He had no liking for diagnostic hair-splitting,

and he made it plain, year in and year out, that he regarded the distinction between neurotic and psychotic, or between endogenous and reactive, as artificial; this was, of course, a theme to which he referred in many of his published writings, dwelling particularly on the gradations and essential continuity of the various depressive conditions. He was similarly sceptical about the bolder reports of therapeutic triumph, being (like his father) of the opinion that 'the argument from results . . . was riddled with fallacies', the simplest instance of which was seen when 'the improvement existed only in the mind of the person who claimed to have brought it about'. He derided 'therapeutic chanticleers'. In the Bradshaw Lecture he spoke scornfully of the 'search for unitary causes and unitary cures for (psychiatric) syndromes, which is as naïve and as futile as the quest for the elixir of life'. In his Presidential Address to the Listerian Society in 1937 he caustically remarked that 'those who see many of the alleged cures (by psychotherapy) at present are apt to be reminded of the missionary who regretted his inability to cure his flock of cannibalism but claimed that at least he had taught them to eat with a knife and fork'. Mapother quoted with approval an aphorism of Hughlings Jackson: 'the tendency to appear exact by disregarding the complexity of factors is the oldest failing in medical history.'

Another tenet to which he adhered was in regard to the agents of progress.'I hold that properly critical research will never come from those who are in practice or bound for it. The only hope for the sort of dispassionate long-term research which psychiatry needs is the creation of teams of investigators guaranteed careers, with rewards comparable to those which similar abilities would command if otherwise marketed. Most of the members of such teams should not primarily be psychiatrists at all, but real experts in various branches of science, who have brought its technique to the service of psychiatry and then received enough training in this to enable them to see its problems . . . Then we should get progress, not potboiling'.

Before I came to the Maudsley I had received my psychiatric education in two main schools, under the influence of two outstanding men—

149

Adolf Meyer at the Johns Hopkins and Karl Bonhoeffer at the Charité. I had also learnt a great deal from Macfie Campbell in Boston and Beringer in Heidelberg. I expected, from what I was told, that at the Maudsley I might have to readjust my modes of thought to a somewhat insular, rigidly materialist and old-fashioned model, of which Mapother would be the exponent. In fact I found it quite otherwise. The fundamental standpoint of Meyer was very close to that of Mapother, though more profound and less intelligible; the clinical principles of Bonhoeffer and the brilliant group around him—such men as Kronfeld, Birnbaum, Thiele—were readily adaptable to the Maudsley climate, allowance being made for the greater erudition of the Germans. Certainly Denmark Hill was not a psychiatric backwater to someone recently educated in Baltimore and Berlin, and Mapother's influence was no less pervasive and justly respected within its range, than that of of the better known leaders abroad.

Mapother's contributions to the lasting literature of his subject would undoubtedly have been greater if he had not devoted so much time to planning and administration. Knowledge of his achievements in this field led to his being consulted by the Macmillan Commission, the Government of Ceylon, the Ministry of Health and the Home Office, the Commonwealth Fund, and other public bodies. But, of course, the chief exercise of his administrative abilities fell within the work at and for the Maudsley. At times this brought him into conflict with the Board of Control. The chief dispute turned on the legality of retaining in the Maudsley as a voluntary patient someone who had after admission lapsed into a stupor and thus become 'non-volitional'. It is now a dead issue, but at the time it was important and was fiercely debated. Mapother's lack of veneration for the Board of Control is manifest in the following comment of his on their injunctions about 'non-volitional boarders' and the certifiable voluntary patient: 'both (these rulings) are moss-grown absurdities invented by the Board of Control'. '(there are) fresh indications that the Board is restarting on its historic mission of backing the wrong horse'.

Mapother also took strong exception to the proposal that there should be wards in general hospitals for early and recoverable patients. Only the prejudiced could, he said, regard this as preferable to a psychiatric clinic on the Maudsley pattern spanning the whole range of mental illness. He made his position abundantly clear in various papers. In 1929 he said 'there are no substitutes for the psychopathic clinics; wards in general hospitals, whether municipal or voluntary, can no more replace them than cottage hospitals can do the work of the medical schools'. And in 1934, with the added experience of running a ward (Pantia Ralli) in King's College Hospital, he elaborated his objections. In the Quinquennial Report in 1936 he wrote in the same strain: 'it is essential to emphasise that the quite real success of this experiment (the ward in King's College Hospital, staffed and controlled by the Maudsley) is no argument whatever for the theory that in respect either of early treatment or of teaching any material advance can be made by admitting mental cases to the wards of a general hospital under ordinary circumstances'. Although the reasons he gave for this uncompromising stand still have some force, I think it is certain that under the condition now prevailing he would welcome the development of adequately functioning comprehensive psychiatric units in general hospitals, and particularly in teaching hospitals. But it is also certain that in his lifetime he neither foresaw nor favoured them. Indeed he felt very strongly about it, as is evident in his note on the neuropsychiatric unit to-be: 'King's College Hospital is very interested, and would indeed like to induce the L.C.C. to place the proposed Unit upon some spare ground which King's College Hospital has not the money to utilize. I should entirely disagree with this proposal; I am sure the Unit in such circumstances would lose its efficiency in research and advanced post-graduate teaching, and that the neurology studied there would cease to be of the kind directly relevant to psychiatry.'

It is pleasant to record that on Mapother's retirement at the end of 1939 because of ill-health, the Chairman of the Board of Control, Sir Laurence Brock, wrote regretting this and adding 'it would be absurd to suggest that we were always in agreement or that you had ever given me ground for regarding you as a passionate admirer of our Board. But, however much we may have disagreed from time to time, I always found discussion with you extraordinarily stimulating even if the stimulus—forgive me for saying so—was occasionally tinged with exasperation.' Mapother wrote a charming reply, and sent copies of memoranda on outstanding projects which would have to go into cold storage during the war: he hoped Brock and Hubert Bond would keep them alive.

PERSONAL TRAITS

No account of Mapother's efforts and successes would be appropriate without some reference to his personality, which was distinctive and unmistakably consistent. He was not at first sight impressive: his slight build, restless movements, and sometimes his troubled breathing caught one's attention. But this was soon forgotten, or rather shifted to his lively, humorous face and pithy conversation. He was intensely distrustful of anything that seemed to him humbug, and he disliked sentimentality almost as much. Anything that savoured of professional commercialism was likewise anathema. His own integrity was beyond question in small matters as well as large ones. He insisted on strict, at times austere, standards of clinical probity.

His intellect was sharp and shrewd, with a touch of legal inquisition, and at its best when examining a complex issue or—in a very different way—making the case for some Maudsley need. His wit served as an astringent partner to his zest for controversy: he began a lecture on mental hygiene—in itself a calm enough theme—with the characteristic promise: 'in order to render this discussion fruitful, it is essential to shun the noble but nebulous platitude, to be concrete at all costs, and provocative if possible.' And provocative he certainly was: many examples come to mind: 'the eel seems indicated as the totem animal of the whole community of psychologists'; or, on another favourite topic, 'the explanation is only satisfactory to those who regard as science a process of circular argument consisting of restatement of observed fact in terms of animis-

tic entities . . . more briefly, the translation of platitudes into jargon'. Fundamentally the temper of his mind was partisan, in the good sense; he was not serene and detached, but eager, pertinacious, argumentative, scathing in criticism and powerful in reasoned support. With all his enjoyment of swordplay and iconoclasm, he remained hopeful and positive, by no means a cynic (even though he said that psychology awaited its Voltaire).

He was energetic and expected others to be so. Surprisingly, Bernard Hart told me that as a young doctor at Long Grove Mapother had the reputation of being lazy: it is hard to credit; there must have been a critical change in his interests or character after that. He was courageous in meeting the recurring threat to his life from his fibrosed lungs and the attacks of asthma every winter. Capable of impetuous outbursts of anger, he was regretful and generous afterwards, and showed no rancour. Deceit angered and upset him: I remember being struck by his furious discomposure on the morning of the Hoare-Laval disclosures in 1935.

He had some foibles. He was absent-minded in things that did not concern the Maudsley: for example on sitting down after he had read a paper to the Eugenics Society he immediately joined heartily in the applause. He was prone to shuffle and reshuffle his correspondence and papers until he had the greatest difficulty in disinterring what he wanted. He worked through his mid-day meal, interviewing people and drinking endless cups of cold tea. He was unpunctual, no doubt because he crowded so much into each day, and often had a queue waiting in the corridor outside his door to see him.

Perhaps these trivialities are unworthy of mention, but they are prominent in our recollection of him. There are other, more important features of his life which he would not have talked of, nor shall I. I refer to his wife, upon whom he leant heavily for support. She spent herself in the same causes as he did, and her self-denial in the last years of her life in order to fulfil his dreams and hopes left a lasting memorial in the Mapother Fellowship.

I know there is much more to be said about this single-minded, upright, creative man: I

151

hope it will be said by subsequent Mapother Lecturers. It is fitting that I conclude by quoting from the farewell letter written to him on his retirement by R. H. Curtis, the Chief Officer of the Mental Hospitals Department of the L.C.C: 'it will be for a successor to help in the rebuilding of what you have seen thrown down; but your successor, whoever he is, will have the advantage in that task of the foundations which you have helped to lay' . . . No one is in a better position than I to know how true that is.

Paranoia and paranoid: a historical perspective

AUBREY LEWIS

From the Institute of Psychiatry, De Crespigny Park, London

SUMMARY   The history of the words paranoia and paranoid is traced from the Greeks to the present day and their fluctuations of usage and concept are explored.

The words paranoia and paranoid have become part of common literate speech. Some people think their meaning is sufficiently clear. But, like 'hysterical', 'sadistic', and a good many other terms that have passed from psychiatry into ordinary usage, their technical meaning has wavered, and their everyday meaning become correspondingly loose.

In Greek literature 'paranoia' and the verb *paranoeo* were used as loosely as we are accustomed to use 'crazy' or 'out of his mind'. They occur in Euripides, Aeschylus, Aristophanes, Aristotle, and Plato. Hippocrates applies 'paranoia' to the delirium of high fever; several other writers put it in a context where it denotes senile deterioration, justifying action by the patient's son, according to Attic law. However, 'paranoia' did not always refer to madness or dementia, or other severe disturbance, but sometimes meant 'thinking amiss', 'going astray', 'folly'. In any case it was not a technical term, as melancholia was, and was not preserved in medical writings. Its revival in the 18th century, to meet classificatory needs, was therefore practically a rebirth. This was effected by Boissier de Sauvages.

In his *Nosologia Methodica* (1763) de Sauvages gave paranoia as the Greek equivalent of amentia: 'Amentia, Graecis paranoia; Latinis dementia, fatuitas, vecordia; Gallis imbecillité, bétise, niaiserie, démence.' Some years earlier, in his *Pathologia Methodica* (1759) he had tersely described it as 'universale mite chronicum sine febre delirium': In the *Nosologia* he expanded the characteristics of paranoia as a 'delirium particulare mite sine furore et audacia cum morbo diuturno. Est ineptitudo ad recte ratiocinandum et judicandum'. Clearly he had dementia in mind.

R. A. Vogel, while treading in de Sauvages's footsteps (1772), enlarged the scope of the Greek term, making it equivalent to *vesania*, or *morbus mentis*, which should include mania and melancholia, *fatuitas, stupiditas, amentia, oblivio.*

William Cullen (1783–84) who had great respect for Vogel, accepted without reservation his use of the term as equivalent to *vesania*: 'vesaniarum ordinem hic instituere velim quae cum classe Vogelii nona Paranoiae inscripta eadem omnino sint'. Cullen cited as their main features impaired judgment and afebrile course; he excluded hallucinations and 'erroneous appetites' or *morositas.*

HEINROTH

In spite of the ascendancy which was enjoyed by Vogel in Germany and Cullen in Scotland, their classification of mental disorders did not command general assent, and paranoia did not figure in succeeding diagnostic schemata. It was only after a retirement of 40 years that it was launched on a second career, destined to be much more troubled, mutable, and insecure than its sponsor could foresee. The sponsor was Heinroth (1818), consciously harking back to Vogel and Cullen: 'Cullen beschäftigte sich, mit Ausschuss dieser (Halluzinationen, Morositates) unter der Rubrik der Seelenstörungen bloss mit den von ihm genannten Vesaniis die Vogel Paranoias genannt hatte.'

Heinroth's system is a significant part of the history of psychiatry, and cannot be briefly stated or grasped without regard to the philosophy that underlay it. He initiated the German practice of treating paranoia and *Verrücktheit* as

153

completely interchangeable synonyms. Since German writers have been chiefly responsible for the exceptional gymnastics through which the term paranoia passed on its way to Nirvana, the relevant German concepts command disproportionate attention.

Of his three great classes of mental disorder, Heinroth regarded *Verrücktheit* (paranoia) as falling within the first class, the exaltations or hypersthenias, and affecting the understanding predominantly. He recognized, however, that pure types are rare and that mixtures with disorders predominantly of the will or the affects are the rule. These he regarded from the Linnaean standpoint as species, and to describe them he devised Greek and Latin terms which he evidently felt he must defend: 'Die Form selbst wird jedesmal die Bezeichnung, wenn gleich neu und auffallend, rechtfertigen. Die Not trieb zur eigenen Wahl, wo sich kein Vorgänger fand; und der Reichtum der griechischen Sprache bei der Armut der römischen führte die Mehrzahl der griechischen Benennungen herbei.'

His schema is the logical expression of his religio-biological outlook and convictions, in which spiritual freedom was equated with mental health. He defined paranoia as 'Unfreiheit des Geistes mit Verstandesüberspannung in Verkehrtheit der Begriffe und Urteils'. Perception is unaffected. There are four species of paranoia: *ecnoia*, *paraphrosyne*, *moria*, and *paranoia catholica*. In *ecnoia* a single false idea is responsible for gross distortion of a subject's relation with the outside world, and corresponding practical activity on his part: there are three varieties of the disorder. In *paraphrosyne* there are delusions about the supernatural; *moria* is a sort of megalomania; and *paranoia catholica* a general mixture of emotional, cognitive, and volitional aberrations.

Heinroth did not regard delusions as indicating disorders of mood but of the understanding; nevertheless he recognized the importance of emotion in generating delusions: 'Der in Leidenschaft Befangene täuscht sich über die Gegenstände und über sich selbst; und diese Täuschung, und der daraus springende Irrthum heisst Wahn. Der Wahn ist kein krankhafter Zustand des Gemüthes sondern des Verstandes; aber im Gemüthe, nämlich in der Leidenschaft, liegt der Grund des Wahns.' He tended to equate passion, vice, and delusion as three stages in a progressive disorder.

In associating paranoia with a particular form of delusional state, Heinroth was to some extent anticipating future developments. His psychology, however, was so intimately interwoven with metaphysics and his clinical syntheses that it alienated many psychiatrists: thus Bucknill and Hack Tuke, after quoting in their *Textbook* (1874) a paragraph in which Heinroth alleged that insanity is the loss of moral liberty, burst into unrestrained invective: 'It would seem impossible to compress within a single paragraph a larger amount of false and mischievous psychological teaching. . . . It should only be retailed after being duly labelled Poison!'

Heinroth's views attracted some of his contemporaries, such as Ideler, and prepared the way for the vigorous debates about the wholly psychogenic or wholly somatogenic nature of mental illness. Paranoia, however, did not occupy a place in the front line of the polemics or in the textbooks which were appearing in increasing numbers during the first half of the 19th century.

KAHLBAUM'S CLASSIFICATION

The concept of paranoia entered on a new and bolder phase when Kahlbaum (1863) proposed a system of classification which depended not on theoretical schemata but on the methods found most suitable in the natural sciences and empirical medicine. Full observations of clinical phenomena, pathology, causation, and course and outcome were the basis on which he delimited symptom complexes. Griesinger had proposed (1845) that the term *Partial Verrücktheit* should be reserved for an incurable disorder, in which there were prominent ideas of persecution and of grandeur and which was always secondary to a preceding acute or primary mental illness; *General Verrücktheit*, he held, was a severe state of confusion in which the patient is active but demented. Kahlbaum likewise distinguished between partial and general, placing the 'family' Paranoia among the partial *vecordias* which, in his system, were as a class 'primary' or 'original' in that they would remain essentially unchanged during a lifetime, in contrast to the general or complex disorders (*vesanias*) which passed through four stages, a

154

delusional condition of the same form as *Verrücktheit* sometimes preceding the final stage (dementia). Kahlbaum, like some other psychiatrists of the 19th century, was not attributing a meaning to the term paranoia because of a passion for labelling, but in order to denote a logical concept of mental disease different from that generally held or propounded by outstanding contemporaries. It is difficult to do justice to the changes advocated in the meaning of paranoia or its synonym without embarking on a history of 19th-century psychiatry, which would lead far from the bare facts of linguistic usage.

Kahlbaum had been influenced by the French psychiatrists Morel and Guislain in laying great weight on the course and outcome of a mental disease, as distinct from a mere symptom complex. Although at first his proposals did not find ready acceptance, the central question had to be answered: was 'paranoia' to be exclusively the name of a persistent chronic condition or could the same clinical picture be produced as one rather late stage in the *vesania typica*—that is, as a secondary feature supervening on the way to dementia?

The restriction of the term to an independent or 'primary' delusional condition thenceforward gained ground. In 1865 a prominent exponent, Snell, suggested (following Esquirol's terminology) that the condition should be named *Primäre Monomanie*: two years later he abjured this, and wrote about *Primäre Verrücktheit*. He stressed the systematic nature of the delusional structure, which is sharply imprinted and firmly held. Another prominent contemporary, Sander (1868), substituted the adjective *originäre* for *primäre* and maintained that this *Originäre Verrücktheit* (paranoia) was a hereditary disease in which intelligence remained intact, but the patient had delusions of persecution and self-aggrandisement, indicating abnormal judgment about the relation between self and outer world.

For the next half-century the words and the concept they denoted were given so many shades of meaning that, although the delusional core was always there, the diagnostic application varied enormously, and there was general discontent. A firm effort to tidy the semantic confusion was made by Westphal in 1878. He laid it down that paranoia (*Verrücktheit*) was always an independent 'primary' psychosis, which could begin with a hypochondria or acute hallucinosis, or show from the outset the features described by Sander. The clinical picture and course varied with the degree of involvement of formal thinking and motor behaviour. It was primarily an affection of the intellect, never secondary to melancholia (as Griesinger had thought it at first): 'Das Wesentliche bei der Verrücktheit ist der abnorme Vorgang im Vorstellen; in der Sphäre der Vorstellungen (mit oder ohne Sinnesdelirien) spielt sich der Vorgang ab und der allgemeine Inhalt dieser krankhaften Vorstellungen bleibt sich immer gleich.'

'THE PARANOIA QUESTION'

Important contributors to the discussion of (what came to be called) the 'paranoia question' were Meynert, Mendel, Wernicke, Krafft-Ebing, Schüle, Neisser, Cramer, Arndt, and Kraepelin. Krause said in 1897, with general approval, that there was hardly any problem in psychiatry that had for the last few decades been so much debated and led to such extreme differences of opinion among the leading authorities as this. The apparent frequency of the condition consequently varied greatly. In reports from many hospitals paranoiacs constituted 50% of all admissions, while at the other extreme Weygandt, for instance, said that he had diagnosed paranoia on only three occasions, out of 3,000 patients he had seen. His reluctance was prescient.

Mendel and Werner had a considerable share in getting 'paranoia' more widely used than the synonym *Verrücktheit*. Mendel had advocated the exclusive use of 'paranoia' in 1880, Werner took the same standpoint in 1891, and *Verrücktheit*, though it did not entirely fall out of currency, was regarded generally as an old-fashioned, ambiguous term.

The nosological position of the litigious 'querulant' became a controversial matter which went on for 20 years: a subdivision, *paranoia querulantium*, was created for it. Other refinements of classification within paranoia were proposed: the arguments bespeak much subtlety and sharpness but have a very musty odour now. It is hardly possible to speak of a consensus amid the wrangling, but the nearest approach to one in the 1890s was provided by Snell, who in 1890 reformulated his definition: paranoia is a chronic disease whose essential feature is delusions of influence (*Beeinträchtigung*) and persecution, based on hallucinations and usually accompanied by delusions of grandeur. The content of the delusions was given varying weight in the delimitation of the disease. Neisser (1891) insisted that the delusions should be logically articulated, internally consistent, and lasting unchanged till death: the delusional system is a product of the essential disease, of which the invariable immediate expression is heightened self-reference (*krankhafte Eigenbeziehung*). In other respects Neisser's views were out-of-step and excessively comprehensive: they harked back to the notions of paranoia prevalent in the '50s and '60s. Almost all writers during this period stress that in paranoia consciousness is clear, thinking is formally correct, and it is not until the senium (or last stage) that dementia may supervene.

KRAEPELIN'S VIEWS

Because of the great influence he exercised and the clarity and honesty with which he expressed his changing views, Kraepelin is the best guide to central opinion. In 1892 he affirmed his strong adherence to Kahlbaum's criteria for delimiting mental diseases, which relied on community of cause, course, duration, and outcome; and he urged that the term paranoia should be restricted to a chronic, persisting, incurable delusional system, on a constitutional basis. He specifically rejected 'acute curable paranoia' as a tenable concept.

In the 1896 edition of his textbook, Kraepelin again insisted on the overriding importance of course and outcome. He accordingly treated dementia praecox, catatonia, and dementia paranoides as three distinct degenerative diseases (*Verblödungsprozesse*). Paranoia he classified as a further and distinct disease, with a different course and outcome.

In the next edition of the *Textbook* (1899) he fused the three 'degenerative processes' into the one disease, 'dementia praecox'; and put into it (as 'dementia paranoides') all conditions that are initially thought to be paranoia but which dement quickly and in other ways show that they are forms of dementia praecox. The reasons for this change had been explained in an address he gave in Heidelberg in 1898. He could not include in paranoia conditions in which there were mood-swings, peculiarities of demeanour (*Haltung*), progressive fading and disorganization of the delusions, pronounced feelings of bodily interference, or hallucinations (except in very rare cases). He added, after the discussion that followed his paper, that this was not just a dispute about names: agreement about such nosological matters was essential.

In a carefully reasoned paper in 1912 he considered whether, in view of its shabby record, paranoia had better be dropped altogether as a legitimate category. He wished to retain it to denote insidious, endogenous development of unshakeable delusions, while the personality remains intact. It is, he held, a psychological malformation, with its roots in a peculiar paranoid disposition: its clinical manifestation in each affected individual is a response to the stresses of life. The differential diagnosis from dementia praecox depended mainly on whether the characteristic features of the latter (disordered thinking, apathy, volitional anomalies, rigid personality) were evident, and it could be very difficult to decide. He chose the term 'paraphrenia' to designate those who have a paranoid disturbance of personality which develops later than in dementia praecox and is milder; they are, in brief, patients who could have been called paranoiac if they had not had hallucinations, especially auditory hallucinations. Kraepelin was prepared to call paranoia a psychogenic disorder, grouped with hysteria. It is clear, from his many changes of posture, that Kraepelin was never comfortable with paranoia: if he had lived a little longer he would perhaps have surrendered it altogether at last.

The trend towards reductive definition of paranoia was evident in many articles that appeared about the turn of the century. Thus in 1901 Gustav Specht, after noting how paranoia had in a few years changed from a very commonly diagnosed condition to a rarity, declared himself to be in complete agreement with the strict and narrow criteria specified by Kraepelin: 'Fälle in denen sich von Anfang an klar erkennbar ganz langsam ein dauerndes unerschütterliches Wahnsystem bei vollkommener Erhaltung der Besonnenheit und der Ordnung des Gedankenganges herausbildet.' The slightest deviation from this formulation, he said, would lead eventually to the inclusion of every so-called functional psychosis in the paranoia group. Specht's paper was important on another count. He dissented sharply from Westphal's generally accepted dictum that paranoia was essentially a disorder of the understanding: he argued that paranoia must be a primary disorder of affect. This contention roused Bleuler, among others, to enter the fray. His monograph (1906) *Affektivität, Suggestibilität, Paranoia* began with a blunt assertion that paranoia is a splendid example of how a psychiatrist who works with unclear concepts can be lost in a bottomless sea. He accepted Kraepelin's definition but not Specht's psychopathology. The bulk of the monograph is devoted to expounding his own view of the psychological development of paranoia, but in the final clinical section he takes up the question of whether hallucinations can be prominent in the disease. He holds that they occur in many cases, are then often of brief duration and in a confusional setting. He regarded it as likely that there are intermediate groups which span the gap between paranoia and dementia praecox. He left the question of a somatic pathology of paranoia open, but concluded that so long as we do not know the fundamental process underlying paranoia, we cannot know whether it is a unitary disease; delusions of grandeur and delusions of persecution may be essentially different diseases: alternatively a number of hallucinatory forms which Kraepelin did not include in paranoia may be identical with the common forms of the disorder.

KRETSCHMER

So long as the delimitation of any mental disease was taken to depend on clinical pattern, course and outcome, Kraepelin's formulation of paranoia stood firm, but when psychopathology (as part of aetiology) was included in the criteria, some awkward readjustments had to be made. The chief exponent of this necessity was Kretschmer. His monograph on *Sensitiver Beziehungswahn* took account of the views of some predecessors, particularly Birnbaum who described *wahnhafte Einbildungen bei Degenerierten* (1908); Friedmann who reported cases of 'mild paranoia' (1905); and Gaupp with his 'abortive paranoia'.

These men put forward evidence in support of their view that a favourable outcome was possible in some forms of paranoia, and that it was in part a psychogenic disorder occurring in people of psychopathic personality (then called 'degenerate'). Kretschmer juxtaposed these conditions with his *Sensitiver Beziehungswahn*, and in detailed review sustained the thesis that there is no disease to be called 'paranoia': 'Dann haben wir die Lösung des Paranoiaproblems fertig, wenn wir klar zugestanden haben, dass es Paranoiker, aber keine Paranoia gibt.' He recognized three types: *Kampfparanoiker*, *Gewissensparanoiker*, and *Wunschparanoiker*, with overlapping clinical features but differing aetiology. It is hardly possible to give in brief summary the complicated reasoning with which Kretschmer explained and defended his position. It is noteworthy that in spite of the apparently irreconcilable views separating the Kraepelinian from the Kretschmer concepts, Johannes Lange, Kraepelin's pupil and closest associate, was content to say that Kraepelin's paranoia was extremely rare and that it sometimes arose on the basis of a mild schizophrenic defect or schizoid character: or even became evident in the lingering phases of a manic-depressive psychosis. Lange dealt with paranoia broadly as an abnormal reaction, in some respects similar to hysteria. There was very little to choose between Lange's standpoint and Kretschmer's, or indeed even Eugen Bleuler's.

Important observations and hypotheses were put forward by Gaupp and by Kolle. Gaupp over a long period (1914-1939) published his findings on the psychopathology of the mass-murderer Wagner, whom he studied with extraordinary thoroughness, and reviewed other examples and aspects of paranoiac personality. Kolle (1931) analysed a relatively large number of patients with this diagnosis (including those recognized by Kraepelin in the Munich clinic) and came to the conclusion on many grounds that what had been called paranoia was really a rare form of schizophrenia; to add to the semantic confusion he renamed it paraphrenia—the term used by Kraepelin to denote an intermediate group lying between paranoia and dementia paranoides—and as an alternative title brought back Snell's term *primäre Verrücktheit*.

Jaspers' distinction between 'process' and 'personality development' (*Entwicklung einer*

Persönlichkeit) had an obvious relevance for the nosological status of paranoia, just as 'disease' and 'symptom complex' had for the previous generation. Most of the theoretical moves that sometimes enlivened and sometimes desiccated German psychiatry affected the prevalent concept of paranoia, so that it is a recurring theme illustrating or complicating contentious issues. Its shadowy, fluttering existence qualified it for use in darkening counsel.

FRENCH VIEWS

While there was this intense concern with the 'paranoia question' in Germany, a parallel but independent line of development was taking shape in France. It began with Esquirol (1838) who delimited monomania as a *délire partiel*, a chronic affection in which there is some impairment of intelligence, affections, and volition, with one or very few delusional objects, no impairment of logical reasoning, and no abnormal general behaviour. He described several varieties: *folie raisonnante*, homicidal monomania, an erotic form, and impulsive forms—for example, pyromania—which comprehended obsessional acts. Obviously monomania was a heterogeneous class.

In 1852 Lasègue collected all the cases in which delusions of persecution were paramount, and insisted on the frequency and significance of auditory hallucinations in the syndrome. Bearing in mind Morel's views about 'degeneration' he emphasized that in these patients the disorder was 'autre chose que l'exagération d'une tendance naturelle ... c'est un élément pathologique nouveau introduit dans l'organisme moral'. Then Falret (1878) attributed to the disorder a series of phases: incubation (few symptoms or indications); hallucinations of hearing and systematized ideas of persecution; hallucinations of smell and stereotyped delusions; *délire ambitieux* (ideas of grandeur). He held that this last megalomanic stage (on which his contemporary Foville had written a monograph) occurred in only about a third of the patients. Like Lasègue he described the *persécuteurs persécutés* who, as *Querulanten*, had figured largely in the German literature. Falret's views were the subject of very lively debate in the French psychiatric world, and in particular the

clearly expressed and firm proposals of Magnan were to the fore. Magnan (1893) had it in common with Kraepelin that he put great nosological weight on course and outcome. He was acquainted with German writings on the subject; he noted that *Verrücktheit* connoted delusions and hallucinations, and that it corresponded to the French *délire chronique* or monomania (though he thought the Germans at fault in not distinguishing between the *dégénerations* and what Magnan called *délire chronique à évolution systématisée*. He postulated stages: incubation; persecution; grandeur; and then dementia. A sharp distinction was made between this progressive systematized disorder and delusional states which lacked coherent organization or were transitory. He correlated his own scheme with Schüle's (1894) and with Krafft Ebing's (1888). He recognized, however, the pitfalls and difficulties that lay in assuming equivalence of diagnostic terms and, though aware of the growing German preference for the term 'paranoia', he showed no disposition to adopt it instead of his *délire chronique*, nor have French psychiatrists collectively taken to 'paranoia' as a good designation. Exceptions in this respect are Séglas, Génil-Perrin, and Jacques Lacan.

Séglas (1895) defined paranoia as 'un état psychopathique fonctionel, caractérisé par une déviation particulière des fonctions intellectuelles les plus élevées, n'impliquant ni une décadence profonde ni un désordre général, s'accompagnant presque toujours d'idées délirantes plus ou moins systematisées et permanentes, avec hallucinations fréquentes'. He held that it is doubtful whether secondary paranoia occurs: and, in common with almost every contributor to the elucidation of what the term 'paranoia' stands for, he utters a heartfelt protest: 'cette question de délimitation, déjà difficile au point de vue clinique, est d'une étude encore singulièrement embrouillée par l'emploi des dénominations usitées très nombreuses et souvent employées dans des sens différents.' His own discussion of the clinical features of acute paranoia illustrates his complaint.

Among the obstacles to any faithful conversion of the French terms for paranoia into English, pride of place must be given to *délire*. It is the key word in all French discussion of the chronic systematized delusional state, and indeed in all

French discussions of the principles of classification. Henri Ey faces the discrepancy, but complacently rejoices in the French idiosyncrasy on this point. 'Pour nous, psychiatres de langue francaise, . . . il est facile de saisir la continuité des divers degrés des états "délirants" car nous n'avons qu'un mot . . . pour désigner l'idée délirante, le thème délirant, le délire aigu ou le délire alcoolique. Par contre, dans les pays de langue allemande (Wahn et Delirium) ou de langue anglaise (Delusion and Delirium) la tradition (plus que la science) a introduit une sorte de séparation "contre nature" qui a faussé completement le problème.'

To trace the fluctuations of usage and concept in French studies of paranoia at the hands of Sérieux and Capgras, Ballet, de Clérambault, Régis, Ey, and Lacan would be a rewarding exercise, but it would lead too far from the theme of this article, the vicissitudes of the word 'paranoia'—a word never heartily welcomed in France. Italy was more receptive, and from 1882 the term was widely used following the powerful example of Morselli, Tanzi, and Lugaro.

BRITISH PSYCHIATRISTS

British psychiatrists were by no means of one mind about it. Hack Tuke wrote in 1892: 'The use of this word (paranoia) has become very frequent in Germany and in the United States, but it has not obtained favour in Great Britain. . . . The Greek etymology does not render us any assistance in the endeavour to comprehend the particular class of case to which it is applied. It is regarded as synonymous with that very favourite word of the German alienists "Verrücktheit", in respect of which there has been so much difference of opinion and so much change since the time of Griesinger to the present day that a lamentable amount of confusion and obscurity has been introduced into the nomenclature of mental alienation.' Maudsley at about the same time (1895) wrote, rather petulantly, that the systematic insanities 'used to be described under the name of Monomania or Partial Mania; but as these names were thought to limit the area of disorder too strictly, the tendency now is to abandon them in favour of a still worse-conceived name—Paranoia—which means properly nothing less than general insanity. Because monomania expressed too little, though it marked well an essential feature of the disorder, those who are in love with a new term, without understanding it, and run gladly after a new thing because it is new, would supersede it by a name which marks not any special character of the disease, but really means just what it is not—general madness. To christen it mental derangement would appear plain nonsense: to call it so in Greek passes for scientific nomenclature. Thereupon in accordance with precedent, the invention of the new name is supposed to be the discovery or discrimination of a new disease.' He proposed for the condition the name 'primary systematised mania'.

Conolly Norman did not object to the word and treated it (1899) as an exact synonym for 'systematized delusional insanity': 'The peculiarity which has been called the "systematization of organization of delusions", together with fixity of the morbid idea and usually slow development, forms the characteristic note of paranoia.' His account shows familiarity with the main German and French writings on the subject since the middle of the century.

Clouston (who had used the term without comment in 1890) became ill-disposed towards it (1904), partly because different authors meant different things by it, but partly because, by some undisclosed reasoning, he had evidently come to regard it as obscene. Citing Ludwig of Bavaria as a typical paranoiac, Clouston remarks on his 'sexual perversion of the most abominable kind' and digresses to say that this 'unsavoury subject, i.e. sexual perversion, has been too fully dealt with by German psychiatrists' and that 'the whole subject of paranoia is allied to the "degeneracy" and the "hysteria" which Max Nordau so vividly describes as influencing our present-day literature and art'. In spite, however, of Clouston's and Maudsley's objections, paranoia made its way into British textbooks until a later turn of the wheel reduced the disease-concept to a 'subject of purely historical interest'.

IN THE UNITED STATES

In the United States a less conservative spirit was abroad. Spitzka adopted the term (1883), and from 1901 onwards Adolf Meyer educated

159

American psychiatrists by his erudite and critical reports of relevant studies in Europe, as well as by his own contributions towards defining the concept and reviewing the psychopathology and treatment. He was greatly impressed—'concepts equally suggestive and helpful'—by Freud's explanation of the dynamics of paranoia.

In 1896 Freud had published a contrast between the mechanisms of obsessional neurosis and paranoia, the latter based on his analysis of a woman whom he referred to as suffering from paranoia, though he later recognized that dementia paranoides would have been a more correct diagnosis. In 1911 his lengthy exposition of the Schreber case appeared. The impact of the Schreber analysis has been great and is not diminished by the emendation of Freud's diagnosis which is now generally agreed upon. As Macalpine and Hunter have pointed out, Freud was not at pains to be consistent in the use of diagnostic terms (although he wrote that 'paranoia' should be kept distinct from 'dementia praecox') and there can be no question that Schreber's illness conformed much more to the clinical picture of schizophrenia than to any of the prevailing notions of paranoia. For the limited purpose of this review it does not call for detailed consideration since it did not affect diagnostic practice or clinical delimitation. What it did affect were the more fundamental questions of the relation between paranoid psychoses and the personality of those who developed such an illness: Lacan's monograph is an instance, as was Bleuler's monograph on *Affectivity and Paranoia*, and Kretschmer's on *Beziehungswahn*.

A number of compound words of Greek origin have been used to refer to mental disorder —paraphrenitis, paraphrosyne, parergasia, parafrenesie, paraphrenia; but only the last of these has survived, by the skin of its teeth. Kraepelin applied it to the uncertain group between his 'dementia praecox' and his 'paranoia'; Freud proposed to substitute it for 'dementia praecox' or 'schizophrenia'; and Leonhard calls one of the atypical schizophrenic psychoses *affektvolle Paraphrenia*, equating it with Kleist's *progressive Beziehungspsychose*. It might be a good thing

for psychiatry if coining names for diseases *ad libitum* were made as serious an offence as coining money without authority. Leonhard's justification lay in his painstaking clinical and genetic studies and the continuity of the theoretical position that had originated with Wernicke and been elaborated by Kleist. This resulted in a self-contained parallel nosological system (which included Kleist's 'involutional paranoia').

Although the rarity of paranoia in the strict Kraepelinian form is constantly referred to and confirmed, few if any writers go so far as to deny that it occurs at all. Moreover the interest in pragmatically justified and clinically correct classification of diseases and syndromes has waned—in America because of the preoccupation with psychoanalytic dynamics, in Europe largely because of the concern with existential analysis. It is now common to find intricate expositions of the psychopathology of paranoid states which either by their silence on the matter take it for granted that everybody knows what is a paranoid state, or indicate that they regard all paranoid states as varieties of schizophrenia. There is much looseness in the use of the noun 'paranoia' and the related adjectives 'paranoiac', 'paranoic', and 'paranoid': obviously what is 'paranoid' should be like paranoia, but with a difference: if there is no difference it is paranoiac. 'Paranoiac' as a noun designating the patient who has paranoia has no substantive counterpart, to denote the patient who has a paranoid disorder. The literary and vernacular use of 'paranoid' as meaning 'resentfully distrustful' is as inexact as the corresponding use of 'hysterical'.

Current German (and Swiss) practice is to view paranoid conditions as reactions or 'developments', arising out of a psychopathic constitution subjected to the strains of daily life. Binder, for example, has extended this (1960) to include catathymic delusional formation. Others—for example, Conrad—stress the paranoid-hallucinatory pattern which may develop in the symptomatic psychoses. Weitbrecht, while regarding paranoid psychosis as a personality reaction, maintains the distinction between paranoiacs whose delusions have grown out of overvalued ideas and paranoid schizophrenics whose personality is intact.

French psychiatrists have been strikingly conservative in this linguistic matter. They either advocate dropping the terms 'paranoia' and 'paranoid' altogether, or they adhere to the traditional classification; chronic delusional psychoses are divided into those in which progressive deterioration occurs (paranoid schizophrenia) and the non-progressive forms of which there are three—namely, systematized (paranoia), hallucinatory, and fantastic. Within the systematized chronic delusional psychoses they continue to distinguish on de Clérambault's lines *délire de révendication* (which includes the *querulants*, the cranky inventors, and the ideological extremists), *délire passionel* (jealousy and erotomania), *délire de relation* (*sensitiver Beziehungswahn*) and *délire d'interprétation* (the *folie raisonnante* of Sérieux and Capgras). Along with this evidence of respect for classical French terminology and subdivisions, there is a reluctance to impute causal importance to past or present events and an emphasis on hereditary determinants which derives from another tradition. 'Ces délirants se montrent en effet profondément perturbés dans leur vie instinctive (caractère endogène de l'affection) par les expériences délirantes aiguës (moments féconds) qu'ils presentent, par leurs antécédents héréditaires assez fréquents, ils imposent bien l'idée que le délire n'est chez eux ni réductible à l'action des évènements passés ou actuels, ni à des phénomènes mécaniques cérébraux localisés' (Ey, Bernard, and Brisset, 1960).

CONTEMPORARY BRITISH AND AMERICAN USAGE

British psychiatrists differ a good deal in their use of the term 'paranoid': 'paranoia' is almost entirely given up. At one end of the spectrum it is maintained that paranoid states are not disorders of the same nosological rank as schizophrenia but are to be distributed according to the symptoms and other characteristics of a particular major disorder which may accompany them; at the other end of the spectrum it is held that the terms 'paraphrenia' and 'paranoid schizophrenia' must be discarded, and the distinction between schizophrenia, on the one hand, and the paranoid states on the other must be sharpened. A very recent textbook treats paranoid conditions solely as a variety of schizophrenia, while another textbook includes the paranoid development, as Weitbrecht, Kehrer, Kahn, and other German writers do, among the morbid reactions which may occur in persons of psychopathic constitution (though the authors reject any separation of the paranoid group of psychoses from the main body of schizophrenia). In the main British psychiatrists eschew the term paranoia, seldom use the term 'paraphrenia' and apply the non-committal adjective 'paranoid' to delusions or delusional states in which the false beliefs include ideas of self-reference that cannot be adequately derived from the prevailing morbid mood (as delusions of impending punishment can be derived, for instance, from self-reproachful depression).

Contemporary usage in America seems to avoid a clear demarcation between paranoia, paraphrenia, and paranoid schizophrenia in favour of a continuum which would make classification and definition of these diagnostic terms a rather superfluous exercise. In the most recent and thoughtful American contribution to the topic, Norman Cameron (1967) expresses the opinion that paranoid states 'are, in effect, mild forms of paranoia that are actually static. They often begin as active paranoid reactions, lose their vigour and progression, and leave the person chronically paranoid'. He also puts forward a view commonly held in the United States that 'biological inheritance appears to play no part in the development of paranoid reactions', and therefore it cannot be declared an endogenous disorder.

It would be informative to survey the usage of these terms in many other countries, but it would call for a wider command of languages, and might reveal only minor variations from what has been evident in the countries referred to above. It might also add to existing causes of confusion. There is at least one Scandinavian centre where 'paranoid' is applied to mild forms of the disorder ('in analogy with schizoid'), and 'paranoia' is used for psychotic forms of the disorder.

There are other aspects of the paranoid state which are more or less implied in the subject of this review—*folie à deux*, for example; alcoholic paranoia; amphetamine psychosis; megalomania; senile paraphrenia; and institutionalized paranoia in other cultures, such as among the Dobu of New Guinea whom Fortune studied. But their relevance to the theme of this survey is not direct and close enough to warrant inclusion.

HOW SHOULD 'PARANOID' BE DEFINED?

How, then, is 'paranoid' to be defined so that it has the least subjectivity and the most tenable basis possible (assuming that we should not accept Kretschmer's dictum that definitions prevent us from getting a clear insight into conditions 'die weder logisch noch symptomatisch sondern nur lebendig sind')?

A paranoid syndrome is one in which there are delusions of self-reference which may be concerned with persecution, grandeur, litigation, jealousy, love, envy, hate, honour, or the supernatural (the list is Kolle's) and which cannot be immediately derived from a prevailing morbid mood such as mania or depression. It may be a symptomatic condition, a toxic condition, or a part of a schizophrenic disorder. The adjective 'paranoid' should not be applied to persons, but may be applied to a psychopathic personality characterized by the same features as a paranoid syndrome except that 'dominant ideas' must be substituted for delusions. Unlike 'paranoiac' it is a descriptive term carrying no implications about chronicity, permanence, curability, presence of hallucinations, integrity of personality, or aetiology. 'Paraphrenia' can be comprehended within 'paranoid'. Recognition of a paranoid syndrome is not a diagnostic act but a preliminary to diagnosis, as would be the recognition of a stupor, or depersonalization. The syndrome will eventually be classifiable in one of the major categories of mental disorder.

BIBLIOGRAPHY

Banse, H. (1912). Zur Klinik der Paranoia. *Zentralblatt für die gesamte Neurologie und Psychiatrie*, **11**, 91–109.
Baruk, H. (1959). *Traité de Psychiatrie*. Masson: Paris.
Berner, P. (1965). *Das paranoische Syndrom*. Springer: Berlin.
Binder, H. (1960). Die psychopathischen Dauerzustände und die abnormen seelischen Reaktionen und Entwicklungen. In *Psychiatrie der Gegenwart*, edited by H. Gruhle *et al.* Band 2. Springer: Berlin.
Birnbaum, K. (1908). *Psychosen mit Wahnbildungen und wahnhafte Einbildungen bei Degenerirten*. Marhold: Halle.
Birnbaum, K. (1915). Zur Paranoiafrage. *Zentralblatt für die gesamte Neurologie und Psychiatrie*, **29**, 305–322.

Bleuler, E. (1906). *Affektivität, Suggestibilität, Paranoia*. Marhold: Halle.
Bucknill, J. C., and Tate, D. H. (1874). *A Manual of Psychological Medicine*. Churchill: London.
Cameron, N. A. (1967). Paranoid reactions. In *Comprehensive Textbook of Psychiatry*, edited by A. M. Freedman and H. I. Kaplan. Williams and Wilkins: Baltimore.
Clérambault, G. (1942). *Oeuvre Psychiatrique*. Presses Universitaires: Paris.
Clouston, T. S. (1904). *Clinical Lectures on Mental Diseases*. 3rd edn. Churchill: London.
Cramer, A. (1895). Abgrenzung und Differenzial-Diagnose der Paranoia. *Allgemeine Zeitschrift für Psychiatrie*, **51**, 286–309.
Cramer, A. (1899). *Die Halluzinationen im Muskelsinn*. Mohr: Freiburg.
Cullen, W. (1783–1784). *First Lines of the Practice of Physic*. 4th edn. Bell and Broadfute: Edinburgh.
Du Saulle, H. L. (1871). *Le Délire des Persécutions*. Plon: Paris.
Eisath, G. (1915). Paranoia, Querulantenwahn und Paraphrenie. *Zentralblatt für die gesamte Neurologie und Psychiatrie*, **29**, 12–78.
Ey, H., Bernard, P., and Brisset, C. H. (1960). *Manuel de Psychiatrie*. Masson: Paris.
Esquirol, E. (1838). *Des Maladies Mentales*. Baillière: Paris.
Falret, J. P. (1878). Du délire de persécution chez les aliénés raisonnants. *Annales médico-psychologiques*, **20**, 396–400.
Freud, S. (1958). *The Case of Schreber. Complete Works*, translated under general editorship of J. Strachey. Vol. 12. Hogarth: London.
Friedmann, M. (1905). Beiträge zur Lehre von der Paranoia. *Monatschrift für Psychiatrie*, **17**, 467–484, 512–560.
Gaupp, R. (1920). Der Fall Wagner: eine Katamnese, zugleich ein Beitrag zu der Lehre von der Paranoia, *Zentralblatt für die gesamte Neurologie und Psychiatrie*, **60**, 312–327.
Gaupp, R. (1938). Krankheit und Tod des paranoischen Massenmörders Hauptlehrer Wagner: eine Epikrise. *Zentralblatt für die gesamte Neurologie und Psychiatrie*, **163**, 48–82.
Gaupp, R. (1942). Zur Lehre von der Paranoia. *Zentralblatt für die gesamte Neurologie und Psychiatrie*, **174**, 762–810.
Griesinger, W. (1845). *Pathologie und Therapie der Psychischen Krankheiten*. Braunschweig: Wieden.
Griesinger, W. (1868). Vortrag zur Eröffnung der psychiatrischen Klinik zu Berlin am 2. Mai, 1867. *Arkiv für Psychiatrie und Nervenkrankheiten*, **1**, 143–158.
Guiraud, P. (1950). *Psychiatrie Générale*. Le François: Paris.
Heinroth, J. C. A. (1818). *Lehrbuch der Störungen des Seelenlebens*. Vogel: Leipzig.
Huber, G. (1955). Das Wahnproblem (1939–1954). *Fortschritte der Neurologie, Psychiatrie, und ihre Grenzgebiete*, **23**, 6–58.
Huber, G. (1964). Wahn (1954–1963). *Fortschritte der Neurologie, Psychiatrie, und ihrer Grenzgebiete*, **32**, 429–489.
Johanson, E. (1964). Mild paranoia. *Acta psychiatrica et neurologica Scandinavica*. Suppl. 177, Munksgaard: Copenhagen.
Kahlbaum, K. (1863). Die Gruppirung der psychischen Krankheiten. Kafemann: Danzig.
Kehrer, F. (1928). Paranoische Zustände. In *Handbuch der Geisteskrankheiten*, edited by O. Bumke. Band 6, Springer: Berlin.
Kehrer, F. (1951). Kritische Bemerkungen zum Paranoiaproblem. *Nervenarzt*, **22**, 121–125.
Keyserlingk, H. (1964). Zur Paranoia-Frage. *Schweizer Archiv für Neurologie, Neurochirurgie und Psychiatrie*, **94**, 154–167.

Kleist, K. (1911). Die Streitfrage der akuten Paranoia. *Zentralblatt für die gesamte Neurologie und Psychiatrie*, **5**, 366–387.

Kleist, K. (1913). Die Involutionsparanoia. *Allgemeine Zeitschrift für Psychiatrie*, **70**, 1–134.

Kolle, K. (1931). *Die Primäre Verrücktheit*. Thieme: Leipzig.

Kraepelin, E. (1896), (1899), (1913). *Lehrbuch der Psychiatrie*. 5th edn., Barth: Leipzig; 6th edn., Barth: Leipzig; 8th edn., Barth: Leipzig.

Kraepelin, E. (1894). Die Abgrenzung der Paranoia. *Allgemeine Zeitschrift für Psychiatrie*, **50**, 1080–1081.

Kraepelin, E. (1899). Zur Diagnose und Prognose der Dementia Praecox. *Neurologisches Centralblatt*, **18**, 91–93.

Kraepelin, E. (1912). Uber paranoide Erkrankungen. *Zentralblatt für die gesamte Neurologie und Psychiatrie*, **11**, 617–638.

Krafft-Ebing, R. (1888). *Lehrbuch der Psychiatrie*. Enke: Stuttgart.

Kretschmer, E. (1927). *Der sensitive Beziehungswahn*. 2nd edn., Springer: Berlin.

Kretschmer, E. (1950). Grundsätzliches zur modernen Entwicklung der Paranoialehre. *Nervenarzt*, **21**, 1–2.

Krueger, H. (1917). *Die Paranoia*. Springer: Berlin.

Lacan, J. (1932). *De la Psychose Paranoiaque*. Le François: Paris.

Lange, J. (1924). Uber Paranoia und paranoische Veranlagung. *Zentralblatt für die gesamte Neurologie und Psychiatrie*, **94**, 85–152.

Lange, J. (1926). *Die Paranoiafrage*. Springer: Berlin.

Lanteri-Laura, G. (1966). Délires chroniques de l'adulte. *Encyclopédie de Médecine-Chirurgie*, 37299. Paris.

Leonhard, K. (1960). Die atypischen Psychosen und Kleists Lehre von den endogenen Psychosen. In *Psychiatrie der Gegenwart*, edited by H. Gruhle *et al.* Band 2, Springer: Berlin.

Lasègue, C. E. (1852). Du délire de persécution. *Archives générales de médecine*, **28**, 129–150.

Lüdeman, N. E. (1897). Die Entstehung, Ausbildung und Verlauf der Paranoia. M.D. Thesis. Greifswald, Sell.

Magnan, V. (1893). *Leçons Cliniques sur les Maladies Mentales*. Bureaux de Progrès Médical: Paris.

Maudsley, H. (1895). *Pathology oꞌ Mind*. Macmillan: London.

Mendel, E. (1880). Paranoia. In *Real-Encyclopädie*, edited by A. Eulenburg. Urban and Schwarzenberg: Wien.

Mendel, E. (1884). Uber sekundäre Paranoia. *Archiv für Psychiatrie und Nervenkrankheiten*, 1884, **15**, 289–290.

Mendel, E. (1890). Uber die psychiatrische Nomenclatur 'Verrücktheit' und 'Wahnsinn'. *Allgemeine Zeitschrift für Psychiatrie*, **46**, 531.

Mercklin, A. (1891). Uber die Beziehungen der Zwangsvorstellungen zur Paranoia. *Allgemeine Zeitschrift für Psychiatrie*, **47**, 628–668.

Meyer, A. (1951). *Collected Papers*. Vol. 2: Psychiatry. Johns Hopkins Press: Baltimore.

Neisser, C. (1891). Erörterungen über die Paranoia vom klinischen Standpunkt. *Centralblatt für Nervenheilkunde und Psychiatrie*, **15**, 1–20.

Norman, C. (1899). Systematised delusional insanity. In *System of Medicine*, edited by T. C. Allbutt. Macmillan: London.

Plato. *Laws*, 929.

Plato. *Theaetetus*, 195A.

Sander, W. (1868). Uber eine spezielle Form der primären Verrücktheit. *Archiv für Psychiatrie und Nervenkrankheiten, vereinigt mit Zeitschrift für die gesamte Neurologie und Psychiatrie*, **1**, 387–419.

de Sauvages, B. (1759). *Pathologia Methodica*. Tournes: Leyden.

de Sauvages, B. (1763). *Nosologia Methodica*. Tournes: Amsterdam.

Schneider, H. (1903). Ein Beitrag zur Lehre von der Paranoia. *Allgemeine Zeitschrift für Psychiatrie*, **60**, 65–110.

Schneider, K. (1920). Zur Frage der sensitiven Beziehungswahn. *Zentralblatt für die gesamte Neurologie und Psychiatrie*, **49**, 51–63.

Schnizer. (1914). Zur Paranoiafrage. *Zentralblatt für die gesamte Neurologie und Psychiatrie*, Referate, **8**, 313–365 and 417–440.

Sérieux, P., and Capgras, J. (1909). *Les Folies Raisonnantes*. Alcan: Paris.

Schüle, H. (1894). Zur Paranoia-Frage. *Allgemeine Zeitschrift für Psychiatrie*, **50**, 298–318.

Séglas, J. (1895). *Leçons Cliniques sur les Maladies Mentales*. Asselin and Houzeau: Paris.

Snell, L. (1865). Monomanie als primäre Form der Seelenstörung. *Allgemeine Zeitschrift für Psychiatrie*, **22**, 368–381.

Snell, L. (1890). Die Uberschätzungsideen der Paranoia. *Allgemeine Zeitschrift für Psychiatrie*, **46**, 447–460.

Specht, G. (1901). *Uber den Pathologischen Affekt in der Chronischen Paranoia*. Böhme: Leipzig.

Spitzka, E. C. (1883). *Insanity*. Bermingham: New York.

Tuke, D. H. (1892). *Dictionary of Psychological Medicine*. Churchill: London.

Vogel, R. A. (1772). *Academicae Praelectiones*. Vandenhaeck: Göttingen.

Weitbrecht, H. J. (1963). *Psychiatrie im Grundriss*. Springer: Berlin.

Werner, C. (1891). *Die Paranoia*. Enke: Stuttgart.

Wernicke, C. (1900). *Grundriss der Psychiatrie*. Thieme: Leipzig.

Westphal, C. (1878). Uber die Verrücktheit. *Allgemeine Zeitschrift für Psychiatrie*, **34**, 252–257.

Wigert, V. (1918). Studien über die paranoischen Psychosen. *Zentralblatt für die gesamte Neurologie und Psychiatrie*, **40**, 1–151.

Zeller, A. (1844). In *Bericht über die Wirksamkeit der Heilanstalt Winnenthal, 1840–1843. Allgemeine Zeitschrift für Psychiatrie*, **1**, 39–42.

Zutt, J. (1958). Vom gelebten welthaften Leibe. In *Proceedings 2nd International Congress for Psychiatry, Zurich, 1957*, Vol. 4. Orell Füssli: Zurich.

Psychological factors in human fertility

Aubrey Lewis

At the time when Professor Essen-Möller wrote his masterly thesis on the fertility of the mentally ill, there was much concern in western countries about the general decline in fertility and ways whereby the birth rate could be raised. Now it is recognised all over the world that the opposite problem confronts us in urgent form. Current methods of limiting fertility and the extent to which they are used successfully are therefore of great social importance. Psychological factors play a large part here, yet psychologists and psychiatrists have added little to the sum of knowledge about these determinants of family size: in contrast to the demographic and technological approach, psychological studies have been disproportionately taken up with dubious beliefs and untested speculations. An exception to this is to be found in the study of the relation between intelligence and family size. A brief review of the present state of knowledge and inquiry bearing on psychological factors in family limitation in the general population seems timely. A survey of the differential fertility of the mentally ill would no doubt be a more satisfying exercise, embracing not only Professor Essen-Möller's classical monograph but also the subsequent thorough investigations by Odegaard and by Stevens, but it would point a less arresting moral.

Attitudes so family limitation

In 1960 two very similar inquiries were made in the United States and the United Kingdom. The American inquiry was carried out, by Whelpton and his colleagues, for the University of Michigan and the Scripps Foundation; the English one by Rowntree and Pierce for the Population Investigation Committee. The numbers of families in the sample was large, over 2000 in each study.

The American women were asked whether they were for or against doing something to limit the number of their pregnancies or to control the time when they get pregnant; only five per cent said they were against all methods of fertility control, including the rhythm method.

In the British study the proportion of women who expressed total disapproval in reply to the same questions was higher than in the American study— 14.9%. The reasons given were religious or moral in 42.6%; "birth control is harmful and unnatural", 28.2%; "love of children", 16.6%. The older women tended to disapprove more, and on somewhat different grounds; whereas 31% of those married before 1929 disapproved of birth control because of their "love of children", only 9% of the women married in the nineteenforties disapproved on this ground. Moreover of the younger women half of those who said they disapproved nevertheless used some method of birth control. It is evident that stated attitude is not a clear indication of practice.

These and other studies in various countries raise two main questions: is there everywhere an increasing readiness to approve and use birth control? and what psychological factors are at work behind the façade of commonsense reasons for approving or disapproving?

As to a change in attitude, even before the advent of the "pill" this was evident, but now more so. Not only have an increasing number of developing countries officially adopted birth control programmes, but the opposition expected from the population of these countries has not been found: attitude studies pointed either towards ready acceptance or neutrality and passivity in individuals. The National Academy of Sciences Report (1963) put it strongly: "almost every survey on attitudes towards family planning, from urban areas in the United States to villages in India, shows that a large proportion of people say they are favourable to the idea of limiting family size, especially after the third or fourth child". But these statements cannot be taken entirely at face value: e.g. in Israel surveys of women in hospital for a confinement seemed to show that about 70% of those born in Israel, Europe or America had considered how many children they wanted, but only 18% of those born in Asia or Africa said they had given thought to the matter: but of all those who said they had never thought about it, more than a quarter said they had nevertheless practised contraception of one form or another.

Rational socio-economic considerations cannot be the sole causes for people's contraceptive behaviour.

A little light is thrown on the less overt factors by workers in Seattle. They studied seventy-two women who were taking Norethynodrel, and their husbands. The women all had strong conscious motives for controlling the size of their family. They were given psychological tests which measure different aspects of personality: they were then followed up at three monthly intervals, at which it was ascertained whether they had forgotten to take their pills. It emerged that the women who occasionally forgot to take the pills were impulsive, immature, and prone to shun responsibility: their husbands were like them in being domineering and fond of the limelight, but contrasted to them in that they were confident and independent; they were sexually in conflict with their wives. The authors of the paper surmise that forgetting the pill is a covert act of revenge against the husband. But the evidence is meagre and contradictory. In the elaborate Indianapolis study of social and psychological factors affecting fertility, no relation was found between marital harmony or discord and effectiveness of family planning; and only a very slight association between successful family planning and the wife's personality. Planning, however, was most successful when responsibility for deciding whether to have another child was regarded as falling on both partners: when each spouse said it was the other's responsibility, the chances of unwanted pregnancy were increased.

Another American investigator found, in a sample of 94 urban working class women, that compatibility in sexual intercourse was closely connected with the attitude to family planning: "a lack of mutuality in the sexual expressions of husband and wife results in long-delayed use of contraception".

Reluctance to use any contraceptive method may arise as a carry-over from attitudes to limitation by abortion and to prophylaxis against venereal disease by the condom, as in Jamaica.

Coitus interruptus is still—or was until recently—a widely used contraceptive method, frowned on because of its supposed harmful effect upon mental health. For this widespread belief Freud seems to have been largely responsible, though it did not originate with him: Preyer had published a monograph on it, with which Freud was acquainted. Freud wrote, in a private document in 1893, that both men and women would develop neurasthenia if they used contraceptive measures—the condom, extravaginal coitus, and coitus interruptus: and of these he declared "coitus interruptus is found to be the most severe, and produces its characteristic effects even in non-predisposed subjects". He added that no contraceptive measures are innocuous to women. Similarly he held coitus interruptus to be the cause also of anxiety neurosis. The problem, he said, is to find an innocuous contraceptive method, but failing this, society is doomed to fall victim to incurable neuroses "which reduce the enjoyment of life to a minimum, destroy the marital relation and bring hereditary ruin on the whole coming generation". He maintained that sexual intercourse with incomplete gratification deflected sexual tension from the psychological field and so provoked anxiety neurosis. Twenty years later he still propounded this explanation of the dangers of coitus interruptus: "practised as a customary sexual regime, it is regularly the cause of anxiety neurosis in men, and even more so in women". However, in 1926 he wrote that he had discarded the hypothesis of the direct transformation of suppressed libido into anxiety. Psychiatrists generally now regard coitus interruptus as a comparatively harmless (though of course contraceptively risky) procedure which may provoke irritation and tension though these do not, in themselves, lead to a neurotic illness. People who are already over-anxious, tense or neurotic may of course use this method but there are countless mentally healthy people who have also used it without detectable ill effects.

It is commonly alleged that the psychological effect of adopting a child is often to make a hitherto sterile woman conceive. The evidence in support of this is mainly anecdotal. However in a study of 256 women who adopted a child because they had not been able to have one of their own, it was found that in the ensuing nine to twelve years 14% of them had subsequently had a natural child, at an average period of three and a half years after the adoption. A third of those who conceived did so five or more years after the adoption. Moreover many of those who conceived had adopted a child because they had multiple miscarriages or stillbirths. No psychological differences could be detected between those women who had later conceived and borne a live child and the others who had remained infertile. It would obviously be desirable to take a suitable group of infertile women, matched with the adopters for age, social circumstances, and duration of infertility, and determine what proportion of them had conceived during the ensuing nine to twelve years, but this has been so far impossible for technical reasons. Anyway, post-adoption conceptions do not at present throw light on the psycho-genesis of infertility.

Another common but mistaken belief is that female frigidity makes conception much less likely to occur: the evidence to the contrary is pretty conclusive.

The effect of emotional states upon the process of ovulation and conception has been much discussed. Aristotle started this hare, in his de Generatione Animalium. The chief theme has been the action of unconscious drives and conflicts, upsetting the physiological cycle. A prolific and influential writer on this subject postulates that in patients whom she had psychoanalysed, conception was prevented because during coitus the woman's maternally passive tendencies were at odds with her aggressive tendencies, interfering with orgasm: "correct insight into the processes of the sexual act helps us to understand many a case of sterility caused by a psychogenic difficulty of conception". This approach to the psychopathology of sterility is linked to a classification of the types of personality supposedly prone to interference with conception because of unconscious fear, guilt, or aggression. The psychoanalyst describes five such types: immature women prone to pregnancy fantasies at puberty, so that they vomit and have disturbances of diet etc.; women who are overmaternal towards their husbands, or who give all their time and thought to the pursuit of some career or ideology; aggressively independent women who are reluctant to admit their feminity; and women who are emotionally disturbed. Confidence in this comprehensive typology is reduced when we are told that some of the types described are also closely associated with "overfertility": "numerous cases (occur) of quasi-compulsive readiness for fecundation... women whose fertility defies every attempt to reduce it... their entire emotional interest is devoted to their struggle against their fertility... sterility and excessive fertility stem from identical sources and merely represent two faces of a psychic Janus".

An intensive longitudinal study made on concurrent endocrinological and psychoanalytic lines was reported to show that "adaptive regression", a passive, receptive, narcissistic state, characterized the emotional aspects of the progesterone phase. This finds expression in repetition of the "developmental relation to the mother"—identification with her and fears and hopes of outgrowing her. The ensuing conflict could be severe. However, the investigators recognised that severe conflicts about childbearing could exist without recognisably affecting the process of ovulation or fertility.

Another joint endocrinological and psychological inquiry in women prone to spontaneous abortion reported that 44% of them had an immature personality, another 44% had obsessional tendencies, and the rest were mostly unstable and neurotic. Emotional crises were accompanied by a fall in urinary chorionic gonadotrophin and oestrogens.

These reports are clearly unsatisfactory. The finding that seems to emerge from them is that many women who seek medical help because they have not been able to produce a child, though no somatic cause for this can be found and their husbands are normal, show unhealthy traits of personality; but whether these can be held partly responsible for causing the failure to conceive is still an open question. So is the role of general and sexual dissension between infertile women and their husbands: in some it may be a cause, in others a consequence. Too little is known about the effect upon the reproductive cycle.

The most revealing comment, so far as the validity of the published findings goes, is in a critical survey of seventy-five relevant papers. It was carried out three years ago with exemplary objectivity by Professor Noyes, an obstetrician and Miss Chapnick, a psychologist. The papers they examined included all the significant material that had appeared in the English language between 1935 and 1963 on the psychological aspects of human fertility, but papers on impotence and amenorrhoea were not included. The analysis showed "enough variety to support almost any preconceived opinion". The writers of these papers had nearly all assumed that psychogenesis could be safely inferred wherever existing methods of examination showed no physical cause for infertility. Far-fetched psychosomatic guesses (e.g. that a strong unsatisfied desire for a child may cause the ovaries to discharge unripe ova) still "haunt the literature". The evidence presented in the papers reviewed by Noyes and Chapnick was, as they show, scanty and poorly analysed, and no adequate grounds were adduced for concluding that a specific psychological factor can alter fertility, although no less than fifty different psychological factors emerged from the 75 reports. Nobody had made a prospective study. On the other hand, undisputed examples of the influence of emotion upon menstruation and other reproductive functions justify and indeed demand further inquiry, through welldesigned experiments, into the possible relation between emotion and infertility via hypothalamus, pituitary and ovaries.

Intelligence

Much attention has been paid to the relationship between intelligence and size of family. Most investigators have found that there is a negative correlation between children's measured intelligence and the number of their siblings. It has been inferred that this must lead to a fall in the intellectual level of the total population. No such fall, however, has been demonstrated. Various explanations have been put forward for the paradox.

The first point is the negative correlation. Most of the available studies deal with the children's I.Q.; but obviously it is more relevant to determine the relationship between the parents' I.Q. and the number of their children. In the few investigations which have done this, significant negative correlations have not been found. In the Princeton study of 145 engaged couples who were followed up after 20 years, the correlation between their intelligence-test score at the age of approximately 25 and the eventual number of live births they produced was .24 for women and .27 for men: the correlations showed a slight tendency for the brighter parents to have larger families.

J. W. B. Douglas's continuing inquiry has clearly shown the usual inverse relationship between the mental ability of children and the size of their family. The Scottish Survey likewise found an inverse relation, but emphasized that if data only from the high I.Q. scorers and the low I.Q. scorers were examined, little if any relationship between children's intelligence and family size within each of these sub-groups would be evident (though the high scorers were largely drawn from small families and the low scorers from larger families). Douglas found, rather to his surprise, that the negative correlation was least evident in the children of the younger mothers in his study; but the difference between the older and younger mothers was not great, and as it ran counter to the tendency noted in the Scottish Survey, Douglas refrained from drawing any conclusion on the point. He did, however, bring forward good grounds for supposing that environmental factors, both psychological and material, contribute appreciably to the relatively poor performance of children from large families. This is in contrast to R. A. Fisher's suggestion that genes for intelligence and for infecundity have become associated in the upper social classes: this biological explanation is surely insufficient in itself, though it may play a part in producing the relationship.

The explanation put forward by Douglas as highly probable attributes the inverse relationship to the detrimental effect of economic, psychological, scholastic and nutritional conditions, and the overcrowding which may be the accompaniments of large families, especially when they are poor. He supposes that deficiencies of parental care as well as material shortcomings may make the child from a larger family less able to score well in intelligence tests, even if the family is a professional one. The same general conclusion is arrived at by the Scottish Survey.

A kindred explanation is afforded by the work of Nisbet in Aberdeen. He showed that the correlation between children's intelligence test score and family size was smaller when the tests were non-verbal than when they required verbal skill, and since one of the most important single factors in language development is direct contact with adults (which will be less in large than in small families) it is inferred that the relationship between children's test-score and family size can be partly accounted for as arising from an environmental effect upon verbal ability.

The changes now occurring in the use of contraception because of the "pill" and the spread of contraceptive knowledge, must affect the relationship between size of family and intelligence. Census and other data show changes in the correlation between family size and occupation which are presumably due to wider use of contraceptive planning in all classes and a tendency for the better educated to have the larger families. As Glass put it, "the most striking fact in the recent history of fertility is not the emergence of differentials but the development of a basic homogeneity within Western societies".

There has been much controversy over the implications of the inverse relationship: why has the general level of intelligence not fallen if the larger families are the less intelligent? Penrose urged that genetic equilibrium for the distribution of intelligence is maintained by the greatest fertility of those with near-average intelligence, whereas there is lesser fertility (diminished fitness) at the two extremes. Higgins in Minnesota has put forward an alternative explanation of the paradox. He collected 1016 mothers, 1016 fathers, and their 2039 children, all of them with measured I.Q.s. The mean I.Q. of the parents was significantly lower than the mean I.Q. of the children. However, when corrections were made for the different ages at which people were tested, the average I.Q. of the children fell between the averages of their parents. The correlation coefficient between the family size and the I.Q. of the children was —0.30. The correlation between family size and the I.Q. of the parents was —0.11 for the mothers, —0.08 for the fathers. But when the unmarried or childless siblings of the parents were taken into account, the negative correlation disappeared: the higher reproductive rate of the persons with lower I.Q. is offset by the large proportion of their siblings who have no children, so that the I.Q. level of the whole population remains fairly stable.

References

Anastasi, A.: Intelligence and Family Size. Psychol. Bull. 1956, 53:187—209.

Anastasi, A.: Differentiating Effect of Intelligence. Eugenics Quarterly 1959, 6:84—91.

Bachi, R. and J. Matras: Milbank Mem. Fund Quarterly, 1964, 42: 38—56.

Bajema, C. J.: Natural Selection and Intelligence. Eugenics Quarterly, 1963, 10:175—187.

Bakker, C. B. and C. R. Dightman: Psychol. Factors in Fertility Control. Fertility and Sterility, 1964, 15:559—567.

Benedek, T., G. C. Ham, F. P. Robbins and B. Rubinstein: Psychosom. Med., 1953, 15:485.

Carter, C. O.: Changing Pattern of Differential Fertility. Eugenics Quarterly, 1962. 9:147—150.

Clark, A. L. and P. Wallin: Population Studies, 1964. 18:165—174.

Dandekar, K.: Vasectomy Camps. in Maharasthra. Population Studies. 1963 17:147—154.

Deutsch, H.: The Psychology of Women. Vol. 2 London 1947.

Douglas, J. W. B.: The Home and the School. London 1964.

Eisner, B. G.: Psychological differences between fertile and infertile women. J. Clin. Psychol. 1963, 19:391—395.

Freud, S.: Über die Berechtigung Angst-neurose abzutrennen. Collected papers. London: 1924, Vol. 1.

Freud, S.: The Origins of Psycho-analysis. Letters to W. Fliess 1887—1902. London: 1954, p. 72.

Freud, S.: Hemmung, Symptom und Angst. Vienna 1926.

Glass, D.: Discussion on Fertility. J. Royal Stat. Soc. Series A, 1966, 129:210—215.

Glass, D.: Differential Fertility. Godfrey Thomson Lectures, Edinburgh 1961.

Higgins, J. V., E. W. Reed and S. C. Reed: Intelligence and Family Size. Eugenics Quarterly 1962. 9:84—90.

Kiser, C. and P. K. Whelpton: Social Psychological Factors Affecting Fertility. Summary of chief findings. Milbank Mem. Fund. Quarterly, 1958. 36:282—329.

Lewis-Faning, E.: Family Limitation. London: 1949.

McKeown, T.: Influence of Increased Expectation of Life. Proc. Internat. Congress Human Genetics. Copenhagen 1957, p. 213—226.

MacLeod, A. W.: Fertility and Sterility. 1964. 15:125.

Menninger, K.: Psychiatric Aspects of Contraception. Bull. Menninger Clinic, 1943: 7:36.

Michel, W.: Bull. Fed. Soc. Gynae. Obst. Francais, 1962. 14:666.

National Academy of Sciences. Publ. 1091. The growth of World Population. Washington 1963.

National Academy of Sciences. The growth of U.S. Population. National Research Council, Washington 1965.

Noyes, R. W. and E. M. Chapnick: Literature on Psychology and Infertility. A Critical Analysis. Fertility and Sterility 1964. 15:543—558.

Penrose, L. S.: Problems of Intelligence and Heredity. Edinburgh 1959.

Quensel, C. T. E.: Population Studies 1958. 11:234—250.

Rainwater, L.: And the Poor Get Children. Chicago 1960 (abstracted in Social Abstr. Vol. 8 8515).

Rowntree, G. and R. M. Pierce: Birth Control in Britain, Part i. Population Studies 1961. 15:3—31.

Scottish Mental Survey. London: 1953.

Scott, E. and J. D. Nisbet: Intelligence and Family Size. Eugenics Review 1955, 46: 233—235.

Stycos, J. M.: Milbank Mem. Fund. Quarterly 1958. 36:145.

Swain, M. D. and C. Kiser: Interrelation of Fertility and Ego-centred Interest in Children. Milbank Mem. Fund Quarterly. 1953. 31:51—84.

Weinstein, E. A.: Adoption and Infertility. Amer. Sociol. Rev. 1962. 27:408—412.

Westoff, C. F., E. G. Mischler and E. L. Kelly: Preferences in Size of Family. Amer. J. Sociol. 1957. 62:491—497.

Whelpton, P. K., M. A. Campbell and J. E. Patterson: Fertility and Family Planning in U.S.A. Princeton 1966.

Wittkower, E. D. and A. T. Wilson: Dysmenorrhea and Sterility, Personality Studies. Brit. Med. J. 1940, 2:586.

'Endogenous' and 'exogenous':
a useful dichotomy?

AUBREY LEWIS

From the Institute of Psychiatry, De Crespigny Park, London

SYNOPSIS Within a few years of their introduction into psychiatry in 1893 the terms 'endogenous' and 'exogenous' were widely used. The development of the two words and the semantic uncertainty which surrounded them is traced in this article.

Since they were introduced into botany by Candolle in 1813, the contrasted terms, 'endogenous' and 'exogenous' have been adopted in some other sciences. Their advent into psychiatry was effected in 1893 by P. J. Möbius. He was dissatisfied with the current classification of mental disorders which made a primary distinction on grounds of pathology. 'It is now customary', he wrote, 'to distinguish between organic and functional nervous disorders, in the sense that in the former changes in the affected tissue are visible after death, but not in the latter. This differentiation is useless, because it is to a large extent dependent on the methods of investigation: the pathological findings are always being added to by advances in histology.' On rather different grounds—insufficient data, and lack of demonstrable connection between lesions and disorders of function—Kraepelin (1887) had likewise rejected the pathological differentiation six years earlier. But Kraepelin at the same time weighed ætiological classification in the balance and found it wanting, whereas Möbius made it the cardinal feature of his classification. 'Here for the first time that classification has been carried out which alone can satisfy logical and practical requirements: it is classification by causes. Thereby the whole organization of the material and form of presentation is altered.' Möbius made the primary dichotomy one between endogenous and exogenous conditions, and in defining the terms he recognized the difficulty created by multiple and subsidiary causes.

'We say that a poison is the cause of the disorder when it is the *conditio sine qua non*. . . .' 'Every circumstance that can be harmful to human beings can be a contributory cause. . . . Every disease has its own cause, but all the causes of these diseases can be contributory factors. The doctor's task is first to discover the main cause, secondly to determine the chief subsidiary causes, in order of importance. The main cause is irreplaceable, the subsidiary causes can be substituted for one another; the former works qualitatively, the latter quantitatively. If a main cause is demonstrated which must impinge on the individual from without if the disease is to ensue, them we have an exogenous disease before us. But if there are only quantitative factors, of one sort or another, then the chief factor must be in the individual himself, it must be a predisposition; and we call the disease an endogenous one.'

Möbius insisted that the one indispensable condition for developing an endogenous disorder was a certain innate proclivity: 'if this is present, very varied circumstances can evoke the illness'. His consistent application of these principles led to some strange diagnostic bedfellows: in his list of endogenous disorders Huntington's chorea, progressive muscular dystrophy and myotonia congenita figure alongside hysteria, neurasthenia, migraine, hypochondria, and melancholia.

The terms 'endogenous' and 'exogenous' were quickly incorporated into the daily language of psychiatry in Germany, though rarely with explicit acknowledgment to Möbius, or close adherence to his concepts. In this, Kraepelin

173

was an exception: he credited Möbius with the differentiation, and emphasized the relatively stable and uniform patterns and progression of the exogenous syndromes in contrast with the highly variable and erratic endogenous ones: 'but a strict differentiation is obviously impossible: all possible mixtures can occur in the relationship of internal to external causes. The same external noxa can have a very different impact according to the patient's internal state which is essentially unknown to us.'

Möbius's dichotomy was within a few years so widely used that he felt obliged to complain: 'As far as I know, nobody before me had drawn the distinction between "endogenous" and "exogenous" diseases, but of late (1898) the terms are used freely, as though it were an old story.' The meanings attached to them, however, developed on divergent lines. 'Endogenous' was from the beginning equated with 'hereditary', and, in accordance with prevailing ideas, closely linked to 'degenerative'. The views of Morel (1857) and Magnan (1890) were espoused by prominent German psychiatrists, and degeneration (in the sense of progressive deterioration in successive generations) was declared to be the *conditio sine qua non* for an endogenous disease. This cluster of loosely defined concepts was subscribed to by Möbius; and in spite of criticism, particularly by Rumke, 'degenerative' forms of mental illnesses were confidently designated by leading authorities such as Birnbaum (1909) and Kleist (1921).

EXOGENOUS REACTION TYPES

Application of the term 'exogenous' followed quite different lines. In 1909 Karl Bonhoeffer put forward his conception of exogenous reaction types, as the modes of response by the brain to injury. Since he could not find a direct relationship between a particular trauma or toxin and the mental disorder it occasioned, he postulated intermediate products (*ätiologische Zwischenglieder*) which were formed in the body and were responsible for delirium, twilight and confusional states, hallucinosis, and the Korsakow syndrome. Subsequent controversy regarding the exogenous reaction types turned on the interpretation of 'external', and on the diagnostic significance of responses to external injury

which did not fall into any of the familiar exogenous reaction types. Both these issues were thorny. If, in the first of them, the 'external' injury is taken to be 'external' to the affected person's body, those conditions are excluded which arise within the body—for example, uraemia, exophthalmic goitre—yet the clinical features of this large group of 'symptomatic' psychoses are indistinguishable from the exogenous reaction types described by Bonhoeffer. It would be indefensible to classify them separately: the interpretation of 'external' must therefore be modified. The favoured change is to construe 'external' as 'external to the brain', so that what Kleist called somatogenic disorders remain within the exogenous fold. Although a useful working interpretation, this leaves some ambiguities, as in the case of a mental illness attributable to a cerebral tumour.

WEAKNESS OF 'EITHER/OR' APPROACH

Not so much a semantic as an ætiological problem is the categorization of a syndrome which is in its clinical features (including its course) indistinguishable from an endogenous disorder—for example mania—but has been evoked by an extraneous noxa. Foreseen by Möbius and faced by Bonhoeffer, this problem throws into relief the weakness of a rigid dichotomy, based on an implicit assumption that the (main) cause of a mental illness must be either exogenous or endogenous, when it can be, and often is, both. The patient who presents a typical picture of melancholia in the early stage of his dementia paralytica, or the manic patient with pernicious anaemia illustrates the dilemma. It was the focus of Specht's polemical contribution in 1913.

A further difficulty is presented by the purely psychological noxa: it is extraneous, no doubt, but does not fit into the framework of conventional classification as giving rise to an exogenous reaction type, especially if, like Bumke (1929) we substitute 'organic' for 'exogenous'. Kraepelin (1926) and Weygandt (1902) classified psychogenic disorders as exogenous. More recently, Faergeman holds that 'psychogenic' is the antithesis of 'endogenous'. To cope with the difficulty, Ewald (1948) proposed a trichotomy: exogenous, endogenous, and psychogenic.

While much was said and written about the categorization of exogenous disorders, relatively little was put forward to clarify or modify the concept of endogenous conditions. This had a simple explanation: the external causes which justified the term 'exogenous' were manifest, identifiable, and even measurable; the internal causes of 'endogenous' disorders were hypothetical, intangible, elusive predispositions, constitutional or hereditary forces which could be conjectured but not demonstrated. Pedigrees and genetic studies might justify general statements about the probably endogenous factors in a particular mental disease or syndrome, but (with rare exceptions) nothing valid could be said about the individual patient's intrinsic causes. Johannes Lange (1926) put the point bluntly: 'The fine talk about the endogenous, autochthonous origin of the individual attack only hides our almost complete ignorance.' The nihilistic avowal—made by many others besides Lange—would have been less sweeping if applied to the forms of innate metabolic anomaly associated with mental defect, in the light of present knowledge: but in the period so far considered it justified the proposal to call the group of disorders 'cryptogenic' or 'idiopathic'. Although it was accepted by most authorities that the endogenous concept, though logically requisite, was really a cover for a purely negative approach representing as internal causes what was left when all external causes had been eliminated, a few sought to clothe the concept more substantially by defining endogenous disorders as those in which coarse anatomical changes in the brain were improbable, the intensity of the clinical phenomena varied greatly, the most important mental functions remained intact in spite of lengthy illness, and disappearance of the symptoms would not leave any residual impairment (Aschaffenburg, 1915). The defects of this formula were apparent when it was applied to the much-debated question whether schizophrenia was an endogenous or an exogenous disorder. However it was a lone effort: the consensus was in favour of a frank acknowledgment of ignorance regarding internal 'endogenous' causes, with the consequence that it was difficult or impossible in such cases as 'psychically provoked', 'reactive' depressions to decide whether they are endogenous or not (Lange,

1926). Bonhoeffer's original standpoint remained the only tenable one: 'We cannot be absolutely certain what is endogenous in the final analysis. ... In fact we shall hardly ever be able to deal with pure types of exogenous and endogenous etiology. ... We cannot differentiate sharply and completely between the exogenous clinical features and those we have been calling endogenous.' Sometimes, as Ewald (1948) pointed out, external noxae might evoke a syndrome which nevertheless strongly suggested an endogenous disorder by its clinical characteristics and especially by its following a seemingly preordained course irrespective of whether the precipitating external noxa still operated or not. In such a case the distinction tended to be arbitrary.

BRITISH INTERVENTIONS

So far none but German psychiatrists have been cited. Explicit discussion of the theme was for 30 years practically confined to them. The words 'endogenous' and 'exogenous' did not appear in English psychiatric writings until the late '20s of this century, and then in the context of a review of German contributions. Thus R. D. Gillespie in his lengthy article in 1929 on the clinical differentiation of types of depression, quotes Lange freely and states that 'the tendency, reinforced by Kraepelin's influence, has been to regard the symptoms once they had developed, as endogenous and more or less static'. The word 'endogenous' is used without quotation marks, as though it were self-explanatory, and as though synonymous with 'autonomous'.

Devine, surveying recent advances in 1933, wrote that 'it is clear that the endogenous factor in a psychogenetic psychosis has at least equal importance to the exogenous (psychic trauma), as regards causation'. Henderson in 1936 quotes Lange: 'a pupil of Kraepelin took up the matter in a more determined way but not with any greater success. In addition to the constitutional or endogenous types and the psychogenic depressions he produces the "psychically produced melancholias. . . ." He has sought to make a differentiation where none exists, and his attempt is most superficial and arbitrary.' At various points in his exposition, he dwells, like Devine, on the futility of trying in the individual patient to distinguish sharply between endogenous (or constitutional) and exogenous (psychogenic or environmental) causes. He followed his teacher, Adolf Meyer, in deprecating emphasis on the hereditary nature of affective psychosis, because 'the recognition that the affective disorders are dependent mainly on constitutional or endogenous factors is apt to create a fatalistic attitude and a spirit of therapeutic nihilism'. Ironically, it was an energetic innovation in the treatment of 'functional' psychoses that gave the 'endogenous' classification of depression a new lease of life in countries like England where it had previously had only a tenuous and rather apologetic existence. From this time it was unusual for 'exogenous' to be paired with 'endogenous' as antonym or polar opposite. The commonest linguistic pairs were 'endogenous–reactive', 'endogenous–neurotic', and 'psychotic–exogenous'. They were applied to depression but not to mania or schizophrenia (which were explicitly or tacitly assumed to be always psychotic and therefore to fall outside the area of current argument).

A SEMANTIC DISPUTE

The controversy, so far as British psychiatrists moulded and maintained it, was in part a semantic dispute about the meaning of 'endogenous' (equivalent to 'cryptogenic or 'hereditary'?); 'exogenous' (equivalent to 'psychogenic' or to 'organic'?), and 'psychotic' (fundamentally distinct from 'neurotic' and 'reactive' or an imprecise term for a phase in a continuum?). 'Functional', 'biogenic', 'autonomous', 'idiopathic', and 'reactive' contributed also to the semantic uncertainty. But at bottom the dispute (which could as readily have been about 'anxiety' as about 'depression') turned on discrepant notions regarding the principles and method of psychiatric classification, as well as on assumptions about a necessary association between causes, clinical picture, pathology, course ('natural history'), and response to treatment. In the present decade American writers (Friedman, Cowitz, Cohen, and Granick, 1963; Blinder, 1966; Rosenthal and Gudeman, 1967; Mendels, 1968) have joined in the fray, which has become a lively field of Anglo–American

interest, mostly using statistical methods, as in Kendell's recent monograph (1968).

Since this paper is intended to deal with the terms 'endogenous' and 'exogenous' rather than with the forms and nature of pathological depression, the course of the controversy will not be reviewed nor any attempt made to evaluate the contributions. It is, however, necessary to insist that no use of the words 'endogenous' and 'exogenous' could be regarded as legitimate if it did not denote primarily a causal distinction—which, in the case of depression, carries with it the complexities entailed by multiple causes and meagre knowledge about aetiology in the individual patient. Julien Rouart (1950) and, more recently, Kräupl Taylor and others have examined these complexities, which in turn involve acceptance or rejection of the customary dualist concepts.

While British and American psychiatrists were disputing about the divisibility of depression into an endogenous and a neurotic form, German psychiatrists were taking for granted an endogenous cyclothymic variety, and a reactive or psychogenic variety, and a somatosis in which the depression was the visible accompaniment or product of (hypothetical) bodily changes. Schneider (1932) has been the chief proponent of the last of these, while Kleist (1921) has tried to differentiate further the atypical forms. Some writers, like Ederle (1958), find grounds for discarding the endogenous–exogenous dichotomy. But all rely on theory and argument to clarify the use of the terms, rather than on systematically collected further evidence. This is very plain in the expositions of Tellenbach (1961) and Weitbrecht (1963). Weitbrecht recognizes, as do almost all German authorities, that 'exogenous' and 'endogenous' reaction types are not mutually exclusive as a strict dichotomy would require; and that a definition of 'endogenous depression' by its symptoms, psychopathology, and course, though not formally defensible, is used in the present state of our ignorance, pending fuller knowledge of the genetic or the somatic basis of a distinguishable variety of depression. 'It is customary to relate the substrate of endogenous disorder, however indefinite its nature, closely to inheritability and consequently to the body. ... Admittedly that tells us nothing about the essential nature of "endogeny" because special talents, temperaments, types of reaction, characters, and bodily features can be inherited also.' Tellenbach is more recondite. He postulates an 'Endon' as an additional area of causation, besides Soma and Psyche. He holds that (translation is hardly feasible) 'das Endogene (ist) das Stabile, das vom Fliessen getragene Verweilen im So-sein-müssen, Sich-night-entrinnen können: die vorgegebene Prägung der Individualität, ihr Gefüge. Endogen ist all das am Menschen was sich als Einheit der Grundgestalt im Geschehen immer wieder hervorbeingt, zeitigt, seine Selbigkeit.' The distance between this interpretative exercise and the empirical statistical approach of Anglo–American psychiatrists is obviously great. Some French psychiatrists, who use the term 'constitutional' with a generous width of meaning, describe a 'constitutional melancholia' or 'constitutional neurasthenia' which they are prepared to subsume under 'anxiety neurosis'. Others, like Guiraud (1950), equate 'endogenous' with 'genetic': Guiraud, in fact, substitutes 'genetic' for 'endogenous' and argues that since genes have a physical existence, 'genic' disorders are organic. This ingenious logic does not seem to have led to acceptance of the conclusion. The standpoint of Ey (1954) seems to have become more general: he asserts that it is apropos of melancholia that all the major problems of psychiatry have been generated, and he instances the separability of depressive neurosis and depressive psychosis; he believes a radical distinction between them to be impossible.

ALTERNATIVES AND DIFFICULTIES

It is difficult to examine the meaning and usefulness of the terms 'endogenous' and 'exogenous' without reviewing in detail the concepts they embodied and the contention to which they contributed. There is a respectable body of opinion which is now in favour of dropping the terms altogether, or dropping 'endogenous'. If 'endogenous' is to be retained, it should be openly linked to presumptive evidence of a powerful hereditary factor in causation; and it should be buttressed by conjoined use of the terms 'pathogenic' and 'pathoplastic'. If it is to be dropped because it presupposes knowledge about causation which we do not yet possess, it

might be advantageous to substitute for it a term which refers to the clinical characteristics hitherto meant by those who employ the term— namely, insomnia, severely depressed mood, slowness, guilt, loss of weight, delusions, visceral discomfort, agitation, loss of interest in daily affairs, diurnal fluctuation, well-adjusted premorbid personality, and mental health between attacks (cf. Astrup, Fossum, and Holmboe, 1959; Rosenthal and Gudeman, 1967). For this, Heron's (1965) suggestion might be put into effect—that is, substituting 'primary' for 'endogenous'. But in that case the contrasted or complementary term (to replace 'exogenous') could not be 'secondary' as would be expected. Probably the traditional terms 'psychotic', 'reactive', and 'neurotic' best serve the needs of those who do not mind the difficulties which such distinctions entail for rigorous studies and exact communication.

BIBLIOGRAPHY

Aschaffenburg, G. (1915). Die Einteilung der Psychosen, in *Handbuch der Psychiatrie.* Leipzig.
Astrup, C., Fossum, A., and Holmboe, F. (1959). A follow-up study of 270 patients. *Acta Psychiatrica Scandinavica,* Suppl. 135, **34**, 1–62.
Birnbaum, K. (1909). Zur Lehre von den degenerativen Wahnbildungen. *Allgemaine Zeitschrift für Psychiatrie,* **66**, 19–41.
Blinder, M. G. (1966). The pragmatic classification of depression. *American Journal of Psychiatry,* **123**, 259–269.
Bonhoeffer, K. (1909). Zur Frage der exogenen Psychosen. *Zentralblatt für die gesamte Neurologie und Psychiatrie,* **20**, 499.
Bonhoeffer, K. (1917). Die exogenen Reaktionstypen. *Archiv für Psychiatrie und Nervenkrankheiter,* **58**, 58.
Bumke, O. (1929). *Lehrbuch der Geisteskrankheiten.* Bergmann: München.
Devine, H. (1933). *Recent Advances in Psychiatry.* Churchill: London.
Ederle, W. (1958). Über exogene und endogene Symptomatik bei Psychosen, in *Mehrdimensionale Diagnostik und Therapie.* Thieme: Stuttgart.
Ewald, G. (1948). *Lehrbuch der Neurologie und Psychiatrie.* Urban und Schwarzenberg: Berlin.
Ey, H. (1954). *Étude Psychiatrique.* Tome 3. Desclée de Brouwer: Paris.
Friedman, A. S., Cowitz, B., Cohen, H. W., and Granick, S. (1963). Syndromes and themes of psychotic depression. A factor analysis. *Archives of General Psychiatry,* **9**, 504–509.
Gillespie, R. D. (1929). The clinical differentiation of types of depression. *Guy's Hospital Reports,* **79**, 306–344.
Guiraud, P. (1950). *Psychiatrie Générale.* Le François: Paris.
Henderson, D. K. (1936). The affective reaction type, in *Psychiatry for Practitioners.* Edited by H. A. Christian. Oxford University Press: London.
Heron, M. J. (1965). A note on the concept endogenous-exogenous. *British Journal of Medical Psychology,* **38**, 241–245.

Kendell, R. E. (1968). *The Classification of Depressive Illnesses*. Oxford University Press: London.

Kleist, K. (1921). Autochthone Degenerationspsychosen. *Zentralblatt für die gesamte Neurologie und Psychiatrie*, **69**, 1.

Kraepelin, E. (1887). *Psychiatrie*. Abel: Leipzig.

Kraepelin, E. (1896). *Psychiatrie*. Barth: Leipzig.

Kraepelin, E. (1910). *Psychiatrie*, Vol. 2. Barth: Leipzig.

Lange, J. (1926). Über Melancholie. *Zentralblatt für die gesamte Neurologie und Psychiatrie*, **101**, 293–319.

Magnan, V. (1890). *Leçons cliniques sur les Maladies Mentales*. Lecrosnier: Paris.

Mendels, J. (1968). Depression: the distinction between syndrome and symptom. *British Journal of Psychiatry*, **114**, 1549–1554.

Mendels, J., and Cochrane, C. (1968). The nosology of depression: the endogenous–reactive concept. *American Journal of Psychiatry*, **124**, 1–11 (Suppl.).

Möebius, P. J. (1893). *Abriss der Lehre der Nervenkrankheiten*. Abel: Leipzig.

Morel, B. A. (1857). *Traité des Dégénérescences Physiques, Intellectuelles et Morales de l'éspèce Humaine*. Baillière: Paris.

Rosenthal, S. H., and Gudeman, J. E. (1967). The endogenous depressive pattern. An empirical investigation. *Archives of General Psychiatry*, **16**, 241–249.

Rouart, J. (1950). Y a-t-il des maladies mentales d'origine psychique? in *Le Problème de la Psychogenèse des Névroses et des Psychoses*. Desclée de Brouwer: Paris.

Schneider, K. (1932). Über Depressionszustände. *Zentralblatt für die gesamte Neurologie und Psychiatrie*, **138**, 584–589.

Specht, G. (1913). Zur Frage der Exogenen Schädigungstypen. *Zentralblatt gesamte für die Neurologie und Psychiatrie*, **19**, 104

Tellenbach, H. (1961). *Melancholie*. Springer: Berlin.

Weitbrecht, H. J. (1963). *Psychiatrie im Grundriss*. Springer: Berlin.

Weygandt, W. (1902). *Atlas und Grundriss der Psychiatrie*. Lehmann: München.

178

16

AN INDICTMENT OF AUTONOMOUS MAN—SIR AUBREY LEWIS ON THE IDEAS OF B. F. SKINNER

Utopias are broadly of three kinds—descriptions of an ideal state, satires and working models. Professor Skinner is concerned with the last of these. In 1948 he wrote *Walden Two*, a design for community living cast in the form of a novel. He intended it to be a feasible design and, as he wrote 20 years later:

I receive a steady trickle of letters from people who have read *Walden Two*, want to know whether such a community has ever been established, and if so how they can join. At one time I seriously considered an actual experiment. It could be one of the most dramatic adventures in the 20th century. It needs a younger man, however, and I am unwilling to give up the opportunity to do other things which in the long run may well advance the principles of *Walden Two* more rapidly.

Professor Skinner called *Walden Two* his *New Atlantis* ('I have followed Bacon in organising my data') and thenceforward wrote with increasing conviction on the need for fuller knowledge of how to control human behaviour. *Beyond Freedom and Dignity* is the latest statement of his position. He has been bitterly attacked on the grounds that he is in conflict with Western democratic ideas and belittles the role of the individual: to which he rejoins that he accepts the end of a democratic philosophy but disagrees with the means most commonly employed to attain them. 'I believe that man must now plan his own future and that he must take every advantage of a science of behaviour in solving the problems which will necessarily arise. The great danger is not that science will be misused by despots for selfish purposes but that so-called democratic principles will prevent men of good will from using it in their advance towards humane goals. Possibly our only hope of maintaining any given way of life now lies with science, particularly a science of human behaviour and the technology to be derived from it.' Clearly Professor Skinner believes that a workable Utopia is within our reach if we renounce what he calls the pre-scientific traditional views that centre on the autonomous individual rather than on the environment.

Professor Skinner is the most distinguished exponent of Behaviourism in its modern scientific form as a product of strict analysis and experiment. He has no patience with the phrases that conceal our ineptitude in the areas where we are desperately in need of assured development and application. He points to the contrast between the subjective language of those who are concerned with human affairs and the confident, precise language of physics and biology. Centuries of mentalist assumption have led to the rooted notion that there is an autonomous 'inner man' who initiates behaviour. Feelings are rated as causes, not as by-products and accompaniments, and this distinction holds good for evolutionary and other selection:

The contingencies of survival responsible for man's genetic endowment would produce tendencies to act aggressively, not feelings of aggression. We can follow the path taken by physics and biology by turning directly to the relation between behaviour and the environment and neglecting the supposed mediating states of mind. Physics did not advance by looking more closely at the jubilance of a falling body, or biology by looking at the nature of vital spirits, and we do not need to try to discover what personalities, states of mind, feelings, traits of character, plans, purposes, intentions or the other perquisites of autonomous man really are in order to get on with a scientific analysis of behaviour.

This sweeping declaration of war is the prelude to an authoritative review of the broad conclusions to be drawn from experiment. Although Skinner explains and interprets the interaction between environment and operant behaviour, the reader making his first acquaintance with the matter might not realize, from the deceptively simple account he gives, how varied have been the arranged contingencies and how elaborate and detailed the schedules of deprivation or reinforcement.

Professor Skinner is a determinist and he holds that human behaviour is inherently predictable. Genetic influences and modifications of the environment in appropriate ways, rather than the exercise of free will and self-control, are, he maintains, among the most important causal forces involved in man's behaviour. It follows that man is not responsible for his conduct and is not the proper recipient of praise or blame, reward or punishment. In Professor Skinner's scheme of things it is not the individual who is to be credited or discredited, but the environment which has shaped his corresponding conduct. To illustrate this, Professor Skinner takes the age-old struggle of mankind for freedom. Commonly this is attributed to a will to be free, and fulfilment is characterized by a feeling of freedom. Professor Skinner finds this misleading insofar as the 'literature of freedom' assumes that all control of one man by another is bad. (This might be contrasted with Mill's dictum that the only freedom which deserves the name is that of pursuing our own good in our own way, so long as we do not attempt to deprive others of theirs, or impede their efforts to obtain it.) It is unprofitable, in Professor Skinner's view, because it does not take into consideration all the consequences and does not lead to useful distinctions, freeing men from certain sorts of control but not from others. The struggle for freedom is to be analysed in terms of avoidance or escape from an 'aversive' environment: such an environment should make way for other kinds of control which serve desirable ends. This is to go 'beyond freedom', just as giving credit to those features in the environment which deserve respect and admiration is to go 'beyond dignity'. This can be brought about by positive reinforcement, equivalent to a reward.

He then turns to the concept of punishment. In some form, he considers, punishment is ubiquitous. It is designed to remove unwanted behaviour in the expectation that the person punished will be unlikely to behave in the same way again, but its effect will be felt as shame, guilt or a sense of sin. In order to avoid this, neurotic reactions may develop or the affected person may avoid situations in which punished behaviour is likely to occur. There has been a slow and erratic alleviation of aversive features in the environment. Most alternatives to punishment, such as permissiveness or guidance, are at best weak. Effective change is to be brought about by alterations in contingencies of reinforcement. If behaviour can be, or ought to be, controlled, the questions must be insistently asked: who is to devise and exercise the control? What is the end to which the control is to be directed? Clearly this is a question of values. For the Behaviourist the answer lies in positive reinforcement, bringing about good consequences: bad things derive from negative reinforcers. Verbal operants are effective when accompanied by other, specific reinforcers. Causal analysis is then a matter of identifying the controlling contingencies. Much will depend on the individual's repertoire of operant behaviour. But there is also the customary behaviour of whole peoples—their culture—to be taken into account.

\ Culture is the resultant of genetic endowment and natural and social contingencies. Professor Skinner draws the parallel between biological and cultural evolution: the biological is, of course, transmitted by the chromosome gene mechanism, whereas cultural transmission is in the Lamarckian style. The practices that make up a particular culture have been selected by contingencies of survival: indeed, survival is the only value according to which a culture is eventually to be judged. The good of the culture can be worked for by its members according to an explicit design: 'Since a science and a technology of behaviour make for better design they are important 'mutations' in the evolution of a culture; if there is any purpose or direction in the evolution of a culture it has to do with bringing people under the control of more and more of the consequences of their behaviour.'

Professor Skinner is well aware that he exposes himself to violent attack. He quotes prominent writers who call his study a monumental triviality, spinning psychology into a modern version of the Dark Ages; its language, they say, is pedantic jargon and its laboratory apparatus—the Skinner box—a mere contraption; it shows 'innate naivety and intellectual bankruptcy'. He comments mildly that there are signs of emotional instability in those deeply affected by the 'literature of freedom', and he does limited justice to the force of their objections and the risks of undue reliance on the effectiveness of counter-control. On the main issue he makes no concession: 'Man has not evolved as an ethical or moral animal. He has evolved to the point at which he has constructed an ethical or moral culture. He differs from the other animals not in possessing a moral or ethical sense but in having been able to generate a moral or ethical social environment.'

We have ample evidence that putative controllers have to be watched: the more so, as the technology of behaviour control comes to be at their disposal. It is not the good intentions of the controller that should be scrutinized but the contingencies under which he controls. While emphasizing this, Professor Skinner dwells on the risk that the interchange between control and counter-control which is essential to the evolution of a culture may be disturbed by the literature of human rights (such as freedom and dignity) which requires that constructive counter-control should, like control itself, be disguised or minimized:

This could be a lethal cultural mutation. Our culture has produced the science and technology it needs to save itself. It has the wealth needed for effective action. It has, to a considerable extent, a concern for its own future. But if it continues to take freedom or dignity, rather than its own survival, as its principal value, then it is possible that some other culture will make a greater contribution to the future.

In this final chapter Professor Skinner briefly examines some well-known difficulties in the environmentalist position: perception, attention, knowing, thinking (especially abstract thinking), awareness, insight, self-observation, memory, purpose, motivation. He is not a thorough-going environmentalist and gives full weight to man's genetic endowment. He deprecates the kind of environmentalist reform in education, criminology, industry, everyday life and psychotherapy which draws on rich supplies of enthusiasm but is meagrely equipped with knowledge of how the environment works: 'Two hundred years of this kind of environmentalism has very little to show for itself, and for a simple reason. We must know how the environment works before we can change it to change behaviour.' Professor Skinner cites Robert Owen's ill-fated experiment at New Harmony (but would not the history of the Oneida community be an instance pointing in the opposite direction?).

This chapter is an unsparing indictment of 'autonomous' man, the 'homunculus who feels and consequently acts', the man defended by the champions of freedom and dignity. This mythical man's abolition, Professor Skinner insists, has long been overdue. 'Science does not dehumanize man, it dehomunculizes him, and it must do so if it is to prevent the abolition of the human species.' The advantages of behaviourist study of pigeons, rats and other animals, and of transferring some of the findings to human beings, are pointed out. But in regard to peculiarly human behaviour it is the social environment which supplies contingencies of reinforcement, and this is man-made. 'We have no assurance that the environment man has constructed will continue to provide gains which outstrip the losses, but man as we know him, for better or for worse, is what man has made of man.'

It would not be surprising if many readers took this book to be a product of philosophical reflection, traversing some very familiar ground and putting forward provocative speculations unhampered by experience. Such a misconception of the standing and background of a most original and respected psychologist would be due in part, however, to the way in which he writes his books. In 1957 he published two major works. One, on *Verbal Behaviour*, was full of speculation and argument but contained practically no detailed facts. The other, on *Schedules of Reinforcement*, was a massive record (759 pages) of experiments on the pecking behaviour of pigeons, with practically no speculation at all. *Beyond Freedom and Dignity* is an exercise of the same sort as *Verbal Behaviour*. Instead of detailed facts there are observations drawn from everyday life, literature, philosophy and some psychology. There is no reference to Skinner's research into psychopharmacology, programmed instruction (teaching machines), the operant behaviour of psychotic patients, or Project Pigeon (using animals for guided missiles). He has no interest in psychological theories, factor analyses, mathematical models or hypothetico-deduction.

The assault on some of our most dearly prized values such as freedom makes it difficult to consider Skinner's argument dispassion-ately and assess the practicability of his aims and methods. The deter-minants of behaviour in the everyday world may be of an impenetrable complexity, as might be inferred from the language and constructs of an antithetical technique—psychoanalysis. Professor Skinner pleads for the application of scientific principles to social problems: 'The laws of science are descriptions of contingencies of reinforcement.' What seem required are limited, relevant experiments with close safeguards. 'Perhaps we cannot now design a successful culture as a whole, but we can design better practices in a piecemeal fashion. The behavioural processes in the world at large are the same as those in the Utopian community, and practices have the same effects for the same reasons.'

Beyond Freedom and Dignity. By B. F. Skinner. Cape.

'Psychogenic': a word and its mutations

AUBREY LEWIS

From the Institute of Psychiatry, University of London

SYNOPSIS The word 'psychogenic' was introduced into psychiatry in 1894 by Robert Sommer. Many attempts have been made to clarify the concept it denotes and apply it to clinical purposes. These attempts have been bedevilled by unsettled philosophical problems. It is suggested that the word should be decently buried.

The term 'psychogenic' is much used, but seldom defined—its meaning is assumed to be self-evident. It has had a chequered history. It began during the earlier part of the 19th century. Between 1838 and the end of the century 'psychogenesis' was considered to refer either to the origin of mind or to evolutionary development which had been due to the activity of mind in animals and human beings. Tuke in his *Dictionary of Psychological Medicine* (1892) quotes Lloyd Morgan: 'the law of psychogenesis is the elimination of the incongruous in mental development and progress.' With the eclipse of the biological disputes and concepts of which it was partly the expression, this use of the term has become obsolete.

The word was quite independently introduced into psychiatry in 1894 by Robert Sommer, then a privatdocent in Wurzburg. In his book *Diagnostik der Geisteskrankheiten* (Sommer, 1894), published in that year, he wrote:

'With the name "Psychogenesis" (*Psychogenie*) I would single out a definite, practically important group of cases from the huge area comprehended by the collective name Hysteria. ... That the term I have chosen meets every linguistic and scientific requirement I would be inclined to doubt. If anybody finds a better word, it will be welcomed by practitioners and by those theorists for whom language is not just a matter of empty abstract symbols or misleading meanings, but a mode of expression. With the word "psychogenesis" I am trying to draw the proper consequences from the scientific arguments put forward expecially by Möbius and Rieger in Germany concerning the nature of so-called "hysteria", while I also insist that hysteria in its current sense is a wider concept. We are dealing with morbid states (*Krankheitszustände*) which are evoked by ideas (*Vorstellungen*) and can be influenced by ideas.'

Sommer regarded the operative ideas as arising either within the body of the affected person or in his environment

'es entsteht nur meist eine wechselseitige Steigerung zwischen dem psychogenen Individuum und den Aeusserungen seiner Umgebung. . . .' Psychogen in diesem Sinne kann man diejenigen Geisteszustände nennen welche sich κατ' ἐξοχὴν durch das Hervorbringen von äusseren Handlungen, in welchem sich die Geisteszustände ausdrücken, kennzeichnen.'

He stressed the physical factor ('es ist klar dass organisch bedingte Krankheitszustände in dem gleichen Individuum Vorstellungen auslösen können welche ihrerseits auf psychogenem Wege Krankheitszustände bewirken welche das Bild der organischen Erkrankung gewissermassen umhüllen') while making exaggerated suggestibility an indispensable feature of every psychogenic condition ('die pathologische Steigerung der bei jedem normalen Menschen vorhandene Beeinflussbarkeit ist die Grundlage des psychogenen Charakters').

KRAEPELIN

The new coinage was promptly picked up and scrutinized by Kraepelin (Kraepelin, 1896, 1899, 1904, 1910, 1927); successive editions of his textbook draw attention to some of its mutations. In the fifth edition (1896) he admitted the force of Moebius's argument that the decisive Characteristic of hysteria was its translation of ideas into symptoms, but added that he could not accept it unconditionally: 'psychogenesis seems to me peculiar not only to hysteria but to other forms of degenerative insanity as well.' He put the word psychogenesis in inverted commas, as befitted an artefact newcomer. In the next edition (1899) the paragraph was rewritten and 'psychogenesis' does not appear in it. But by 1904, when the seventh edition was published, the term had taken root and Kraepelin, who had previously classified hysteria, along with epilepsy and fear-neurosis, among the general neuroses, now designated them collectively as the 'psychogenic neuroses' which are solely released by affective influences (*lediglich durch gemütliche Einwirkungen ausgelöst werden*). Reverting, however, to the degenerative connotation, he stressed that in the psychogenic neurosis a predisposition, in the form of heightened affective excitability, must be postulated in the affected persons. In the eighth edition (1910) Kraepelin acknowledged that Sommer's definition of the epithet 'psychogenic', though applicable enough to hysteria, was too narrow, judging by current usage: it had established itself as denoting 'caused by psychological factors'. Kraepelin added that some writers talked imprecisely of psychogenic disorders when it was not a question of genuine causation but of release (*Auslösung*) by psychological factors. In the posthumous ninth edition (1927) the emphasis had shifted decisively to the mental constitution of the patients: 'experience has taught us that the chief cause here is almost always to be looked for in the mental predisposition of the patient. . . . The psychogenic disorders are very numerous and varied, in keeping with the variety of the psychological causes.' Among the psychogenic conditions he included neurasthenia, anxiety neurosis, psychogenic depression, induced insanity, prison psychoses, paranoid syndrome in deaf persons, and 'traumatic neuroses'.

Kraepelin's influence was considerable. So prominent a psychiatrist as Eugen Bleuler (Bleuler, 1916) followed his lead: thus Bleuler, in the 1916 edition of his *Lehrbuch*, copied Kraepelin's exposition of the matter closely, even to the extent of adopting some of his ill-advised neologisms for the psychogenic disorders—for example, homilopathy, ponopathy. In later editions, Bleuler developed a more independent approach, paying less attention to the nosological status of hysteria and sorting out the psychogenic symptoms in dementia praecox.

GERMAN CLARIFICATIONS

Two other outstanding German psychiatrists—Karl Birnbaum and Karl Bonhoeffer—sought to clarify the concept of psychogenesis. Birnbaum (Birnbaum, 1923) dealt with it as part of his construct of psychosis (*Aufbau der Psychose*). Psychogenic illnesses in the proper sense of the term, he maintained, are disorders of function whose specific character can be traced back to a mental factor, and in which there may also be special predisposing factors (especially a morbid constitution) which act as auxiliary pathogenic influences. Psychogenic disorders, because of their essential accessibility to psychological forces, are to a large extent fashioned by pathoplastic influences, with consequently numerous and varied forms. Birnbaum admitted, however, that there were great gaps in our understanding of the way psychogenic disorders came about.

Bonhoeffer (1911) devoted an exhaustive review to the question whether there are psychogenic morbid processes and conditions which cannot be attributed to hysteria. Setting aside Sommer's definition of psychogenesis, Bonhoeffer laid it down that psychogenic states were those which are regularly evoked by ideas (*Vorstellungen*) of an emotional sort. Like Birnbaum, Bonhoeffer did not consider it essential that the psychological factor should necessarily continue to mould and sustain the psychotic process. He also explicitly rejected states in which the psychogenic causal factor could only be inferred from analysis of hypothetical unconscious data.

'Ich halte es für richtig, bei der Besprechung mich auf solche Krankheitszustände zu beschränken, bei denen das ätiologische Moment offensichtlich ist und nicht erst auf besonderem, analytischem Wege aus dem Unterbewusstsein in mehr oder weniger hypothetischer Weise erschlossen wird.'

First among the non-hysterical psychogenic conditions he ranked the consequences of a sudden catastrophe affecting many people, as had then recently happened in the earthquake of Messina. The clinical picture had been varied and the only common feature was gross autonomic disturbance. This vasomotor symptom complex after a threat to life was, in Bonhoeffer's view, the only psychogenic condition which could occur in persons who had no psychopathic predisposition (alternatively called 'degenerative constitution'). Phobias and obsessions could be psychogenic, but only very rarely; more common are reactive depressive states of psychogenic origin, which develop in constitutionally melancholic persons and usually clear up when the psychological cause is removed. This reactive syndrome does not necessarily differ from the depressive phase of the manic-depressive psychosis, but characteristically ideas related to the psychogenic factor are predominant in its content. Reactive manic excitement is very much rarer.

Next Bonhoeffer included in his non-hysterical psychogenic disorders paranoiac processes developed on a basis of overvalued ideas; he called them processes because of the progressive delusional state, and psychogenic because they rest on affective situations and experiences of a harmful kind. Here, also, however, a psychopathic constitution of an appropriate type is necessarily the accomplice of the psychogenic factor. Reactions to imprisonment and pensionable injury likewise require a 'degenerate' personality to attain their morbid strength. Epileptic disorders of behaviour are ranked as a psychogenic condition, and 'affect epilepsy' is emphatically included because 'there are always external factors of a psychological nature which release the attacks'. Bonhoeffer describes still other states—for example, explosive excitement, fugue—which are, in his use of the concept, psychogenic. Some of them are very similar in clinical form to melancholic or catatonic 'endogenous' disorders from which they can be distinguished by their affective provocation. the dependence of their course upon the continuance or otherwise of the causal psychological factors, and, in some, the admixture of Ganser features.

Bonhoeffer, one of the most influential of German psychiatrists, did not restrict the psychogenic disorders to those which seemed to be chiefly and indispensably caused by an upsetting experience, or series of experiences. He recognized the equally—or more—important part played in the aetiology by unhealthy personality, and he stressed the relation of the course of the illness to the persistence of the noxious psychological agent. The ostensible agent must be such as could be held responsible, on understandable grounds, for an affective unheaval; but, at about the same time, a compromise between this common-sense view and a rather more subtle approach to affective underground influences was offered in the catathymic concept of psychogenesis put forward by H. W. Maier (Maier, 1912), Bleuler's colleague and successor. He recognized that an apparently trifling event might evoke a major disturbance because previous psychological damage, probably no longer within the patient's conscious recollection, had sensitized him.

From that time the leaders of German psychiatry seemed mostly content to use the concept of psychogenesis imprecisely and without regard to the pan-psychogenic formulations of psychoanalysis. Gruhle (1927) stressed the role of motives which by empathy could be understood as causes of psychosis or morbid reaction. Braun (1928) defined the psychogenic reaction as the result of reciprocal interplay between specific disposition to a particular kind of disorder and a psychological experience which evokes or causes the disorder. Even Jaspers (1948) fought shy of defining the term or stating its exact relation to 'hysteria': but he extended and analysed the general concept and clarified the criteria of a psychogenic reaction (or reactive psychosis). As elsewhere in his exposition. he distinguished emphatically between understandable relations and genuinely causal relations. His list of psychogenically operative troubles includes senile changes, prolonged imprisonment, collapse of comforting illusions, and restrictions through poverty and despair. A contemporary view (Binder, 1960) traverses the same ground: predisposition and poorly integrated personality play a pathoplastic part in the aetiology of psychogenic disorders, while the environmental noxa or noxae are pathogenic factors.

The meaning attached to the term 'psychogenesis' by German authorities deserves chief attention since it was German psychiatrists who invented the word and have since devoted much

187

critical attention to it. In other countries it had a more belated career, and initially was discussed only by writers who had met it in the German literature. First among these was the Geneva psychiatrist, Theodore Flournoy (Flournoy, 1900). In 1900 he published his dramatic study, *Des Indes a la Planéte Mars*, and in it he several times wrote the word 'psychogènèse' without inverted commas, as though it were in current use. Evidently he employed it in two senses: to name a normal psychological phenomenon, and as designation of the mode of origin of a medium's spirit 'guide' ('aussi peut on distinguer trois phases dans la psychogenèse du guide de Mlle Smith'.)

ANGLO–SAXON VIEWS

The word took longer to reach English-speaking countries. It was not until the late 1920s that it gained currency unobtrusively, almost always in a review of the German concept it denoted, and with special reference to Kraepelin, Lange, Bleuler, or Birnbaum. Bernard Hart (Hart, 1929) used it without comment on its meaning in 1929, and by 1933 it was fairly established, so far as British usage went—but still undefined. In the United States psychiatrists of European origin and schooling adopted the term with full awareness of its German history but with some reluctance to restrict its meaning as much as Kraepelin did. In this August Hoch and Adolf Meyer were dominant influences. Hoch wrote in 1907 a paper on 'The psychogenic factors in the development of psychoses', and he could safely refer in 1910 to 'disorders such as hysteria, certain simple paranoid states and some psychoses of degenerates—that is, conditions in which the psychogenic nature of the symptoms is now scarcely questioned by anyone'. The applicability of the term to psychotic conditions of uncertain aetiology was much canvassed at this time, as in Adolf Meyer's paper on the role of the mental factors in psychiatry, in which he says we have 'in Lady Macbeth's dream states a marvellous picture of a psychosis of the type which just begins to play a more prominent part in psychopathology—the psychogenetic disorders' (Meyer, 1908). In this context Meyer drew attention to the way Bleuler (and to some extent Jung) interpreted certain of the symptoms of

dementia praecox as secondary and psychogenic. Morton Prince (Prince, 1915) referred to 'the antecedent psychogenetic factors which led to the development of particular ideas and complexes'. A more explicit definition (much indebted to Kraepelin) was put forward by MacCurdy in 1925:

'Psychogenic disorders are those in which the symptoms appear as psychological reactions to mental events. The symptoms may be the direct expression of the mental causes or they may represent them indirectly through the mediation of morbid psychological processes—the diseased personality.'

THE LAST 30 YEARS

ORTHODOX

During the last 30 years three main approaches may be discerned (apart from the psychoanalytic) 'orthodox', 'nihilist', and 'catholic'. The orthodox has the German imprint: it is well represented by the Danish psychiatrist Strömgren (1958), who wrote: 'Unter psychogenen Psychosen verstehen wir Krankheiten, für deren Entstehung ein Konflikt oder ein Trauma seelischer Natur die wichtigste Voraussetzung ist.' Three forms are described—the emotional; the paranoid; and the confusional, which affects object consciousness. Since Wimmer published his exhaustive review Scandinavian psychiatrists have taken a special interest in the problem. Faergeman's (1963) monograph has indicated in what sense the term 'psychogenic psychosis' is used and cherished in that part of the psychiatric world. Jörgensen (1956) expressed a frankly critical standpoint, verging on nihilism: 'some consider that psychogenic means "caused by a situation"; others hold that the designation "psychogenic" can be applied only when psychic symptoms develop without any demonstrable external cause . . . There exists no universally valid definition of the concept "psychogenesis". . . Purely external psychic causes do not exist.' The implied stricture seems justified when one reads Faergeman's assurance that 'psychogenic' can mean 'growing out of innate constitutional factors' or 'psychopathic condition caused by environmental factors with which the organism cannot cope. . . .' He concludes that 'psychogenic can refer equally well to something caused or

188

produced by the psyche as to some alteration in the psyche due to situational or environmental—particularly interpersonal—factors.'

NIHILIST

A penetrating and sophisticated but ultimately negative study of the problem has come from the French school, and especially from Henri Ey. At the outset of a three-day conference on the subject in 1946 Ey threw his glove into the ring: 'je répudie tout psychogenèse, toute causalité psychique des troubles mentaux; j'éstime que le psychogenèse définit le plan d'activité psychique normale.' The argument harks back to Jaspers's distinction between understanding and explaining the notion of causality, and to the legitimacy of Cartesian dualism inherent in the terms.

CATHOLIC

The 'catholic' standpoint does not shrink from applying the concept of psychogenesis to all mental disorders, including schizophrenia on the one hand and 'psychosomatic' conditions on the other. How close this comes to acceptance of Freudian postulates is evident in Adolf Meyer's papers in the first decade of this century on the problems of mental reaction types, mental causes and diseases. Devine (1933) went so far as to write that 'psychogenetic confusions may be properly included in the toxic-infective group of psychoses', and that an 'emotional situation' may elicit 'severe psychoses of the confusional type which in predisposed individuals may even develop into intractable schizophrenic conditions'. More recently a standard textbook (Noyes, 1953) states that not only the psycho-neuroses but also schizophrenia, manic-depressive psychosis, involutional psychosis, and the various paranoid states are psychogenic disorders in which psychodynamic factors are largely or solely operative. Henri Ey (1954) regrets the 'extension quasi infinie du domaine des névroses considerées comme des réactions psychogènes' but he and his co-authors (Ey, Bernard, and Brisset, 1960) see advantages (as well as objections) in viewing mental disorders from the standpoint of 'psychosociogenesis'—a term which can be supposed to cover all the vicissitudes of human existence as causes of mental

illness. Psychogenic is one of the terms applied to schizophreniform attacks of brief duration (Labhardt, 1963).

The role of this concept in the theoretical discussion of almost all forms of mental disorder is so widespread, so loosely interpreted, and so intimately entangled with assumptions about causation and psychopathology that concise review is impossible and outside the scope of this note. This holds good particularly where phenomenological and existential points of view prevail.

A vast amount has been written about the legitimacy of the concept—or, rather, of the various concepts—which are meant when the words 'psychogenesis' and 'psychogenic' are used. Hardly anything fresh has been said, however, for a good many years. Neither have the vagueness and laxity of usage been rectified: psychogenic and neurotic, psychogenic and reactive, psychogenic and 'non-organic' are by some writers substituted for one another as though they were synonyms. These are surface difficulties; at bottom there are the mind–body problems, and admitted ignorance about aetiology.

CONTEMPORARY DEFINITIONS

The present shoddy state of the term can be seen in more or less contemporary definitions. 'Psychogenic disorders of personality are those that seem to arise largely because of disturbed interpersonal relations, social maladjustments and the like' (Cobb, 1941); '. . . we shall consider "psychogenic causation" as implying causation by exogenous mental influences' (Kind, 1966).

'If the integrative disturbances arise in the field of inner psychic experiences and situations the disorders are called psychogenic. In the psychogenic mental disorders the direct effects of structural, biochemical and physiological factors are minimal or absent, while psychological and social factors are maximal . . . there is very little scientific basis for the distinction between the psychoneuroses and other psychogenic mental disorders. . . .' (Noyes, 1953).

'Psychogenic disorders, clinical as well as experimental, are caused by need-linked stimuli which, unlike all other aetiological factors are merely perceived by the organism.' 'The psychogenic disorders of man are in fact sociogenic' (Wolf, 1966).

189

'Ce que nous trouvons comme dénominateur commun à tous les facteurs psychogénétiques c'est qu'ils constituent des réactions intentionelles et significatives ... notre vie de rélation n'est pas autre chose qu'une série psychogénétique infinie d'actes de finalité capables d'assurer notre adaptation au réel, d'accomplir notre destin. C'est cela qui constitue le contenu concret de la notion de psychogenèse (Ey, 1950).

'Psychogenic, term usually employed of disorders which originate in mental conditions' (Drever, 1952).

'Expressions indiquant le rôle déterminant et parfois exclusif que jouent les processus purement psychiques dans la production et le developpement des névroses et des psychoses. ... Sous le nom de processus psychogènes on désigne les mécanismes par lesquels une perturbation initiale de la vie affective va declencher une série de désordres sécondaires et de répercussions sur la personnalité' (Porot, 1952).

There are more definitions having the same shimmering ill-focused quality as those just quoted. Perhaps the most tell-tale is Faergeman's:

'Psychogenic can mean: 1. born by the mind, that is, growing out of innate constitutional factors as, for example, the psychopathies, the manic-depressive psychosis and at least some of the schizophrenias; or 2. it can mean psychopathologic conditions caused by environmental factors which which the organism cannot cope with the employment of normal defence mechanisms and discharge channels. We can conclude that "psychogenic" can refer equally well to something caused or produced by the psyche as to some alteration in the psyche due to situational or environmental—particularly interpersonal—factors.'

Robert Sommer rendered psychiatry a disservice when he coined the word 'psychogenic' and so gave currency to a confused but speciously attractive and convenient concept. The subtle arguments of French and German disputants have shown it to be at the mercy of inconsistent theoretical positions touching on the fundamental problems of causality, dualism, and normality. It would be as well at this stage to give it decent burial, along with some of the fruitless controversies whose fire it has stoked.

REFERENCES

Binder, H. (1960). Die psychopathischen Dauerszustände. In *Psychiatric der Gegenwart*. Springer: Berlin.
Birnbaum, K. (1923). *Der Aufbau der Psychose*. Springer: Berlin.
Bleuler, E. (1916). *Lehrbuch der Psychiatrie*. Springer: Berlin.
Bleuler, E. (1926). Zur Unterscheidung des Physiogenen und des Psychogenen bei der Schizophrenie. *Allgemeine Zeitschrift für Psychiatrie*, **84**, 22–37.
Bonhoeffer, K. (1911). Wie weit kommen psychogene Krankheitzustände und krankheitprozesse vor, die nicht der Hysterie zuzurechnen sind? *Allgemeine Zeitschrift Psychiatrie*, **68**, 371–386.
Braun, E. (1928). Psychogene Reaktionen. In *Handbuch der Geisteskrankheiten*. Edited by O. Bumke. Springer: Berlin.
Cobb, S. (1941). *Foundations of Neuropsychiatry*. Williams and Wilkins: Baltimore.
Devine, H. (1933). *Recent Advances in Psychiatry*. 2nd edn. Churchill: London.
Drever, J. (1952). *A Dictionary of Psychology*. Penguin: Harmondsworth.
Ey, H. (1950). *Le Problème de la Psychogenèse des Névroses et des Psychoses*. Desclée de Brouwer: Paris.
Ey, H. (1954). *Études Psychiatriques*. Desclée de Brouwer: Paris.
Ey, H., Bernard, P., and Brisset, C. (1960). *Manuel de Psychiatrie*. Masson: Paris.
Faergeman, P. M. (1963). *Psychogenic Psychoses*. Butterworth: London.
Flournoy, T. A. (1900). *Des Indes à la Planète Mars*. Atar: Geneva.
Gruhle, H. W. (1927). Geisteskrankheiten und Strafrech. In *Handwörterbuch der Rechtswissenschaft*. de Gruyter: Berlin. Reprinted (1953) in *Verstehen und Einfühlen*. Springer: Berlin.
Hart, B. (1929). *Psychopathology*. 2nd edn. 5th edn. 1962. Cambridge University Press: London.
Hoch, A. (1907). The psychogenic factors in the development of psychoses. *Psychological Bulletin*, **4**, 161–169.
Hoch, A. (1910). Constitutional factors in the dementia praecox group. *Review of Neurology and Psychiatry*, **8**, 463–474.
Jaspers, K. (1948). *Allgemeine Psychopathologie*. 5. Aufl. Springer: Berlin.
Jörgensen, E. G. (1956). On the concepts psychogenesis and psychosomatics. *Acta Psychiatrica Scandinavica*, Suppl. 108, 135–149.
Kind, H. (1966). The psychogenesis of schizophrenia. A review of the literature. *British Journal of Psychiatry*, **112**, 333–349.
Kraepelin, E. (1896). *Psychiatrie*. (8 Auf. 3 vols. 1909–1913.) Barth: Leipzig.
Labhardt, F. (1963). *Monographien aus dem Gesamtgebiete der Neurologie und Psychiatrie*, Heft 102. Springer: Berlin.
MacCurdy, J. T. (1925). *The Psychology of Emotion, Morbid and Normal*. Kegan Paul: London.
Maier, H. W. (1912). Über katathyme Wahubildung und Paranoia. *Zeitschrift für die gesamte Neurologie und Psychiatrie*, **13**, 555–610.
Meyer, A. (1908). The role of the mental factors in psychiatry. *American Journal of Insanity*, **65**, 39–56.
Noyes, A. P. (1953). *Modern Clinical Psychiatry*. 4th edn. Saunders: Philadelphia.
Porot, A. (1952). *Manuel Alphabétique de Psychiatrie Clinique, Thérapeutique et Médico-Legale*. Presses Universitaires de France: Paris.
Prince, M. (1915). *The Unconscious*. Macmillan: New York.

Sommer, R. (1894). *Diagnostik der Geisteskrankheiten.* Urban und Schwarzenberg: Wein and Leipzig.

Strömgren, E. (1958). *Mehrdimensionale Diagnostik und Therapie Festschift zum 70. Geburtstag von E. Kretschmer.* Thieme: Stuttgart.

Tuke, D. H. (1892). *A Dictionary of Psychological Medicine.* 2 vols. Churchill: London.

Wolf, E. (1966). Psychogenic disorders and interpersonal behaviour. *Journal of Psychosomatic Research*, **10**, 119–126.

CLASSIFICATION AND DIAGNOSIS IN PSYCHIATRY: A HISTORICAL NOTE

SIR AUBREY LEWIS

A PROMINENT German psychiatrist of the last century, Heinrich Neumann, ranked classification high: 'It expresses our insight into the essential nature and development of the object classified' (Neumann, 1883). He propounded a classificatory schema based on symptoms and the stages through which they pass; one comprehensive disease taking different forms. 'This way of looking at the matter', he wrote, 'is important for psychiatric progress. Consider its bearing on statistics. A prime requirement for any statistic is that the units on which the calculation rests should be identical. If a statistical problem is to be solved, the result of the calculations is precisely nil, if the units are not identical. Indeed it is worse than nothing because its errors are paraded and spread in the resplendent attire of mathematics.'

Here, two crucial, still unsettled issues are stated: first, the 'diagnostic entity' problem; and secondly, how to ensure that in observation and enumeration we deal with identical units, permitting epidemiological comparison.

The setting up of an orderly and consistent table of 'diagnostic entities' has long been a bugbear of psychiatry. 'The wit of man', wrote Hack Tuke, 'has rarely been more exercised than in the attempt to classify the morbid phenomena covered by the term "insanity".' Classification has remained a battlefield, strewn with conflicting notions of 'disease', 'syndrome', 'type of reaction', 'symptom complex', and the like. Neumann, in agreement with Zeller (1844) and Griesinger (1845), plumped with simplifying ardour for one mental disorder, or disease, which changed shape as it progressed: beginning as depression, it could turn to mania (*Tollheit*), delusional forms (*Wahnsinn, Verrücktheit*), and finally to dementia (*Blödsinn*).

The concept of one comprehensive mental disease (*die Einheitspsychose*) thus launched a century ago has maintained a sporadic life, with various modifications, into the present time (Llopis, 1954; Conrad, 1959; Menninger, 1963). It no longer allocates diverse forms of the single illness to diverse stages but now leans heavily on psychopathology. Still, with rare exceptions, its proponents concede the necessity to classify the phenomena, whether the process is called diagnosis or not.

U 8445

A classification schema will fail if it has been intended to serve conflicting purposes. Neumann foresaw the consequences that might ensue from muddled parameters: 'Better no classification than a bad one.' This was too radical a view, as the course of events has shown; some classification is essential, to escape chaos. But reviews like those of Ey (1954), J. E. Meyer (1961), Brill (1966), Zubin (1967), and Cohen (1970) record the intellectual straits to which the necessity to classify has reduced many thoughtful and erudite psychiatrists during the last two centuries.

An aetiological classification of mental illnesses was the ideal for which many psychiatrists vainly longed. Arnold wrote in 1782, 'When the science of causes shall be complete we may then make them the basis of our classification, but till then we ought to content ourselves with an arrangement according to symptoms' (Arnold, 1782). Prichard, not long after, declared that 'an aetiological classification is the only mode of terminology and arrangement that can be of any practical advantage, and this is all we have to consult' (Prichard, 1835). Gradually it came to be recognized that there are here two major obstacles: the aetiology of many important forms of mental illnesses is not known, and the causes of every mental illness (where they are known) are multiple. Among the multiple causes one may be singled out as necessary, or immediate (precipitating), or preponderant, or genetic; but to make it then the sole criterion of a classificatory axis is impracticable.

In spite of the powerful objections to more than one principle of division being applied within one scheme, the current classification (*International Classification of Diseases*, 8) is a hotch-potch of classifications by cause, pathology, course, and clinical pattern. It is an empirical utilitarian scheme such as Hughlings Jackson contrasted with a scientific one. Parented by Kahlbaum (1863) and Kraepelin (1887, 1927), it was—and to some extent still is—influenced by somatic paradigms. It flies in the face of taxonomic rectitude, but persists for lack of anything better which would be generally acceptable. Its defects could be lessened by direct action (such as the two World Health Organization programmes) as well as by advances in our knowledge of causes and pathology. More logical classifications (such as Essen-Möller's proposed dual system (Essen-Möller and Wohlfart, 1947)) have failed because they did not accord with ingrained diagnostic habits.

In psychiatry more than in any other branch of medicine it is difficult to delimit what is morbid from what is healthy. On this may turn the decision as to whether treatment is to be instituted, or whether legal sanctions rather than medical therapies are called for. There is, however, much diversity in different psychiatrists' standpoints regarding the boundaries of normality. There is a similar diversity in determining what are the desiderata for assigning an illness to one of the ideal types of reaction, syndrome, pattern, entity, or whatever else it may be called. As Adolf Meyer put it over 50 years ago, 'We should have our concepts and words for the totalities, even if they can never be fully realized as wholly indisputable entities. For both scientific and practical purposes it is however wisest . . . not to sacrifice our progress to the old notion of unitary one-name "diseases" . . .' (Meyer, 1917). The basic problem is now well recognized in respect of somatic disease (Scadding, 1967). As a rule diagnosis represents not identification with the ideal type but approximation to it in key respects. Uniformity of usage is aimed at, rather than refinement and precision.

The essential stages in diagnosis, assuming agreement about the classes in the total system, are observation, interpretation, and class allocation. Each has its pitfalls.

Observation is skilled selective perception. It is influenced by observer variation and observer error. Observer variation was first recognized as the 'personal equation' occasioning discrepancy in visual recording. It was initially thought to be due to carelessness but was later studied in relation to reaction time and latterly has been held to account for discrepancies between clinical recordings by equally competent clinicians (Fletcher and Oldham, 1964; Feinstein, 1967). Error would be the wrong word for this; it depends on personal experience, expectation, affect, vigilance, and purpose: in short, as perception is always selective and never total, the likelihood of variability in observing the complex phenomena of behaviour is high, and bias almost inevitable. Observer error is an appropriate term for discrepancy due to plain ignorance on the psychiatrist's part (e.g. not knowing how to test for cognitive impairment, or ignoring gross cultural differences).

Inter-observer variation may be due to differences in style of response, or to some systematic bias. The individual observer's emotional needs and conflicts may also have to be taken into account, as well as his manner of conducting the exploratory inquiry into mental state and history. Studies such as those of Shepherd, Brooke, Cooper, and Lin, 1968; Grosz and Grossman, 1968; and Katz, Cole, and Lowery, 1969, demonstrate the subjectivity which may mar or distort primary observation of psychiatric abnormality.

The interpretative stage, at which the data of observation are translated into the language of organized constructs (e.g. depersonalization, obsessive compulsion, anxiety) gives wide scope for inter-psychiatrist divergencies arising out of differences in theoretical position, especially in respect of psychopathology. It has been less studied than observer variation, perhaps because it is so frequently encountered and so glaringly obvious.

The final stage in diagnosis consists in fitting the observed and interpreted data to an agreed (diagnostic) type. A complete fit is impossible but a close approximation is attainable if the definition of the type or types in question is adequate, especially when it is elaborated in a glossary and includes a statement of the indispensable minimal requirements for the relevant diagnosis.

To minimize the bias, omissions and subjectivity which beset the clinical interview and other means of observation, a systematic schedule is invaluable.

Its merits, however, are not unquestioned. In one of the most widely used current textbooks of psychiatry the student is warned against it: 'While one should not follow a rigid scheme of examination, and much less convey to the patient the impression that he is being asked a fixed list of questions, yet one must have a certain orderliness in one's approach to the mental examination' (Noyes, 1953). This is no new attitude. Sixty years ago a German manual on psychiatric examination and diagnosis showed the same half-heartedness: 'Diese eigenartigen Verhältnisse der psychiatrischen Exploration bringen es mit sich dass die Einhaltung eines bestimmten Schemas nur in groben Umrissen möglich sein kann. . . . Dennoch ist es für den Anfänger wünschenswert dass er eine Art Schema hat, nach welchem er bei seinen Beobachtungen und Fragen vorzugehen sucht und in das er die erlangten Resultate einordnet.' ('These peculiar features of psychiatric examination make adherence to a definite schema possible only within the broadest outlines. . . . Nevertheless it is desirable for the beginner to have a sort of schema which he tries to follow in his observations and questions, and in which he arranges his findings.') (Raecke, 1910.)

Recent studies have shown that it is possible to construct reliable systematic procedures for observing and recording the present mental state of patients and to employ them with confidence for the purpose of epidemiological comparisons (Wing, Birley, Cooper, Graham, and Isaacs, 1967; Spitzer, Fleiss, Burdock, and Hardesty, 1964). Supervised training in their use is essential, but well within the compass of basic psychiatric education. It is, however, significant that it is only comparatively recently that guidance in psychiatric examination has been included as a necessary feature of standard textbooks. This holds good particularly for English, American, and French texts; German authors were more sophisticated: they began to pay regard to this need towards the end of the last century. Kraepelin devoted 20 pages of his textbook in 1887 to the matter; by 1927 it had swollen to more than 100 pages. In the earlier edition he wrote that the methods available for examining the present mental state were extremely inadequate because the only aids at our disposal were those provided by the practical experiences of life; he looked forward to the development of more precise, revealing, and objective techniques. His optimism has been only meagrely confirmed, as yet; his disparaging appraisal of techniques available in his time betrays an attitude strikingly different from that which is now often inculcated (Redlich and Freedman, 1966; Ripley, 1967).

The second or hermeneutic stage in the diagnostic process is dependent on the theoretical standpoint of the diagnostician; his interpretation of his data must be a consequence of his system of psychopathology (and, it may be, his system of somatic pathology).

The final state in diagnosis is an exercise in refined clinical judgement. It can be regarded also as a task for which the computer will prove valuable when the essential diagnostic features have been unequivocally established.

In the meanwhile, 'the best rule, however, for everybody to observe when attempting to form a judgement on any particular case of insanity, is to take care and preserve his own faculties clear, and as free from the mysticisms of speculative philosophy as from the trammels of nosology' (Burrows, 1828).

Manfred Bleuler's *The Schizophrenic Mental Disorders*[1]: an exposition and a review

AUBREY LEWIS

Institute of Psychiatry, University of London

Eugen Bleuler's *Dementia Praecox oder die Gruppe der Schizophrenien* was published in 1912. Thirty years later an erudite historian of psychiatry referred to it as an epoch-making monograph, a product of many years of careful research—'the most important contribution to psychiatry made in the 20th century'. It was a bold prediction, and he could hardly have foreseen that in another 30 years there would be another product of many years of careful research into schizophrenia, again providing a classic of psychiatry, the work of yet another Bleuler. There have been many instances of son following father in the psychiatric career but in none of them have father and son tilled the same wide field with the same assiduity and unremitting mastery as these.

The main purpose of the investigation here reported was to deepen our knowledge of the protracted course of the various forms of schizophrenia and to trace the connection between the history of the patients and their relatives. A secondary aim of the inquiry was to compare schizophrenias at a given time and place with the outcome of comparable investigations at other times and in other places. The sample of patients consisted of 208 schizophrenics who were admitted between 1942 and 1943 to the psychiatric university clinic of Burghölzli and whose condition has been followed, together with that of their nearest relatives, for more than 20 years. About 66 of them were initially seen during their first admission to a psychiatric hospital. The great majority came from the Canton of Zurich; their average age was 40 years, and half of them were single.

They represent an unselected group of all schizophrenics admitted to the Burghölzli from 1942 to 1943. The diagnosis of schizophrenia was made with much care, emphasis being laid on the conjunction of severely disturbed mental life and formality of thinking, eccentricity and remoteness of what were essentially affective phenomena, depersonalization, delusions and hallucinations with particular colouring, catatonic symptoms, and hallucinations of memory. Cases in which the illness was recognizably related to bodily changes were excluded and diagnosis was never made to turn on irreversibility. The criteria were strictly applied, and a number of case histories are supplied which enable the reader to judge whether he would concur in the diagnosis. Cases given the benefit of the doubt could perhaps have been diagnosed as a schizoaffective psychosis, a chronic alcoholic hallucinosis, a paranoia. So many changes in the patients' symptoms occurred during the years of observation that classification as sub-types (paranoid or catatonic) would have been arbitrary.

The follow-up data were collected with exceptional thoroughness and success. Professor Bleuler was able to obtain full social and medical information about the 208 patients, their parents, sibs, spouses, and children up to the time of their death or the end of the systematic investigations, which was in the years 1964–65. Several subsidiary studies were made to check the representative character of the sample; material for these was drawn from various New York and Swiss data. In a characteristic dry note, Professor Bleuler mentions that he and his colleagues at Burghölzli had over the years tried to keep in touch with the whole of the international schizophrenia literature; they took account of 9,884 publications. It might be said that just as

[1]DIE SCHIZOPHRENEN GEISTESSTÖRUNGEN IM LICHTE LANG-JÄHRIGER KRANKEN-UND FAMILIENGESCHICHTEN By M. Bleuler. With a contribution by A. Uchtenhagen. (Pp. 673; 32 illustrations, 118 tables; DM 128.) Thieme: Stuttgart. 1972.

197

everything King Midas touched turned to gold so everything in the schizophrenia literature which Professor Bleuler touched became at once extensive and intensive.

Preliminary consideration raised the question of physical disease in relation to schizophrenia. Inquiry made it clear that there is a fundamental distinction to be drawn between acute schizophrenias and schizophreniform disorders which can be attributed to somatic conditions which precede them. This applied in particular to endocrine disorders, to the study of which Professor Bleuler has made such a notable contribution.

The chief problem which Professor Bleuler set before himself 20 or more years ago was concerned with the interplay between the patients' lives and those of their nearest relatives. To this end he maintained close touch with the relevant persons, recognizing that very few previous studies covered the long life-period and maintained intimate contact through time. In his view, the psychopathology, phenomenology, psychodynamics, and pathological anatomy of schizophrenia had been so thoroughly investigated from many standpoints that until there are fundamentally new techniques or valid hypotheses no important advances can be expected in these areas. From the outset he recognized that the essential yield of the inquiry would be facts, but not the interpretation of the facts; on the other hand, he saw that it was inevitable that someone like himself reflecting for decades on the essence of the schizophrenias could hardly hope to suppress his thoughts on the subject when he came to report his findings from the present study:

'Few will share my ideas about the essential nature of schizophrenia. They will think that I am either too little psychodynamic, or insufficiently somatic, in orientation.'

In a more lengthy review of the points in favour of the diagnosis of schizophrenia, it was first required that general signs of a psychosis (which are specified) must be forthcoming; if, however, an endocrine, toxic, or other organic syndrome was in evidence the case was ruthlessly rejected from the series. What Professor Bleuler regarded as especially significant for the diagnosis of schizophrenia were: 'double bookkeeping';

characteristic schizophrenic thought disorder; abstraction from all affective phenomena in voice, motor behaviour, and rapport; depersonalization in several guises; severe catatonic phenomena in the muscular system, *Beziehungswahn* and kindred delusional ideas and hallucinations as well as severe secondary illusions of memory, and hallucinations. The course of the psychosis was in no circumstances utilized for diagnosis. Professor Bleuler admits that he would regard himself as in a quandary if he had to consider under this rubric cases that were of quite short duration—a matter of days only—but no cases of this kind were admitted to the clinic and he was therefore spared the awkward decision. He was, however, confronted with a not dissimilar problem in regard to the elderly who have their first schizophrenic attack late in life; he excluded them when the illness was intermingled with evidence of an amnesic syndrome. Another diagnostic crux was provided by the separation of admixed manic-depressive or schizoaffective symptoms.

'I have always made the diagnosis of schizophrenia when a patient had experienced one phase of schizophrenic symptomatology, particularly if there were clearly manic or depressive phases then or later. Stupor and delusions in depressions and ideas of grandeur in a manic setting did not bother me and seemed to me to lend no support to the diagnosis of schizophrenia. It is my view that stupor in a euphoric setting, ideas of persecution or wrong-doing in depression, transition from mere flight of ideas to confusion, and hallucinations which do not correspond to the mood all seem to me suspicious of schizophrenia.'

Summing up the particular considerations, Professor Bleuler is confident that almost all Swiss psychiatrists would confirm his diagnosis and that among them he would be regarded as one who has the most exacting requirements for diagnosis of schizophrenia.

Seven detailed case histories are provided indicating how the diagnostic issue has been handled. As an example of the scrupulous care employed the final opinion of the diagnosis of one of these may be quoted. It concerned a man who had, in all, four psychotic phases. In the first of these his symptoms were typically schizophrenic, with confusion and hallucinosis. At the height of the second and third phases there were exacerbations in which the patient was much hallucinated and inaccessible; in short, he showed a classical, very severe schizophrenic picture. He was therefore included in the series, although there were features which suggested manic-depressive psychosis. In his second phase there were manic features interwoven with the hebephrenic. Towards the end of the third phase and the fourth phase the picture was more conspicuously manic and the schizophrenic features receded from the foreground. The basic course was like that of a manic-depressive and left no demonstrable traces in the personality except perhaps a certain resignation and gloom. In an additional note the family history is recalled; his father and one of his sisters had a psychosis like his, another sister had attacks of depression without any schizophrenic colouring. In view of the numerous manic-depressive features, it would not have been wrong, Bleuler comments, if the diagnosis of mixed (schizoaffective) psychosis were to have been made. There were in the sample nine patients who had a considerable manic-depressive element, three in whom the first illness had occurred after the 60th year of life, three whose illness resembled chronic alcoholic hallucinosis, six psychedelic reactions, and one possible paranoia.

It is difficult to convey in a short review a notion of the painstaking thoroughness with which the work has been carried out. As Director of Burghölzli, Professor Bleuler was able to distribute his time as he thought best: he relates that

'the foundations of the book were provided largely by the daily routine work in the clinic with the patients. I also set aside a considerable amount of my daily time exclusively for this work during a period of 28 years. On leave several times for a period of one to four months I was able to give my whole time to the work, and altogether my expenditure of time in the investigation and the writing up of the total material must have been equivalent to well over four years.'

CLINICAL FEATURES

FINDINGS IN THE PARENTS

Among the parents of the probands 5 to 7% presented either certain or highly probable schizophrenia. Incidence of schizophrenic mothers was twice as frequent as of schizophrenic fathers, no doubt because on the average women marry earlier than men. In affected parents the schizophrenia was late in onset and mild. Manic-depressive psychoses were more common among the parents of schizophrenics than among the general population, though less frequent than among the parents of manic-depressives. Senile psychoses appeared more frequently among the parents of the probands than in the general population. An increase of suicide among the parents of schizophrenics could be demonstrated.

The frequency with which schizophrenic *children* in the sample had been prematurely deprived of one or other parent was a question that could be answered only on larger numbers. An *ad hoc* inquiry was set in motion and data collected on, in all, 1,319 patients; particular attention was paid to the problem because of the way in which such information about their childhood had been construed by one group as indicative of hereditary predisposition; by others as pointing to psychogenesis. Premature loss of a parent was not much more frequent among the schizophrenics than in the general population, and it is more frequent among patients with other illnesses than the schizophrenic. As between the sexes, it was found that schizophrenic women had lost a parent through death more frequently than schizophrenic men and more frequently than healthy persons: in particular, mother-deprivation in early life is not found to be an apparent cause of schizophrenia, but Bleuler postulates a heightened predisposition to the development of schizophrenia in women who have suffered this privation. He points out that much of the contention as to whether an unfavourable milieu promotes mental illness or conversely rests on a false premise—namely, that man is always placed in a milieu in whose structure he has not had any say. The environment influences the child; the child influences the environment. The relationship which the schizophrenic patients had had with their father was in about half the cases unsatisfactory (partly because of the frequent alcoholism of the father). Professor Bleuler had formed the impression that more important than the attitude of the parents to the child was the effect of the child on the parents and their attitude towards him. He could not provide statistics on the point, nor would he make undue claims to precision.

SCHIZOID PSYCHOPATHY

It was often formerly taken for granted that schizoid psychopathy was an inherited feature of constitution. But in the 208 Burghölzli cases, 50 had schizoid features, which in 37 of them had shown themselves during their school days. Twenty-nine of the 50 probands who had this anomaly came from homes in which conditions were appalling: from Professor Bleuler's material it is concluded that there is a statistically significant correlation between appalling conditions in childhood and morbid schizoid constitution. The misery endured during childhood leaves the impress of an attitude which forms the basis for schizophrenia in later life. It is, however, doubtful whether the positive correlation between terrible experience in childhood and schizophrenic illness occurs in those who have pre-psychotically normal character. There appears also to be a sexual difference. Horrible conditions in childhood dispose girls and boys to unfavourable personality development, but only girls are predisposed to schizophrenia in such cases.

SEXUAL BEHAVIOUR

This feature was inquired into as far as was practicable. There was no evidence of strong deviation before the onset of the schizophrenic illness.

PROTRACTED COURSE

Study of the course of illness in schizophrenic psychoses is well known to be frustrating. The dogma that schizophrenia was incurable stood in the way of any serious inquiry. The advent of active somatic therapy in the 1930s presented a new situation, with better understanding of the spontaneous prognosis. On the other hand, enthusiasts who were unaware of the variety of courses which schizophrenia might follow attributed to therapy the improvement which was part of the course of the illness. Other obstacles were too short a follow-up period; assessment on only one occasion (on admission to hospital); the error due to small numbers; account not being taken of the possible choice of probands on grounds of prognosis.

SOCIAL FACTORS

Professor Bleuler directs attention to the conclusion drawn by Faris and Dunham, Redlich, and Hollingshead, and other students of the demography of schizophrenia that the condition is more frequent in people of low social and economic status. In opposition to this, he records that in his material the schizophrenic patients' occupational standing was like that of their fathers and of the average population before the beginning of their psychosis; when, however, the illness had made itself manifest there was an occupational decline.

END-STATE

Most schizophrenics whose illness has lasted for years, possibly for decades, reach a fairly stable state. Professor Bleuler, however, insists 'that it [end-state] cannot be construed as referring to a completely final and unchangeable condition'. In his use of the term, it applies to recovery as well as to chronic psychosis. The figures show that in the last few decades very severe end-states (called 'dementias') have become much less common, medium and mild end-states have increased, while the recoveries among the end-states have remained constant. These changes he attributes to the advent of more effective treatment. He found that in an enlarged population of patients (including some from New York) about two-thirds to three-quarters of the schizophrenics run a favourable course and only one-third to one-quarter are malignant. Of those schizophrenics who had been in an end-state for several years, only one-quarter to one-third eventually have a long lasting recovery. The number of one-quarter to one-third relates to the recoveries which have lasted for years and are stable, though possibly interrupted by single psychotic phases. In one-tenth to one-fifth of all schizophrenics who have been once admitted to hospital the illness ensues in severe chronic psychosis.

With the passage of time there was a sharp recession in the number of patients whose schizophrenia began with an acute attack which immediately passed into a lasting severe condition; the credit for this recession must go to modern treatment.

Of patients in the series who had been admitted to hospital for the first time in this attack, about one-third subsequently recovered, sometimes after several transitory attacks. The number of those who developed a chronic schizophrenic psychosis in the course of the final years of study was larger than in the earlier years, but the number who passed into a severe chronic psychosis was smaller.

Even after decades many schizophrenics showed distinct improvement but one group proved to be an exception to this rule. Improvement was never found to occur in patients whose schizophrenia continuously passed into the most severe chronic form of the illness. First-admission probands who were still living at the end of the period of observation showed a good or relatively good outcome: 50% were able to live independently in the community and to earn their own living and only 22% were under care in a mental hospital.

The figures lent no unmistakable support for the view that there is a correlation between unhappy conditions in childhood—for example, a 'broken home'— and a deteriorating course. The expected correlation was found between personality and end-state but, though positive, it was less pronounced than clinical experience would suggest.

The probands' reaction to the death of their parent was investigated and appeared to show that the impact was greater in girls and women than in boys and men. In seven patients their condition improved after the death of their mother or father towards whom they had a pronounced ambivalence; in 22 probands, however, the parents' death led to aggravation of the patients' condition corresponding to his dependence on the parent.

EFFECT OF TREATMENT

Heightened expectations on this score are not ratified:

'There is no support for the view that the therapeutic methods available result in the avoidance of those appalling forms of the illness in which it begins insidiously and progresses steadily. If in an illness with an acute onset treatment is promptly instituted and recovery occurs, in a large proportion of such cases the recovery would have taken place without any treatment . . . the investigation did not show that any particular technique of treatment is of

decisive importance. It seems that all forms of treatment are beneficial which aim skilfully, patiently and with inner conviction at the following objectives— rehabilitating the patient so that he can bring into play his natural abilities; an emotional storm at the right time; relaxation and sedation when he is too excited.'

PROBANDS' DEATH

In the years between 1942 and 1965 there were frequent cases of death which occurred suddenly and inexplicably. The risk of suicide in schizophrenics is high and is not limited to the initial stages. Tumours as a cause of death are much rarer than in the general population.

PROBANDS' SIBLINGS

The patients had 818 brothers and sisters all of whom were thoroughly investigated. Approximately 9% of these had schizophrenia. Other psychoses were no more frequent than in the general population. Between the two members of a schizophrenic sibship the differences might be considerable in respect of end-state, type of course, age at onset, and prepsychotic character; nevertheless there was evidence of an intrinsic similarity in their symptomatology except for those in whom the course was a highly malignant one. The old assumption that more severe schizophrenics were those with whom the hereditary factor was the most important one was not corroborated: the different types of course in schizophrenia are not conditioned by different particular hereditary factors but by the totality of inherited factors and the experiences to which the patient had been exposed in the course of his life. Possibly because of harmful upbringing, women were more numerous than men among the schizophrenics who had brothers or sisters.

FERTILITY

The 208 patients had, in all, 184 children. Half the probands were single. Children of schizophrenics fell ill with schizophrenia 10 times more frequently than is the case in the general population; those affected ran a milder course than did their parents. There were, however, among the offspring fewer psychopaths. The probands included three who had a schizophrenic spouse;

they gave rise to five children of whom three were mentally healthy: 'Family histories show strikingly that people can remain healthy even if during the greater part of their childhood they have been exposed to their schizophrenic parents.' One hundred and one children of the probands had married and in at least 84 of these the marriage has been happy and successful. Living with schizophrenic parents had a less damaging effect than upbringing under shocking conditions.

'As the majority of the children of schizophrenics lead effective lives it is all the more remarkable when one knows what appalling difficulties they have had to overcome in their childhood. Anyhow many of the children who grow up under miserable conditions do not forget their early distress . . . this darkens the life of many, they have feelings of inferiority and doubt as to their adequacy in marriage.'

OLDER CONCEPTS

A chapter is devoted to reviewing certain cardinal questions—'schizophrenic dementia', psychogenic origin, hereditary background, schizoid psychopathy, one or several groups of schizophrenias. The chronic states which were designated as schizophrenic dementia contained a large autistic element and did not follow an acute psychotic episode. The conspicuous dependence of the course of the illness on psychotherapeutic measures makes it probable that similar influences are of importance in its genesis. Psychogenesis appears to have the least support in the benign acute phasic forms of the illness. The course of the catastrophic schizophrenias which have an acute beginning and gradually pass into a chronic severe form is the product not of hereditary factors but of bad treatment. Bleuler's data also confirm the old rule that schizophrenics who have a premorbid schizoid psychopathy run a particularly unfavourable course; he emphasizes, however, the arbitrary nature of the distinction between schizoid constitutional peculiarity and an imposed schizoid attitude. To the question of whether the data now warrants breaking up the group of schizophrenias into distinct aetiologically independent diseases the answer is an unequivocal no. Some of the old beliefs have to be modified: thus, the malignant form has

almost disappeared. The frequency of chronic progressive psychoses has not diminished, nor has the frequency of long recoveries been increased; instances of essential improvement or lasting recovery have been attained without any prolonged drug treatment.

AETIOLOGY

In a spirit of what may be called proud humility, Professor Bleuler opens his concluding chapter with the following justification.

'If one has treated and cared for schizophrenics over many years, been on intimate terms with them, thought about them, read literature about them, and oneself studied aspects which others have not yet tackled, one can hardly help arriving at a standpoint on the great questions which this group of diseases arouses: what is their essential nature? How do they come about? What is essential and effective in our treatment? In my earlier years I listened, at first without understanding but later with half understanding, to discussions between my father and Binswanger, Freud, Jung, Kraepelin, Meyer, Minkowski and others. Since then I have constantly asked myself how far modern developments in schizophrenia and in medicine generally would have altered the attitude of investigators of schizophrenia. I would therefore like to add my thoughts about these large theoretical questions, although they form perhaps a jarring appendix.'

On the question of the essentially somatic nature of the schizophrenias he maintains a cautious reserve; very many able observers have applied themselves to the demonstration of bodily change but so far to little purpose.

Inheritance also plays its part. Pedigree studies had shown that a simple Mendelian mode of transmission could not be demonstrated either for schizophrenias as a whole or any particular form of schizophrenia.

'For the assumption of one or a few morbific genes as the basis of schizophrenias the only support is a preformed opinion that these exist. In truth, to consider such an assumption today is needless, since no mutation rate is known which is high enough to counteract the lessening of their fertility. In the light of present knowledge inherited conditions for the occurrence of schizophrenia are most probably either a multitude of unfavourable hereditary characters or an unfavourable concurrence (dysharmony) of intrinsically favourable hereditary dispositions.'

There is much that remains healthy in the schizophrenic psyche—good memory, intellectual capacity, and warmth of mood and feeling. Conversely, a healthy person pursues an inner life which can only with difficulty be distinguished from schizophrenic mentation: this is exhibited in dreams, in magic, in archaic thinking, and in autism, as well as in projection tests and in transitory physical disorders.

PSYCHOPATHOLOGY

The older view, that the symptoms of schizophrenia can be divided into secondary and primary, now needs revision, though it is still important to recognize which symptoms (the secondary ones) are a consequence of unfavourable experiences, especially unskilled treatment. Autism can be regarded as the most elementary feature in schizophrenia; what were considered irreducible, 'primary' phenomena of the disorder can now be understood as deriving from the autistic attitudes of the schizophrenic.

'ESSENTIAL NATURE' OF SCHIZOPHRENIC DISORDERS

The inherited features are to be looked for not in metabolic disturbance but in the predisposition in character and mood. Unlike other lines of personality development, this reaches a threshold beyond which the capacity to adapt to the real world is lost; instead, there is a vain effort to create a world which fits their abnormal experience of life: they find refuge in autism. Effective therapy of schizophrenia calls for the same capacity as leads to the harmonious development of personality.

In a declaration of faith, Professor Bleuler doubts the notion that there is something essential and sensational to be discovered, something of which we have at present no conception. With equal or even greater force he proclaims his conviction that discarded theories of schizophrenia without any empirical basis were not merely harmless rhetoric; they did harm and 'anyone who lived through such a disastrous phase can hardly speak of it without bitterness'. He quotes two examples. The first is concerned with heredity: the assertion that schizophrenia would be transmitted on simple Mendelian lines, combined with the 'silly' belief that inherited disorders can never be influenced acted like a frost on every therapeutic enthusiasm. Those who regarded the schizophrenic psychosis as a destructive brain process were certainly not supporting the view, so salutary in treatment, that schizophrenics can think and feel like the rest of us. Along similar lines, Bleuler protests against the World Health Organization's endorsement of the view that deprived children may become schizophrenic or criminal.

RORSCHACH FINDINGS

In the original plan Professor Bleuler meant to apply the Rorschach tests to all his 208 probands and the nearest relatives. One of his colleagues had pointed out to him how often the relations of schizophrenics showed Rorschach protocols suggestive of schizophrenia. His own investigations pointed in the same direction. It was, therefore, tempting to look for latent schizophrenia in relatives, using the Rorschach technique. Experience, however, dictated caution in judging what a Rorschach finding suggestive of schizophrenia really meant. Lack of time prevented him from investigating the matter personally. It was, therefore, taken over by Dr. Uchtenhagen. He reports his findings and their interpretation in a remarkably restrained fashion. He studied 218 Rorschach protocols, of which 122 were obtained from populations of schizophrenics and 96 from patients with brain damage. The results speak volumes for the integrity of the investigator: Professor Bleuler puts it tersely:

'[Uchtenhagen's] findings show that a Rorschach protocol suggesting schizophrenia in no wise justifies the assumption of a latent schizophrenia. Such findings can derive from the emotional attitude of the tested person to the test situation.'

Dr. Uchtenhagen is likewise quite outspoken:

'The unconscious conflicts whose activation can lead to the picture of a schizophrenic psychosis or of schizophrenia-like behaviour are not in the least specific for the disease schizophrenia. They cannot be correlated with clinical pictures; on the contrary, the responses often show the greatest similarity to the Rorschach performance of healthy people.'

203

It is impossible in a brief review to do justice to so massive a work as Professor Bleuler's monograph. The present cursory notice, for example, gives no inkling of the painstaking statistical treatment or of the conscientious assiduity with which possible objections are examined. In method and in interpretation it is a model of how follow-up studies should be reported (though few will be found with the intellectual and moral stamina required for such an undertaking as this has proved to be).

A report of this sort always runs the danger of being dry-as-dust, but this charge cannot be levelled at the monograph, which is informed by the humane spirit that is one of the legacies of Eugen Bleuler to his son. In 1931 Manfred Bleuler read a summarized version of his father's work in psychiatry to an American audience. In it, he said:

'He has a great tendency to sympathize with the schizophrenic patients and to share their fears and worries. He is happy when he feels that something in a schizophrenic patient's mind responds to his attention. I believe that all his conceptions about schizophrenia have been due directly to this attitude. Both the basis and the results of his work with psychiatric patients have been the conviction that it is worth while to give them individual interest and personal sympathy.'

Like father, like son.

Psychopathic personality: a most elusive category

AUBREY LEWIS

From the Institute of Psychiatry, De Crespigny Park, London

SYNOPSIS For 150 years the diagnostic concept at first called 'moral insanity' has been troubling psychiatric nosologists. Initially emphasis was laid on the affective disturbance in this condition, which was unaccompanied by intellectual impairment. Then its conformity to the idea of a degenerative process became prominent. At various times its relation to epilepsy, hereditary disease, and vice and crime has held the stage. Latterly little advantage has been taken of the information provided about personality by the investigations of psychologists.

Psychopathic personality is one of a cluster of terms which have been used, interchangeably or successively, in the last 150 years to denote a life-long propensity to behaviour which falls mid-way between normality and psychosis. Mania *sine delirio*, moral insanity, moral imbecility, psychopathy, degenerate constitution, congenital delinquency, constitutional inferiority—these and other semantic variations on a dubious theme have been bandied about by psychiatrists and lawyers in a prodigious output of repetitious articles.

In 1801 Philippe Pinel described a condition which he called *manie sans délire*. Its specific features were absence of any appreciable alteration in the intellectual functions—perception, judgment, imagination, memory—but pronounced disorder of the affective functions, blind impulse to acts of violence, even murderous fury. Illustrative cases which he cited included some which would not now be regarded as explosive forms of psychopathic personality. In 1818 a German psychiatrist, Grohman, delimited 'moral diseases of the mind' which he said depend upon physical anomalies in the brain; he posited three subgroups—moral dullness (*Stumpfsinn*), congenital brutality, and moral imbecility (*Blödsinn*). He subscribed to faculty psychology, and took his stand on the somatic theory of psychopathology in the polemic then prevailing between Nasse and his colleagues on the one hand, and Heinroth, the pan-psychological champion, on the other. In France, Esquirol (1838), after some hesitation, confirmed Pinel's observation that intact understanding in these patients can coexist with periodic excitement, and he included the condition among the monomanias, which were likewise a disputed category at the time.

MORAL INSANITY

The next psychiatrist to deal specifically with this topic was J. C. Prichard. In a textbook of his which appeared in 1822 he gave his reasons for dissenting from Pinel's view regarding *manie sans délire*. When, however, in 1835 he produced a riper work, *A Treatise on Insanity and other Diseases Affecting the Mind*, he declared himself convinced of the rightness of Pinel's opinion. With the designation 'moral insanity' he enlarged and generalized Pinel's '*manie sans délire*'. He saw it as a 'morbid perversion of the natural feelings, affections, inclinations, temper, habits, moral dispositions and natural impulses, without any remarkable disorder or defect of the intellect or knowing and reasoning faculties and particularly without any insane illusion or hallucination'.

The sharp distinction that Prichard drew between 'lesions of the understanding' and 'affective lesions' rapidly became a controversial question. On the one side were authorities like Henry Maudsley, who put their standpoint unambiguously:

'As there are persons who cannot distinguish certain colours, having what is called colour blindness, so there are some who are congenitally deprived of moral sense' (Maudsley, 1874).

Equally weighty opinion to the contrary was expressed by Griesinger, J. P. Falret and others.

A DEGENERATIVE PROCESS

Interest shifted from this argument when in the middle of the century Morel (1839) put forward his persuasive views about degeneration: 'degeneration is a morbid deviation from the normal human type, transmissible by heredity, and evolving progressively towards extinction.' His clinical experience as head of a mental hospital stirred his interest in the theoretical and social aspects of degeneration:

'What are asylums but places where the chief kinds of human degeneration are concentrated. The ever growing number of suicides, crimes, offences against property and the person, the appalling precocity of young criminals, the degradation of the race—these are indisputable facts. I had to find out whether the increasing proportion of the insane (or, if you prefer it, the more hopeless complications of their condition) were the outcome of a complex of general causes.'

Treatment, he found, was mostly ineffectual, especially in his class of patients with 'hereditary insanity' (monomania, 'nervous temperament', eccentricity, 'dissolute immorality').

Degeneration, as Morel conceived it, had two essential features: hereditary transmission, and increasing severity in successive generations, leading to extirpation of affected individuals, families, or groups. It did not carry with it the opprobrium which attaches to the word in common speech. The intrusion of moral judgments, which had been evident in Prichard's terminology and that of many other 19th-century psychiatrists, is partly to be attributed to the equivocal meaning of the word 'moral' in French: though mainly used with the same significance as in English, sometimes it refers to every mental function that can be subsumed under the general term 'affective'. Hence it came about that 'moral insanity' and 'moral imbecility' were often treated as synonyms of emotional abnormality (délire emotif) or of constitutional proclivity to vice and crime. English psychiatrists

had less linguistic temptation to this, though they were much influenced by Morel. Maudsley, for example, wrote in 1874 that

'there is an insane temperament which without being itself a disease may easily and abruptly break down into actual disease under a strain from without or from within; moral feeling like any other feeling is a function of organization; an absence of moral sense is an occasional result of descent from an insane family'.

As recently as 1932 Henderson and Gillespie wrote:

'Under the term "mental defect" we propose to include not only intellectual defect in its various grades, but also emotional and moral defects which have been present from an early age. . . . For "emotional instability" and "moral deficiency" or "moral imbecility", as it has unfortunately been called, we shall use the wider term "constitutional psychopathic inferiority".'

After Morel, modification of the concept came chiefly from Magnan and his disciples in Paris. He described a large category of 'héréditaires dégénerés', within which he included idiots, imbeciles, feeble minded, and 'dégénerés supérieurs' (Magnan, 1893). The latter (dégénerés supérieurs) had average or brilliant intellectual powers, but moral defects. Physical stigmata or degeneracy were numerous in all the four subdivisions; the corresponding psychological stigmata were obsessions, irresistible impulses, dipsomania, coprolalia, kleptomania, sexual anomalies, and some other analogous features. Common characteristics of these phenomena were concomitant anxiety, awareness by the affected individual of his abnormality, and satisfaction following the accomplishment of an impulsive act.

Magnan subscribed to Morel's picture of doomed hereditary descent, proceeding from folie raisonnante or mania in the first generation to idiocy or imbecility in the fourth.

MEDICOLEGAL ASPECTS

Much controversy centred on these views, especially in France and Germany (Bumke, 1912). In England the medicolegal aspect which had engaged Prichard's interest continued to be the dominant issue. Maudsley (1874) exemplifies this:

'moral insanity', he wrote, 'is a form of mental alienation which has so much the look of vice or crime that many persons regard it as an unfounded medical invention ... the symptoms are mainly exhibited in the perversion of those mental faculties which are usually called the active and moral powers —the feelings, affections, propensities, temper, habits and conduct ... (the individual) has no capacity of true moral feelings; all his impulses and desires, to which he yields without check, are egoistic ... his affective nature is profoundly deranged, and its affinities are for such evil gratifications as must lead to further degeneration and finally render him a diseased element which must either be got rid of out of the social organization or be sequestrated and made harmless in it'.

Maudsley pleaded that when such a person has committed an offence 'the truest justice would be the admission of a modified responsibility'.

The Italian contribution was for a time influential; Tanzi and Lombroso (Wolfgang, 1960) were the standard bearers. Tanzi pointed out the objections to regarding degeneration as a cause of moral insanity—which he preferred to call 'constitutional immorality'. He detached it from the forms of ethical failings which are a symptom of disease supervening in a previously normal person, and from the supposed 'epileptic personality' on which Lombroso and, following him, Maudsley and others laid stress. Tanzi also criticized the so-called stigmata of degeneration, reputed to be especially common in psychopaths.

The impact of Lombroso's boldly proclaimed views was more positive. In the 'anthropological' period of his output (1872–85) he proclaimed that the 'born delinquent' with his physical stigmata was the atavistic incarnation of 'moral insanity'. In his second period pathological criteria (chiefly of epilepsy) were to the fore. The born criminal with his evidence of arrested development and his deficiency of altruistic feelings, exhibits, Lombroso maintained, an 'epileptoid' state, a predetermined adversity of character.

French, German, and Italian psychiatrists vied with each other in proposing alternative names for the condition, but most English psychiatrists continued to call it moral insanity while deploring the shortcomings of such a term. Savage

(1881) considered that it was easier to describe what the condition is not than to come to a comprehensive definition of it: moral insanity could be a '"secondary" state or stage of mental disease and not a fixed or permanent condition itself' whereas in the primary or essential form peculiarity of character and eccentric behaviour are present from early childhood. Tuke (1892) declared that the wide difference of opinion on this subject among 'mental physicians' was mainly due to 'the want of definition of the terms employed'.

CLARIFICATION OF TERMS

A determined and sustained effort to clarify the relevant terms was made by Koch (1891). He introduced the plural form 'psychopathic inferiorities' which, he said, would include

'all mental irregularities whether congenital or acquired which influence a man in his personal life and cause him, even in the most favourable cases, to seem not fully in possession of normal mental capacity, though even in the bad cases the irregularities do not amount to mental disorder'.

By the term 'psychopathic' Koch intended to stress the presumptive physical basis of the condition.

'They remain always psychopathic in the sense that they are caused by organic states and changes which lie on the far side of the limits of physiological normality ... they rest on a congenital or acquired inferiority of brain constitution.'

He admitted, however, that this could not be demonstrated anatomically or chemically. He held that congenital psychopathic disposition or diathesis is essentially recognizable as sensitiveness (*Zartheit*); the effect of congenital psychopathic taint (*Belastung*) appears as eccentricity, egotism, violent outbursts; and congenital psychopathic degeneration can take a severely antisocial or asocial form, midway between mental disorders and mental normality: neither fish nor flesh, nor good red herring.

Koch's orderly and emphatically confident presentation led to the adoption during the ensuing 20 or 30 years of some of his terminology and much of his theorizing. Müller in 1899 wrote

207

that moral insanity is only a prominent symptom of a psychopathic state: the term had been under heavy fire but might be retained for forensic use. Tiling in 1896 offered 'perversion of character' as an equivalent for 'congenital moral degeneration'. The term 'inferiority' did not last long, however, probably because it connoted a value-judgment which medical usage repudiated. For a considerable period 'psychopathic' was not open to this objection. As Gruhle (1953) kept repeating, the concept of psychopathy implies nothing more than that a person's disposition or temperament deviates appreciably from the average. Gradually, however, this ethically and socially neutral significance was submerged so that a psychopath came to be classified as 'antisocial', or was renamed 'sociopath'.

KRAEPELIN'S CHANGING EMPHASIS

The plainest indicator of the changing notion of this condition is provided by the successive editions of Kraepelin's textbook. In his second edition (1887) he put insanity in the group of congenital defects (*Schwachsinn*); it consists in 'deficiency of those forces which restrain the individual living in society from reckless gratification of his immediate egotistical inclinations'. Impulsive insanity and obsessions are included in the same group. In considering the role of heredity and predisposition, he gives the views of Morel much weight. Nine years later, in his fifth edition of 1896, Kraepelin places psychopathic states among the constitutional disorders; they are life-long morbid personalities, 'mental dystrophies' (*seelische Entwicklungshemmungen*). In this formulation the influence of Lombroso is discernible. The next edition of Kraepelin's textbook (1899) presents psychopathic states as a form of degeneration, along with 'impulsive insanity', obsessions, constitutional depression, and sexual perversions. Harking back to Koch, Kraepelin enlarges the class of 'psychopathic inferiorities' to fill the extensive intermediate territory between indisputable insanity and mental health.

In the 7th edition (1903–1904) the emphasis is on degeneration.

'In the great area of degenerative insanity (*Entartung-sirresein*) it is practicably impossible to delimit

definite varieties: the artificially contrived groups overlap at every point. We will therefore keep two big divisions separate—"original states" and "psychopathic personalities". . . . We will designate as psychopathic personalities those peculiar morbid forms of personality development which we have grounds for regarding as degenerative'.

Kraepelin, however, was uneasy about his far-flung concept of degeneration:

'The characteristic of degeneration is a lasting morbid reaction to the stresses of life, an inappropriateness in thinking, feeling or willing throughout life': but, he added, 'if we were to regard degeneration as the source of all those congenital attributes that interfere with the attainment of the general purposes of life, we would find traces of it everywhere.'

The 8th edition (1909–1915) describes psychopaths as showing inferiority in affect (*Gemutsleben*) or in the development of mature volition (*Willensausbildung*). They can be divided into those with the stamp of morbid predisposition (obsessional neurosis, impulsive insanity, and sexual deviation) and those with the stamp of personal peculiarity.

It is plain that Kraepelin found the classification of these conditions defeating, as he frankly admits. Successive editions show him struggling, with little success, to cope with the task of shaping categories out of the rich variety of human character and conduct. His efforts and his failure are characteristic examples of the frustration which besets students of personality when they aim at precision. 'All typologies place boundaries where boundaries do not belong. They are artificial categories . . . each theorist slices nature in any way he chooses, and finds only his own cuttings worthy of admiration' (Allport, 1938).

An approach from the standpoint of dynamic psychopathology has not been helpful. It might be expected that psychoanalytical formulations would be illuminating; but they do not attempt a thoroughgoing classification. Alexander (1952) minimized the difficulty:

'This group of behaviour disorders has long baffled psychiatrists and the diagnosis psychopathic personality has come to be considered a waste-basket diagnosis. From the psychodynamic point of view, however, this diagnosis is not more difficult to make than any other diagnosis of a neurosis. The differential criterion is neurotic acting-out versus neurotic symptoms.'

Edward Glover (1955), on the other hand, regards the condition as prepsychotic or larval; but

'until more detailed subdivisions are effected there is something to be said for the otherwise vague caption psychopathy, provided of course we recognize three main subgroups: (a) sexual psychopathy ... (b) "benign" psychopathy in which social incapacity is the main feature, accompanied, however, usually by psychosexual disorder, and (c) antisocial psychopathy of a more malignant type in which delinquent outbursts associated with a variable degree of sexual maladjustment develop in an otherwise unstable ego'.

Kraepelin's adoption of 'psychopathic personality' led to general decline in the use of 'moral insanity' and 'moral imbecility', but Prichard's terms did not suffer total extinction. There was, moreover, an appreciable lag before 'psychopathic personality' became the accepted designation in English speaking countries. This occurred in the 1920s.

Mercier in 1914 had contemptuously referred to forms of chronic insanity which 'may be divided into two important classes or subtypes, and a rabble of others which need not be considered here'. But in 1922 Smith, a progressive prison doctor, wrote under the heading 'psychopaths', that

'there exists a class of persons who are not insane nor mentally defective ... their mental condition is such that they are unable to make proper adjustments to the demands of society ... the group is of very mixed character and it is not easy to settle on any satisfactory classification. We have practically no form of classification of them in this country. So the author proposes to adopt the classification suggested by the Surgeon General of the United States Army.'

Among the subdivisions of psychopathy, Smith listed inadequate personality, emotional instability, paranoid personality, pathological lying, and sexual anomalies. A separate class of offenders, the 'constitutionally infirm' are 'unbalanced and their power of inhibition is lessened. Their conduct is impulsive and variable'.

Smith borrowed from American psychiatrists who in their turn had borrowed from the German writers, especially Kraepelin.

It is not easy to account for the persistence of the term 'moral insanity' (though in a dwindling degree) when so many influential authorities, especially in Germany, pointed to its demerits. The chief sustaining factors seem to have been its use in the courts, and its place in legislation covering the commitment of mentally defective persons (Anderson, 1962). In the 1913 Act 'moral imbeciles' were defined as 'persons who from an early age display some permanent mental defect, coupled with strong vicious or criminal propensities on which punishment has had little or no deterrent effect'. The 1927 Amending Act defined 'moral defectives'. In the Mental Health Act 1960 the slate was wiped clean and 'psychopathic disorder' was given official recognition; it was defined as

'a persistent disorder or disability of mind (whether or not including subnormality of intelligence) which results in abnormally aggressive or seriously irresponsible conduct on the part of the patient, and requires or is susceptible to treatment'.

Among the many criticisms of this definition the most obvious centres on the clause which runs 'requires or is susceptible to treatment'; the opinion of psychiatrists or other competent experts as to who requires or is susceptible to treatment will inevitably tend to be subjective and inconsistent.

THE LAST 50 YEARS

There have been many comprehensive reviews of the state of opinion about psychopathic personality during the last 50 years. In Great Britain Henderson (1939), Curran and Mallinson (1944), and Craft (1966); in Germany Schneider (1958), Birnbaum (1926), Kahn (1936), Dubitscher (1936), and Binder (1960); in France Trillat (1965), and Delmas (1943); in the United States Jenkins (1960), Gurvitz (1951), Robins (1967), Carlson and Dain (1962), Maughs (1941), McCord and McCord (1956). These reveal a preoccupation with the nosological status of the concept (latterly influenced by Jaspers), its forensic implications, its subdivisions and limits;

the propriety of identifying psychopathic personality with antisocial behaviour; semantic niceties—for example, the distinction between dyssocial and asocial; cerebral damage as a cause; genetic factors, especially sex chromosome anomalies. The effect of reading solid blocks of this literature is disheartening; there is so much fine-spun theorizing, repetitive argument, and therapeutic gloom ('to me therefore the psychopath, no matter what his age, is a child delinquent, who has never profited by experience, has rarely been benefited by medical, social or punitive measures. He is so unpredictable in his reactions that he is the most dangerous member of society': Henderson, 1939).

The majority of fairly recent writers on the subject deplore the looseness and bias which vitiate attempts at defining it: 'discussion of the prognosis and treatment of all these various types of vulnerable, unusual, abnormal and sociopathic characters, now all lumped together as psychopathic personalities, must embrace so many factors that it cannot profitably be undertaken before more agreement has been reached on questions of definition and delimitation' (Curran and Mallinson, 1944). The difficulty is not evaded by making the definition short and sweet:

'abnorme Persönlichkeiten die an ihrer Abnormität leiden oder unter deren Abnormität die Gesellschaft leidet [People of abnormal personality who suffer through their abnormality or cause society to suffer through it]' (Schneider); 'der Begriff der Psychopathie besagt nichts weiter als dass die Anlagen eines Menschen vom Durchschnitt erheblich abweichen [The concept of psychopathy amounts to no more than that the predisposition (*Anlage*) of a man deviates appreciably from the average]' (Gruhle, 1953).

Detailed definition is likewise unsatisfactory:

'Diese psychopathischen Konstitutionen hängen ursächlich und wesensgemäss mit jenem Erscheinungskreis zusammen den man biologisch als Entartung zu kennzeichnen pflegt i.e. eine von der Norm ungünstig abweichende biologische Degenerationsform von erblichem Charakter [These "psychiatric constitutions" belong in causation and essential nature, to that class of phenomena which we are accustomed to designate as degenerative—that is, as a form of hereditary degeneration which shows

adverse departure from the biological norm]' (Birnbaum, 1926).

An inherent problem is how to agree on the range of the normal personality and the tenable criteria of mental illness. Failure in this is attested by the absurd discrepancies between different people's estimate of the prevalence of psychopathy (Wallin, 1949).

For the purposes of the WHO classification of diseases a provisional definition might run

'Psychopathic personality is a condition in which ingrained maladaptive patterns of behaviour are recognizable by the time of adolescence or earlier, and are continuous throughout life; the personality is abnormal in the balance and quality of its components.'

Like every other attempt at defining psychopathic personality this is open admittedly, but perhaps inevitably, to criticism on several counts. Neither 'maladaptive patterns of behaviour', nor 'balance of the components of personality', nor their quality are matters of direct observation: individual investigators will no doubt differ rather widely in judging them. The definition might, moreover, be thought too inclusive; it would, for example, cover the postencephalitic behaviour disorders and might be taken to embrace also sexual perversions. But the main difficulty is occasioned by our unsuccess in nailing normal personality down, either as a whole or in its components.

CONCEPTS OF PSYCHOLOGISTS

It is surprising that psychiatrists have paid little attention to the methods and concepts of psychologists in this field. The reason may be practical:

'Many personality qualities can be measured or diagnosed fairly effectively, but the methods are far too elaborate and time consuming, or far too dependent on the skill and experience of the psychologist, to be generally applicable for any practical purposes, or to be used by anyone not specially trained. True, it is possible to suggest some improvements on the unreliable methods that the layman habitually employs' (Vernon, 1953).

In a similarly cautious and tolerant vein Gordon

210

Allport concluded that there is no one-and-only method for the study of personality

'in respect to accuracy and reliability some of the segmental methods are to be preferred; in respect to adequacy of approach the various synthetic or relational methods are better . . . it is something of a struggle to strike a balance between excessively rigid and perfectionalistic standards (that accomplish nothing but a sterilization of research, limiting it to worthless fragments of behaviour having no essential bearing upon personality) and loose standards that permit wanton assertions and extravagant claims to go without check or proof' (Allport, 1938).

Some psychologists who have concerned themselves with the measurement of factors affecting psychopathy have, like some psychiatrists, put psychopathy essentially on the same footing as delinquency: 'the psychopath presents the riddle of delinquency in a particularly pure form'. Eysenck, commenting on the tendency of the psychopaths to exhibit traits of extraversion, makes it pungently clear that in his view if there is a failure of correlation between questionnaire and psychiatric ratings, this indicates 'faults in the psychiatric ratings, both as regards validity and reliability, and it might further be suggested, not that the questionnaire has no value as a clinical tool but rather that the psychiatric diagnosis has no value as a clinical tool' (Eysenck and Eysenck, 1969). The extensive studies of Quay and his associates on adolescents yielded two large factors, one of which, betokening impulsiveness, rebelliousness and lack of emotional involvement, they called 'psychopathy': it correlated with recidivism, institutionalization, and crimes against the person.

Another assiduous inquirer into this problem (Foulds, 1965) has maintained that

'egocentricity, lack of empathy, and treating others as objects, in the absence of the necessary and sufficient conditions for making a diagnosis of personal illness, are themselves necessary and sufficient conditions for the identification of psychopaths, at least when they are present in such degree that they lead the individuals concerned to conflict with the law or to their being brought for treatment'.

Foulds touches on a crucial issue when he puts forward his argument that traits and attitudes emphasize the continuity of behaviour, whereas symptoms and signs of illness emphasize the discontinuities. Attacks of illness or violence may punctuate the course of psychopathy, but cannot be intrinsic and necessary features of it.

The conclusion of the whole matter is somewhat gloomy. The diagnostic groupings of psychiatry seldom have sharp and definite limits. Some are worse than others in this respect. Worst of all is psychopathic personality, within its wavering confines. Its outline will not be firm until much more is known about its genetics, psychopathology, and neuropathology.

REFERENCES

Alexander, F. (1952). *Dynamic Psychiatry.* University of Chicago Press: Chicago.
Allport, G. W. (1938). *Personality. A Psychological Interpretation.* Constable: London.
Anderson, E. W. (1962). The official concept of psychopathic personality in England. In *Psychopathologie Heute*, pp. 243–251. Herausg. von H. Kranz. Thieme: Stuttgart.
Binder, H. (1960). Die psychopathischen Dauerzustände und die abnormen seelischen Reaktionen und Entwicklungen. In *Psychiatrie der Gegenwart*, pp. 180–202. Edited by H. W. Gruhle, R. Jung, W. Mayer-Gross, and M. Müller. Springer: Berlin.
Birnbaum, K. (1926). *Die psychopathischen Verbrecher.* 2. Aufl. Thieme: Leipzig.
Bunke, O. (1912). *Über nervöse Entartung.* Springer: Berlin.
Carlson, E. T., and Dain, N. (1962). The meaning of moral insanity. *Bulletin of the History of Medicine*, **36**, 130–140.
Craft, M. (editor). (1966). *Psychopathic Disorders and Their Assessment.* Pergamon: London.
Curran, D., and Mallinson, P. (1944). Psychopathic personality. *Journal of Mental Science*, **90**, 266–286.
Delmas, F.-A. (1943). Les constitutions psychopathiques. *Annales Médico-psychologiques*, 101e année, **1**, 219–232.
Dubitscher (1936). Der moralische Schwachsinn. *Zeitschrift für die gesamte Neurologie und Psychiatrie*, **154**, 422–457.
Esquirol, J.-E.-D. (1838). *Des Maladies Mentales.* 2 vols. J.-B. Baillière: Paris.
Eysenck, H. J., and Eysenck, S. B. G. (1969). *Personality Structure and Measurement.* Routledge: London.
Foulds, G. A. (1965). *Personality and Personal Illness.* Tavistock: London.
Glover, E. (1955). *The Technique of Psycho-analysis.* Baillière: London.
Gröhmann (1818). Psychologie der Verbrecher aus Geisteskrankheiten oder Desorganisationen. *Zeitschrift für psychische Aerzte*, **1**, 174–189.
Gruhle, H. W. (1953). *Verstehen und Einfühlen.* Springer: Berlin.
Gurvitz, M. (1951). Developments in the concept of psychopathic personality (1900–1950). *British Journal of Delinquency*, **2**, 88–102.
Henderson, D. K. (1939). *Psychopathic States.* Chapman and Hall: London.
Henderson, D., and Gillespie, R. D. (1932). *A Text-book of Psychiatry:* 3rd edn. Oxford University Press: London.
Jaspers, K. (1965). *Allgemeine Psychopathologie.* 8. Aufl. Springer: Berlin.
Jenkins, R. L. (1960). The psychopathic or antisocial personality. *Journal of Nervous and Mental Disease*, **131**, 318–334.

Kahn, E. (1936). The psychopathic personalities. In *The Oxford Medicine*, Vol. 7, *Psychiatry for Practitioners*, pp. 239–255. Edited by H. A. Christian. Oxford University Press: New York.

Koch, J. L. A. (1891). *Die psychopathischen Minderwertig-keiten*. Maier: Ravensburg.

Kraepelin, E. (1887). *Psychiatrie*. 2nd edn. Abel: Leipzig.

Kraepelin, E. (1896). *Psychiatrie*. 5th edn. Barth: Leipzig.

Kraepelin, E. (1899). *Psychiatrie*. 2 vols. 6th edn. Barth: Leipzig.

Kraepelin, E. (1903–1904). *Psychiatrie*. 2 vols. 7th edn. Barth: Leipzig.

Kraepelin, E. (1909–1915). *Psychiatrie*. 4 vols. 8th edn. Barth: Leipzig.

Magnan, V. (1893). *Leçons Cliniques sur les Maladies Mentales*. Battaille: Paris.

McCord, W., and McCord, J. (1956). *Psychopathy and Delinquency*. Grune and Stratton: New York.

Maudsley, H. (1874). *Responsibility in Mental Disease*. King: London.

Maughs, S. B. (1941). A concept of psychopathic personality. *Journal of Criminal Psychopathology*, **2**, 329–356; 465–499.

Morel, B.-A. (1839). *Traité des Dégénérescences Physiques, Intellectuelles et Morales de l'Espèce Humaine*. J.-B. Baillière: Paris.

Müller, E. (1899). Ueber 'moral insanity'. *Archiv für Psychiatrie*, **31**, 325–377.

Mercier, C. A. (1914). *A Text-book of Insanity*. 2nd edn. Allen and Unwin: London.

Partridge, G. E. (1930). Current conceptions of psychopathic personality. *American Journal of Psychiatry*, **10**, 53–99.

Pinel, P. (1801). *Traité Medico-philosophique sur L'Aliénaiton Mentale*. Richard, Caille et Ravier: Paris.

Prichard, J. C. (1835). *A Treatise on Insanity*. Sherwood, Gilbert, and Piper: London.

Quay, H. C. (1964). Personality dimensions in delinquent males as inferred from the factor analysis of behavior ratings. *Journal of Research in Crime and Delinquency*, **1**, 33–37.

Robins, E. (1967). *Anti-Social and Dyssocial Personality Disorders. A Text Book of Psychiatry*, pp. 951–958. Edited by A. M. Freedman and H. Kaplan. Williams and Wilkins: Baltimore.

Savage. G. H. (1881). Moral insanity. *Journal of Mental Science*, **27**, 147–155.

Schneider, K. (1958). *Psychopathic Personalities*. Translated by M. W. Hamilton. Cassell: London.

Smith, M. (1922). *The Psychology of the Criminal*. Methuen: London.

Tiling, Th. (1896). Ueber angeborene moralische Degeneration oder Perversität des Charakters. *Allgemeine Zeitschrift für Psychiatrie*, **521**, 258–313.

Trillat, E. (1965). Les déséquilibrés. 3. In *Encyclopédie Medico-Chirurgicale*. Psychiatrie, 37310 A10. Paris.

Tuke, D. H. (editor). (1892). *A Dictionary of Psychological Medicine*. 2 vols. Churchill: London.

Vernon, P. E. (1953). *Personality Tests and Assessments*. Methuen: London.

Wallin, J. E. W. (1949). *Children with Mental and Physical Handicaps*. Staples: London.

Wolfgang, M. E. (1960). Cesare Lombroso. In *Pioneers in Criminology*, pp. 168–227. Edited by H. Mannheim. Stevens: London.

The survival of hysteria

AUBREY LEWIS

From the Institute of Psychiatry, The Maudsley Hospital, London

SYNOPSIS There have been many battles in the last 100 years between those who consider hysteria to be a 'morbid entity' or 'disease' and those who would like to drop it once and for all. The controversy still goes on. It has not been settled by follow-up studies or by applying genetic considerations. Hysteria is a tough subject, unlikely to be killed so long as clinicians find it useful, if not indispensable.

In psychiatry there are forms of illness, with names going back two and a half millennia, which have had sentence of death passed upon them more than once, yet they obstinately survive. Paranoia is one such condition and term, hysteria is another. Hysteria is indeed an extreme case. Built upon a false and absurd notion of pathology, it was inevitably the subject of controversy, ridicule, and denial. Funeral orations upon it have often been delivered in the last 100 years, in language appropriate to the state of psychiatric knowledge. Thus, of English writers on the subject, in 1874 W. B. Carpenter described it as

'a state of the nervous system which is characterized by its peculiar excitability, but in which there is no such fixed tendency to irregular action as would indicate any positive disease.'

A quarter of a century later Ormerod (1899) wrote that the objections to 'hysteria' are obvious:

'not only that it has become etymologically meaningless but also that to many minds it has the disagreeable connotation of a certain moral feebleness in the patient, and of unreality in the symptoms.'

In 1965 another English physician, Slater, expressed forcefully his contemporary objections.

'All the signs of "hysteria" are the signs not of disease but of health ... there is nothing at all consistent in the medical condition of the patients who get diagnosed as "hysterics" ... no evidence has yet been offered that the patients diagnosed as suffering from "hysteria" are in medically significant terms anything more than a random selection.'

These indictments, which have been reinforced by clinical and genetic evidence, are paralleled by similarly destructive arguments put forward by notable French, Swiss, and German psychiatrists. There is a long series of these, worth recalling. In 1902 Hoche said roundly, 'Hysteria is not a syndrome [*Krankheitsbild*] but a special form of mental disposition'. Dubois (1904) put it on record that 'il est inutile de s'efforcer de donner à l'hystérie le caractère d'une entité morbide'. Steyerthal (1908) predicted

'within a few years the concept of hysteria will belong to history ... there is no such disease, and there never has been. What Charcot called hysteria is a tissue woven of a thousand threads, a cohort of the most varied diseases, with nothing in common but the so-called stigmata, which in fact may accompany any disease.'

Gaupp (1911) said

'Nowadays the cry is ever louder: away with the name and the concept of hysteria: there is no such thing, and what we call hysteria is either an artificial, iatrogenic product, or a melange of symptoms which can occur in all sorts of illnesses and are not pathognomonic of anything'.

Bumke (1925) reviewed the neuroses and declared 'There was once a disease hysteria, just as there was hypochondria, and neurasthenia. They have disappeared. The syndrome has replaced the disease entity.' Kraepelin (1927) said: 'Hysteria is not a sharply delimited syndrome but a special way of dealing with affective tensions; it can occur in very different morbid conditions in

213

which inner excitement is not adequately kept under control.' Moerchen (1929) simply entitled his diatribe 'Hysteria is not a disease'. Kranz (1953) concluded that

'hysterical phenomena are only modes of reaction which fundamentally are available to everybody and are not in themselves abnormal, but become so in that they last unduly long, become fixed, or are excessive. . . . It is reasonable to ask that we should at least drop the word "hysteria" in favour of "hysterical reaction", and in the end give up this term too, loaded as it is with moral value-judgments: we can make ourselves understood by psychiatrists without it. But in spite of all that "hysteria" will not disappear altogether from psychiatric vocabulary for a long time to come.'

Rouquier (1960) confidently wrote on 'la fin de l'hystérie'. And in the most recent French textbook (1964) Pierre Marchais adjures us 'si nous conservons le terme "hystérique", étant donné son caractère traditionnel, il faut bien reconnaître qu'il mériterait d'être abandonné pour deux raisons essentielles'.

UPHOLDERS OF THE TERM

This is an imposing cloud of witnesses. Many more could be cited who testify similarly. But opposite this array there are the upholders of the term, who believe it to be a significant and justified designation of a diagnostic category that has equivalent title-deeds to that of obsessional neurosis and anxiety state. Charcot stated his position unequivocally: hysteria is a mental disorder par excellence. Before him Briquet (1859) had seized the bull similarly by the horns:

'l'hystérie est loin d'être une affection composée de phenomènes incohérents. . . . Je trouvais au contraire qu'elle constituait une affection dont il état tres facile de comprendre la nature, dont tous les symptômes avaient leurs analogues dans l'état physiologique et n'ayant de bizarre que l'apparence . . . dont le diagnostic pouvait se faire aussi sûrement et avec autant de précision que celui de tout autre maladie.'

Régis (1914) avowed his faith with firm simplicity:

'on connait ces débats retentissants qui ont eu lieu en 1908 sur l'hystérie. . . . Nous croyons donc, pour l'observer de près et impartialement tous les jours

que, quelle que soit la façon dont on l'envisage, sous le jour ancien ou sous le jour nouveau, il y a une hystérie, et que cette hystérie, comme l'épilepsie . . . s'accompagne fréquemment de troubles psychiques.'

Much later (1941) one finds a prominent American psychiatrist, Stanley Cobb, declaring that 'hysteria, in the particular sense in which I believe it should be used, is a fairly clear-cut syndrome'.

DEFINING DISEASE

From this welter of powerful opposing voices two main assertions can be picked out: that hysteria is not a disease; and that hysteria is not a syndrome. Obviously the meaning attached to these two terms 'disease' and 'syndrome' is a cardinal issue in the controversy. Those who refuse the name of 'disease' or 'morbid entity' to any condition that has not been demonstrated to have an anatomical or chemical pathology must clearly now refuse it to hysteria: even if we will not go so far as Hoche, who said that it does not have, and never will have, a basis in pathological anatomy, it is at present in that exposed state. It must, however, also be said that our present ignorance, or limited knowledge, of the somatic pathology of schizophrenia should lead to a similar refusal to call that a disease. This is, of course, not merely a semantic quibble, nor a modern difficulty. Although a few writers, like Szasz, insist that mental illness is a myth, and that the only real illness is bodily illness, the majority of psychiatrists have no desire to adopt this crude standpoint, or to differentiate psychoses from neuroses on the ground that the former have—or must be assumed to have—a somatic basis; they have, however, substituted 'reaction type' or 'syndrome' for 'disease'. Adolf Meyer was largely responsible for this change of language and approach in the English-speaking countries: the same movement occurred in France, as Henri Ey (1954) makes clear in his *Études*. Hysteria, then, in modern usage is not a disease; but neither is schizophrenia or melancholia. The hysterical reaction may be a manifestation of a somatic abnormality, as a paranoid psychosis or a manic excitement may likewise be, and in each such case multi-dimensional analysis will take into account constitutional predisposition as well as environmental and physical

214

influences spread over the lifetime of the affected person.

If by common consent the term 'reaction-type' or 'reaction' is applied to hysteria, the chief opportunity for divergent views will be afforded by the personality. Some will be reluctant, or wholly unwilling, to make the diagnosis of hysteria unless the patient's personality is of the supposedly hysterical pattern; while others—the majority, very likely—will be so familiar with the many varieties of personality that may be found in people with a full-blown hysterical reaction that they will refrain, as Kretschmer and many other psychiatrists have, from expecting or requiring a recognizable hysterical personality when diagnosing hysteria, though certain broad characteristics are remarkably frequent and conspicuous.

FOLLOW-UP STUDIES

If instead of hysterical reactions we speak of the hysterical syndrome, then the questions on which Slater and other writers have dwelt will be to the fore—namely, is the clinical picture uniform? And does the course of the disorder show that its pattern remains consistent? Having made two follow-up studies Slater concluded that there is very little consistency: thus when patients who had been diagnosed at a neurological hospital as having hysteria were followed up seven or more years later a few were found to have organic disease which had not been recognized, and those in whom no evidence of organic disease had been found included two now diagnosed as schizophrenics, an obsessional, and seven depressed patients. The remainder fell into two groups—one of mostly young people with acute psychogenic reactions of the conversion type, and the other composed of patients with a lasting personality disorder and a history of attention-getting, manipulative behaviour, and excess of hospitalization. Slater had obtained somewhat similar results in a follow-up study of patients diagnosed as having 'hysteria' at a psychiatric hospital; and others who have conducted follow-up inquiries into hysteria have, as he indicates, made similar observations. He therefore concludes that there is nothing consistent in the medical condition of patients diagnosed as hysterics; they are medically a random selection

of patients, with many sorts of illness. He compares his findings with those of five other follow-up studies and accounts for their diversity by supposing that the later state of the patients depended not on the natural history of the condition but on the diverse operational definitions of it in accordance with which they had been selected as having hysteria.

I made a comparable follow-up inquiry upon patients in whom the diagnosis of hysteria had been made at the Maudsley Hospital over a five-year period: the follow-up was carried out between seven and 12 years later. There were 73 women and 25 men who could be traced: information about their later condition was obtained by an interview with the patient and with a close relative, or in some cases by correspondence with them or their doctor. The relatively large number of patients traced and interviewed was wholly due to the skill and thoroughness of an experienced psychiatric social worker, Miss Margery Seward.

The results were diverse, but not appreciably more so than when a group of schizophrenic or depressive patients is followed up. Seven of the women had died, three from conditions unconnected with their psychiatric affection, three from a probable affection of the central nervous system, and one by suicide. Forty were well and working, free from disabling or troublesome symptoms. A third of the remainder were consistently better than at the time of original admission, though still troubled; a fifth worse than at admission; the condition of the rest was much the same as it had been eight to 12 years before. In the majority of those who had not recovered their mental health, anomalies of personality and social adjustment had been conspicuous first to last, and the stresses to which they had been exposed during the interim period were steady and continuous or practically identical with those recognized at the initial consultations. Eight of the patients had a depressive syndrome, sufficiently accounted for by their situation and social or other environmental difficulties, and showing a strong tincture of hypochondriasis. In none of the patients did the retrospective diagnosis of schizophrenia seem to be justified.

The male group was smaller, and slightly older: the average age on admission was 33,

2 1 5

whereas that of the women was 31. None of the men had died, and 14 of the 25 were well and working at the time of the follow-up. Of the remaining 11, two were improved, four were much as they had been when first seen, and five had become worse: two of these were in a mental hospital, with diagnoses of schizophrenia, and another, who had had a severe fall, had evidently passed into a state of dementia. In both the men and the women the residual psychiatric illness in those who had not recovered was remarkably close in its main features to the clinical picture presented at the time of original admission. The individual case histories show, of course, special factors and personal vicissitudes which coloured the illness, but in very few did this raise the question of an altered diagnosis; and in none besides those mentioned above did this amount to more than a switch from 'hysteria' to 'depressive hypochondriasis' or 'unstable, maladjusted personality'; in one patient euphoria and lability of mood, which had been present according to his wife for years, could be regarded as a mild hypomania.

A diagnosis made eight or 12 years after an earlier psychiatric assessment is not necessarily more correct than the previous one. It is open to those who have made quite different follow-up observations on hysterics to dispute the diagnoses made here on the later occasion, and to suspect that schizophrenics and manic-depressives may have been overlooked. But the findings do not differ seriously from those arrived at by Ljungberg on a much larger sample. That they are not similar to the findings on patients diagnosed at a neurological hospital is not surprising.

A TOUGH OLD WORD

The later state of these patients cannot be held to gainsay the acceptability of the diagnosis 'hysteria' so long as it is regarded as a reaction. There may be other grounds for annihilating the concept, and it is coming too close to the *argumentum ad hominem* to maintain, as Ajuriaguerra has, that

'tous les médecins ne réagiront pas d'une manière égale devant l'hystérique. Il est trop près de nous pour que nous ne réagissions pas d'une manière sentimentale ou aggressive. La forme aggressive consiste à nier l'hystérie en tant que maladie ayant

les caractéristiques determinées. L'accepter dans la nosographie serait révaloriser l'hystérie, faire rentrer les troubles des passions ou des anormalités proches du vice dans le cadre du pathologique et minimiser ainsi la valeur des vertus.'

One need not impute to those prosecutors who ask for the death sentence on hysteria any but objective grounds for their plea: Slater, for example, has advanced genetic evidence in support of his negative contention. But the majority of psychiatrists would be hard put to it if they could no longer make a diagnosis of 'hysteria' or 'hysterical reaction'; and in any case a tough old word like hysteria dies very hard. It tends to outlive its obituarists.

I am grateful to the editor and publishers of *Evolution Psychiatrique* for allowing this article to be published in English.

REFERENCES

Ajuriaguerra, J. (1951). Le problème de l'hystérie. *L'Encéphale*, 40, 50–87.
Briquet, P. (1859). *Traité Clinique et Thérapeutique de l'Hystérie*. J. B. Baillière: Paris.
Bumke, O. (1925). Die Revision der Neurosenfrage. *Zentralblatt für die gesamte Neurologie und Psychiatrie*, 41, 669–677.
Carpenter, W. B. (1874). *Principles of Mental Physiology*. King: London.
Cobb, S. (1941). *Foundations of Neuropsychiatry*. 2nd edn. Williams and Wilkins: Baltimore.
Dubois, P. (1904). *Les Psychonévroses et leur Traitement Moral; Leçons Faites à l'Université de Berne*. Masson: Paris.
Ey, H. (1954). *Études Psychiatriques*. Desclée de Brouwer: Paris.
Gaupp, R. (1911). Über den Begriff der Hysterie. *Zeitschrift für die gesamte Neurologie und Psychiatrie*.
Hoche, A. (1902). *Die Differentialdiagnose zwischen Epilepsie und Hysterie*. Hirschwald: Berlin.
Kraepelin, E. (1927). *Psychiatrie. 5 Auflage*. Barth: Leipzig.
Kranz, H. (1953). Die Entwicklung des Hysterie-Begriffs, *Fortschritte der Neurologie und Psychiatrie*, 21, 223–238.
Ljungberg, L. (1957). Hysteria. A clinical, prognostic and genetic study. *Acta Psychiatrica et Neurologica Scandinavica*, 32, Suppl. 112.
Marchais, P. (1964). *Psycho-pathologie en Pratique Médicale*. Masson: Paris.
Moerchen, F. (1929). 2. Hysterie ist keine Krankheit! Die Verwirrung des Neurosebegriffs. *Zeitschrift für ärztliche Fortbildung*, 26, 686–690.
Ormerod, J. A. (1899). In *A System of Medicine*, Vol. 8, 88–127. Edited by T. C. Allbutt.
Regis, E. (1914). *Précis de Psychiatrie*. 5th edn. Doin: Paris.
Rouquier, A. (1960). La fin de l'hystérie. *Annales Médico-Psychologiques*, 118, T.2, 528.
Slater, E. (1961). "Hysteria 311." The thirty-fifth Maudsley Lecture. *Journal of Mental Science*, 107, 359–381.
Steyerthal, A. (1908). *Was ist Hysterie?* Halle a. S.: Marhold.
Szasz, T. S. (1961). *The Myth of Mental Illness*. Harper: New York.

216

A note on classifying phobia

AUBREY LEWIS

Late of the Institute of Psychiatry, Denmark Hill, London

SYNOPSIS   The increasing interest in the treatment of phobias underlines the need for clarifying their definition and classification. A brief historical note highlights some of the difficulties which have been, and still are, encountered.

The much acclaimed response of phobic states to behaviour therapy has stimulated interest in these disorders and promoted their classification. The position may be dogmatically stated: 'If ever we are tempted to think that all phobic states are a unity which reflects the same disorder and aetiology, we can quickly dispel this illusion simply by looking at the startling contrast between animal phobias and agoraphobias. These two conditions differ radically in onset, course, symptomatology, response to treatment and psychophysiological measures' (Marks, 1970).

The term 'phobia' is used so loosely that one is uncertain whether it refers to a symptom, a symptom complex or an anomaly of personality. Its nosological relation to obsessional disorder is left unclear; its psychopathology remains controversial. Its use as a technical term in psychiatry may be said to date from 1872, when Westphal's classic article appeared, but the condition to which it refers has been repeatedly put on record from the 5th century onwards; Errera (1962) has listed a number of these. An explicit instance (overlooked by Errera) is an article by Benjamin Rush, published in 1798: 'I shall define phobia to be a fear of an imaginary evil, or an undue fear of a real one. The following species appear to belong to it.' Rush then catalogues 18 species named according to the object of excessive fear or aversion, e.g. dirt phobias, rat phobia.

The appearance of Westphal's clear-cut paper led to lively interest in agoraphobia and, treading closely on its heels, claustrophobia, originally called clitrofobia by the Bologna psychiatrist, Raggi (1877). In 1872 Cordes published an elaborate report of his fairly extensive experience of agoraphobia (which, however, he angrily refused to call by the Greek name). Like Benedict and several other contemporaries, he pointed to Griesinger's account of giddiness associated with acute anxiety attacks (*Schwindelangst,Platzangst*). German psychiatrists followed Westphal's lead, but the introduction of the diagnostic term led to the erroneous idea of a unitary disease, whereas phobic manifestations appear in many different kinds of clinical disorder.

French psychiatrists speedily entered the field. Pitres & Régis (1902) recognized two classes of phobia: the diffuse and the special or systematic. The systematic phobia is fixed to a specific object; it may be remittent or intermittent. There are occupational phobias: phobias of places, of natural elements (e.g. storms), of morbidity (e.g. infections), and of living creatures (e.g. snakes, rats). After naming some 70 of these (bedecked with Greek labels) Pitres & Régis emphasized that they belong to a sort of synoptic table, with no pretension to being a nosological classification.

The relation to obsessions was a crux. Pitres & Régis regarded phobias and obsessions not as distinct conditions but as two degrees of the same condition, differing only in the proportion of the two elements – emotional and ideational – which constitute them. Other distinguished pyschiatrists have, however, included phobias in the larger class of obsessions, e.g. 'Man zählt zu den Zwangsideen auch die Phobien' (Bleuler, 1916).

Janet (1903), following Pitres & Régis (1902), classified the systematic and the diffuse phobias as *agitations émotionelles*, which were taken to be a variety of *agitations forcées*. Recent French writers on phobia use the terms 'symptom', 'neurosis' and 'character' without making any

217

exact distinction (Ey *et al.*, 1974; Perrier & Conte, 1961). They are, however, disposed to make a differential diagnosis between obsessional and phobic neuroses: 'This diagnosis is often difficult but it is very important because it largely constitutes the indication for psychotherapy.' It is stated, though on somewhat shaky evidence, that a definite obsessional neurosis has a poorer response to analytic treatment than a phobic neurosis.

Indications for psychotherapy can hardly be determined with any assurance while classification is so ragged and the course so unpredictable: 'Il peut arriver que la névrose se stabilise, même avec des symptômes génants, si les conduites d'évitement et de rassurement sont assez efficaces et si le jeu des pulsions et des défenses réalise un equilibre au moins précaire.' Epidemiological investigation is chiefly called for.

Some American psychiatrists prefer the term 'phobic reaction', but they too deplore the widespread disarray arising from the general imprecision of language that prevails in this area. The phobic reaction is technically classified under the heading of 'psychoneurotic disorder'. The condition was formerly classified as anxiety hysteria (Freud), and the current designation still reflects terminological confusion: 'Complicating the issue is a general imprecision of language that pervades the field' (Frazier & Carr, 1967).

English writers (e.g. Marks, 1970; Snaith, 1968) approach the problem tentatively: 'One way of classifying phobic states has been presented, but the clinical material could have been subdivided differently...Possibly the best classification would be one which took into account both the nature of the phobic situation and its specificity' (Marks, 1970).

The latest tribute to the importance of diagnosing phobias carefully comes from the forensic quarter. Some months ago a man who was required by the police to provide a blood specimen for estimation of its alcohol content refused to do so because of his fear of needles. Lord Justice Stephenson then laid it down that 'no fear short of a phobia recognized by medical science to be as strong and inhibiting as, for instance, claustrophobia, could be allowed to excuse failure to provide a laboratory test specimen' (*Times Law Report*, 23 May 1974).

REFERENCES

Bleuler, E. (1916). *Lehrbuch der Psychiatrie.* Springer: Berlin.
Cordes, E. (1872). Die Platzangst (Agoraphobie). *Archiv für Psychiatrie und Nervenkrankheiten* 3, 521–574.
Errera, P. (1962). Some historical aspects of the concept, phobia. *Psychiatric Quarterly* 36, 325–336.
Ey, H., Bernard, P. & Brisset, C. (1974). *Manuel de Psychiatrie.* Masson: Paris.
Frazier, S. H. & Carr, A. C. (1967). Phobic reaction. In A. M. Freedman & H. I. Kaplan (eds.), *Comprehensive Textbook of Psychiatry.* Williams & Wilkins: Baltimore.
Janet, P. (1903). *Les Obsessions et la Psychasthénie.* Alcan: Paris.
Marks, I. M. (1970). The classification of phobic disorders. *British Journal of Psychiatry* 116, 377–386.
Perrier, F. & Conte, C. (1961). Névrose phobique. *Encyclopédie Médico-chirurgicale,* no. 37360. Editions Techniques: Paris.
Pitres, A. & Régis, E. (1902). *Les Obsessions et les Impulsions.* Doin: Paris.
Raggi, A. (1877). Tre casi di clitrofobia. *Rivista Clinica di Bologna,* 2nd ser., 7, 257–261.
Rush, B. (1798). On different species of phobia. *Weekly Magazine* (Philadelphia) 1, 177–180. Quoted in R. Hunter & I. Macalpine (eds.), *Three Hundred Years of Psychiatry.* Oxford University Press: London.
Snaith, R. P. (1968). A clinical investigation of phobias. *British Journal of Psychiatry* 114, 673–697.
Westphal, C. (1872). Die Agoraphobie. *Archiv für Psychiatrie und Nervenkrankheiten* 3, 138–161.

William Mayer-Gross: an appreciation

AUBREY LEWIS[1]

Formerly of the Institute of Psychiatry, London

We are grateful to the editor and publishers of *Confrontations Psychiatriques* for allowing this article to be published in the original English.

THE YEARS IN GERMANY

William Mayer-Gross was born in the ancient Rhineland town of Bingen. He attended the Gymnasium in Worms and studied medicine in Heidelberg, Kiel and Munich. He took his final medical examinations in Heidelberg in 1912. He then became an assistant in the Heidelberg Psychiatric Clinic and in 1913 presented his doctoral thesis, which dealt with the phenomenology of abnormal feelings of felicity. On the outbreak of the First World War he was called up and served for a year on the Western front; he was then in 1915 assigned to duties in a base hospital where neurotic soldiers were being cared for.

When the war ended he returned to his ordinary medical and academic duties in Heidelberg. The head of the clinic at that time was Nissel, who had succeeded Kraepelin. Nissel's achievements and interests were centred on neuroanatomy and neuropathology. He was a conscientious clinician but he had little sympathy or understanding for the psychopathological approach to the problems of psychiatry. Nevertheless he collected a group of able young people around him, who recognized the relative sterility of this approach except for the investigation of a condition like general paralysis, and he gave them his puzzled approval to follow their lights. His attitude is well illustrated by the Referee's Report which he wrote on Mayer-Gross in 1918: he emphasized Mayer-Gross's abilities as an organizer, his extraordinary energy, and his

[1] Address for correspondence: Professor M. Shepherd, Institute of Psychiatry, De Crespigny Park, Denmark Hill, London SE5 8AF.

independent mode of thought; but, Nissel added, the young man's clinical research followed a devious line of thought which Nissel could not always accept. The same could be said of his attitude to the whole group of young psychiatrists which included Jaspers, Gruhle, Kronfeld, Wetzel, Beringer, Homburger and Mayer-Gross. Some of these, however, had joined the Heidelberg staff after Nissel left to take up the post which Kraepelin offered him in the Munich Clinic. He was succeeded by Wilmanns, who wholeheartedly supported the kind of research which the young men were pursuing.

Mayer-Gross worked continuously in the Heidelberg Clinic, except for a period of six months (1922/3) which he spent at Raginau, the Mental Hospital of Zurich, where Eugen Bleuler's influence still prevailed. He seized the opportunity during his stay of bringing up to date some brilliant papers on the psychopathology of the end-states of schizophrenia. He did not, however, succumb to the seductions of dynamic psychopathology, preferring the more objective kind of psychological study in mental illness. He and his colleagues were bent on a phenomenological approach, without theoretical preconceptions; they sought to establish their methodology on precise lines leading eventually to reinterpretation of observed phenomena in approximately physiological terms. I was fortunate enough to spend some months at the Heidelberg Clinic in 1928 and I was struck by the progressive and zestful atmosphere. I was attached to Dr Beringer's firm but had ample opportunity to recognize the stimulating forces at work generally.

Critics were not wholly lacking who maintained that Jaspers was too philosophical, Gruhle too hypercritical, Mayer-Gross too buoyant, but although this often blocked the way of preferment through appointment to senior university posts, it did not prevent the influence of the Heidelberg school from permeating German psychiatry (in much the same way as the work of the Tübingen school under Kretschmer's direction was concurrently attaining recognition). The method and the theory underlying it were not as new, as the Heidelberg aspirants sometimes maintained, but its fruits were undeniable and manifest for all to see. The chief of these was a large volume on schizophrenia, in its multitudinous clinical aspects, which was entrusted by Bumke (the general editor of the Handbuch) to the Heidelberg group, foremost among them in quantity of contribution being Mayer-Gross.

It is worth recalling that it was in the Heidelberg Clinic that Kraepelin introduced the methods of experimental psychology for the study of fatigue, dreams and drugs, but the effect of attempting to continue this work at that time was disillusioning. Mayer-Gross in particular stressed what seemed to him the dangers likely to arise from pseudo-philosophical speculation, and the loose use of inappropriate concepts.

In spite of his obvious abilities, which were widely recognized, Mayer-Gross's career did not take care of itself. He had, it is true, been appointed Deputy Director of the Heidelberg Clinic and Privatdozent, and in 1929 he was appointed Extraordinarius (Associate Professor). He was moreover co-editor, with Beringer, of the *Nervenarzt*, a progressive and highly successful journal of neurology and psychiatry which they founded.

Clouds of political prejudice were gathering; so that, when Mayer-Gross was invited in 1932 to take the chair of psychiatry at Groningen, he found that his Jewish origin made an insuperable obstacle. The course of events in Germany in 1932–3 indicated clearly enough there was no future for Mayer-Gross and many others in their native land. It so happened that the Commonwealth Fund of America could make available the money requisite for a clinical fellowship at the Maudsley Hospital. It provided the wherewithal for Mayer-Gross's immigration. In the following year the Rockefeller Foundation

provided the financial facilities for rescuing a number of Jewish psychiatrists as well as other technicians and scientists. A place was found for several of them in the Maudsley Hospital, chief among them being Eric Guttmann, Alfred Meyer, and Mayer-Gross.

THE YEARS IN BRITAIN

On his arrival in England Mayer-Gross's immediate need was to improve his command of spoken English. His written English was forceful and correct, but in conversation or lecturing he was bold and fluent rather than idiomatic.

In spite of these linguistic difficulties, which can weigh heavily upon the psychiatrist, he and Guttmann (who formed an excellent working partnership) turned their attention to the investigation of organic states, Mayer-Gross paying particular regard to apraxia and agnosia. They soon won the regard and liking due to their ability, helpfulness and character. Although their primary concern was clinical research, they also took their share in teaching and case discussions, and they unobtrusively helped colleagues struggling with the problems of research.

The harmonious co-partnership between Mayer-Gross and Guttmann broke up in 1939 when Mayer-Gross became Director of Research at the Crichton Royal Hospital, a well-endowed mental hospital with exceptional facilities. Guttmann continued at the Maudsley and subsequently at Mill Hill (a private school converted into a hospital for neurotic patients) and in the Brain Injuries Centre at Oxford.

The Crichton Royal Asylum was one of the eight royal hospitals established in Scotland between 1781 and 1863. In some of its features it did not differ appreciably from the Heidelberg setting to which Mayer-Gross had so long been accustomed. It had a high level of care for patients and served the needs of a comparatively small rural area (Dumfriesshire). The successive medical superintendents had been distinguished men, much enlightened in their views and ready to support research that they could understand. There were, however, more significant differences. While Heidelberg was securely established over the centuries as a centre of academic learning and counted many lively and productive minds among its doctors and professors, the staff of Crichton had been recruited with an eye to clinical and social considerations. Similarly at the Maudsley Mayer-Gross had found an attitude of eager enquiry and the pressures of a metropolitan centre. The spirit of Crichton was easy-going, devoted to the improvement of patient amenities and tending to be bucolic. The outstanding difference lay in the fact that Heidelberg and London were vigorous university centres, whereas Crichton was neither the seat nor the affiliate of a university. It is obvious that when Mayer-Gross was invited to go to Dumfries he recognized that there might be vested interests and an uphill struggle. These were not the conditions likely to dismay a man with his optimistic and energetic temperament, and he knew that he would have the support of the medical superintendent of the hospital, Dr Peter McCowan, who had himself engaged in clinical research in Cardiff under the enlightened aegis of E. W. Goodall. Mayer-Gross accepted the invitation without demur, knowing that he had made some firm friendships in London and had contributed in no small degree to the advancement of psychiatry both in its theoretical and its bedside aspects. The rural surroundings at Dumfries played their part also: Mayer-Gross was an enthusiastic gardener and lover of countryside activities. As his friend Alfred Meyer put it: 'Seeing him attend with infinite care to the plants in his garden which he had wrested from a derelict and poor soil, one could understand the "biological" workings of his mind and why his writings are so natural, original and convincing.'

During the latter part of his stay at the Maudsley, Mayer-Gross had taken part in the setting up of an 'insulin unit' for the treatment of schizophrenia. The unit was fortunately contrived so that it served the purposes not only of clinical care but also of research; it was established on lines very similar to those devised by Professor Max Müller at Munsingen in Berne. The induction of hypoglycaemic coma and the minute study of its effects over a specified period did not entail any radical change from the lines of research with which Mayer-Gross had been familiar in Heidelberg, largely as a legacy from Kraepelin in the studies which he had modelled on those of Wundt. Mayer-Gross knew that it is extremely difficult to conduct clinical research on somebody else's patients. He therefore took the necessary steps to enable him to carry full responsibility for the people under his care. He passed the qualifying examinations of the Scottish Royal Colleges and he became a naturalized British subject; he even changed his first name formally from Willy to William.

In 1955 he reached the age at which it is compulsory for consultants in the National Health Service to retire. For him, however, there could be no question of reducing his activities and idly sitting by. On the contrary, he enlarged his scope in conformity with his steadily increasing reputation, nationally and internationally. He moved to Birmingham where a Department of Experimental Psychiatry had been launched under the auspices of the University there and the Medical Research Council. However, at an early stage of the project Dr Joel Elkes, with whom he collaborated in its development, left Birmingham to take up a post in the United States and Mayer-Gross, with his rich clinical experience and keenness, was only too ready to take up the burden of clinical direction as Senior Fellow in the Department of Experimental Psychiatry and Director of Clinical Research at the likewise newly created Uffculme Clinic. His collaborator at the Uffculme Clinic aptly wrote: 'New ideas came to Mayer-Gross with astonishing facility and even in old age he remained a visionary with great hopes and plans for the future of psychiatry.' He instituted a successful day-hospital at Uffculme and, inevitably, engaged in research on the patients in the hospital and in the general community.

In December 1949 he had a coronary attack. He recovered from it quickly and was prepared to take risks to fulfil what he regarded as his duty, living a full, productive life. At the end of 1960 he and his wife planned a return to live in Heidelberg, where his property and University post had been restored to him and a psychopharmacological laboratory was waiting to carry out research under his direction.

SCIENTIFIC ACHIEVEMENTS

Mayer-Gross's working life fell into four well-defined periods coinciding with his location: Heidelberg, London, Dumfries, Birmingham.

The direction and impetus of his scientific activities bore witness to his adaptability and readiness to make the most of the facilities of the particular place where he might be located. In the Heidelberg period he chiefly devoted himself to clinical and psychopathological studies. The outstanding characteristics of his work then were his versatility and range: the two major contributions were his critical and exhaustive review of the existing knowledge of schizophrenia in its clinical aspects, and the monograph on oneiroid confusional states.

The schizophrenia volume of the Bunke-Handbuch amounted to some 800 pages; half of these were the responsibility of Mayer-Gross who cheerfully shouldered this giant share of the clinical exposition. Many a stout heart would have quailed before the prospect of so herculean a task but Mayer-Gross not only accepted it, but produced an enviable reminder of the state of German psychiatry before the Nazi blight descended upon it.

Not content, as it seems, with a full account of clinical schizophrenia, he traversed the psychopathology of hallucinations, in conjunction with Johannes Stein. It was a brilliant and detailed exposition, with a strong philosophical flavour.

The communication of his findings in the oneiroid experience was submitted to the university as his doctoral thesis. It was the first series of descriptions of their morbid experience by patients collected according to the methods laid down by Jaspers. He did not hesitate, however, to clarify his own standpoint in vigorous terms. Adverting to the downpour of theoretical papers on constitution which were then appearing in the German psychiatric journals (1924) and the dearth of factual material concerning their relevance he deplored the habit, which had become almost a rule, that when a new standpoint cropped up in psychiatry, the whole field had to be ploughed up afresh and the findings of the past thrown overboard; 'this lack of steady continuity cannot be excused by attributing it to the youth of our science'.

Although at this time of his life Mayer-Gross put forward the phenomenological approach as the appropriate one, it did not lead him to ascribe to psychopathological description too catholic a role. Whereas, for example, the dissertation on Glucksgefühl made copious use

of philosophical religious and psychological data expounded by William James, Geiger, Martin Duber, and of course Jaspers, he gradually turned more and more to experimental and particularly physiological studies with a neurological bent. Self-observation by intelligent patients with encephalitis lethargica and symptomatic psychoses offered abundant material for a down-to-earth psychopathology, which was well illustrated by his study of morbid perception, already alluded to. At the same time, in collaboration with Beringer and Bürger-Prinz, information was accumulated about the disturbances of thinking in people who had been suddenly woken from sleep or who were in the process of going to sleep. It is noteworthy that much of Mayer-Gross's clinical research was carried out like this in conjunction with his contemporary, Beringer. They were men of very different stamp; where Mayer-Gross was optimistic and bustling, ready to make decisions and to act on them, Beringer was a conscientious worrier who took life very seriously on the whole and acted even on small matters only after careful reflection; but in many respects their qualities were complementary, as in reporting a psychopathological study like 'the Hahnenfuss case'; here they joined forces as admirably as when founding their journal, the *Nervenarzt*.

Mayer-Gross, whose contacts reached outside the psychiatric clinic, engaged in collaborative studies with von Weizsäcker in investigations of sensory physiology and pathology. In the period before 1920 Max Weber provided much intellectual stimulus from the sociological side. Mayer-Gross appreciated this, though not himself involved. Gruhle, on the other hand, established steady contact with the sociologists and art historians.

Among matters which he studied with appropriate intensity were the psychopathology of drug addiction, as reported by an addict; the psychosomatic problems raised by the 'neurological' symptoms of encephalitis lethargica; the distinction between primary and secondary phenomena in schizophrenia as outlined by Bleuler; the notion of reaction types; changes in sensation in mescalin intoxication; the characteristics of thinking in primitive people as described or inferred by Levy-Bruhl (whose concept of prelogical collective thinking did not find favour

222

with Mayer-Gross, who collaborated with Lipps in this).

All this work and thought was crowded into the interstices, so to speak, of a busy clinical day, for after Wetzel had left the clinic, Mayer-Gross was responsible for the whole of the female side. Slighter papers from Mayer-Gross's pen dealt with such topics as the psychopathology of hysteria; the difference between understanding and explaining; and the effects of cannabis.

From 1933 onwards this productive, high-level work had to be given up and the surrender was painful. But Mayer-Gross, with his resilient personality and his optimism as well as his strong sense of what would be practicable, was happy to accept the post at Dumfries.

During his Heidelberg period Mayer-Gross had occupied himself *inter alia* with organic disease; the obsessional phenomena of encephalitis invited minute study, as did the relationship between encephalitis and schizophrenia. It was not, however, until Mayer-Gross settled in London that he devoted himself more whole-heartedly to the analysis of cerebral disease syndromes. He and Eric Guttman published a schema of examination for organic disease; they also published a joint paper on the problems of general as against focal symptoms in cerebral lesions. This was a closely reasoned, critical examination of the question at a time when Goldstein's holistic views tended to prevail. At this time too Mayer-Gross devoted himself to a very detailed study of constructional apraxia. He showed cause for emphasizing the disorganization of ability to understand, interpret and reproduce the interrelationship of objects in the whole of space. Professor Oliver Zangwill, a psychologist, was also concerned with this problem at the National Hospital for Nervous Diseases. The spatial disorder is evident in the defective activity-space available to many of those with a parietal syndrome. Closely allied to this were papers by Mayer-Gross on agnosia, pre-senile psychosis, and brain injury. For the last of these subjects an impressive monograph was produced embodying elaborate clinical studies by Mayer-Gross and Erich Feuchtwanger. In only a small minority of cases could the brain injury be regarded as a causal factor of schizophrenia.

In the presidential address which Mayer-Gross delivered to the Royal Society of Medicine Section of Psychiatry in 1955, he has told us with what aims and hopes he entered upon his duties at Crichton Royal.

When I was appointed Director of Clinical Research at the Crichton Royal in 1939, the venture was to me both welcome and attractive. I had come from a teaching post in a German university and had spent six years at the Maudsley Hospital in London. Clinical research, that is research into the causation of disease, study at the bedside seemed to feel very familiar to me.

Scientific work in German teaching hospitals and clinics was to a large extent of the same kind; so much so that the concept of clinical research as a separate branch of study had never been formed and there is no corresponding phrase for it in German.

This is how I formulated my tasks in the time of my appointment: lifting a daily clinical experience into the light of scientific investigation; looking for the unusual, illuminating case; testing scientific methods on clinical material; bringing theoretical problems to the patient's bedside; applying scientific critique to the therapeutic procedure; trying out new therapeutic methods under controlled conditions; collecting clinically well-studied case material for statistical elaboration and follow-up studies; instruction of young specialists in research methods.

To a remarkable extent, Mayer-Gross succeeded in realizing these aims. But before describing his efforts and successes, it is well to review the frustrations which he experienced and faithfully recorded. His first troubles were in establishing the clinical basis on which all the research structure could be reared:

Without full clinical observation, without history and documentation in well-kept case records, clinical research into the course and causation of diseases, owing to the mechanism underlying observed symptoms, is impossible.

This work had to be carried on within the restrictive conditions of wartime. There were shortages of staff, with the result that those who were available tended to rush patients to physical treatment, sometimes without their having been adequately observed beforehand:

The practising psychiatrist, for decades used to prudent contemplation on the effect of time on his patient, became extremely active in applying the new therapies at first opportunity. And the research worker found new difficulties by resisting this hurried tendency to practical success.

The Mental Health Survey entailing fieldwork in a rural area comprising over 56000 inhabitants in the South of Scotland, ran into another sort of difficulty:

Its full results could not be published, and those which have become known have not been heeded to any extent by those who could act on them.

Another field study which seemed necessary and promised well was a follow-up of patients who had been treated by the various physical methods lately introduced:

As long as it lasted its work was most instructive and fruitful for clinician and research worker alike; but it came to an end with the main worker's departure. It should have been resumed recently, but no funds were available to support it.

More heartfelt was the initial disappointment in regard to psychology.

For years the department (of Psychological Research) proved almost inaccessible to clinical questions of research, and seemed surrounded by a high wall of concept and test which did nothing to elucidate the obviously abnormal, quite apart from discovering nothing the clinician had not known beforehand. This wall was only breached when the psychologist was taken as a partner and co-worker into the daily run of the ward, in closest contact with the patient and his treatment.

Mayer-Gross also deplored the lack of

academic vivacity, conviviality and competition which is to be found even in the smallest university or school of medicine as a natural by-product of the gathering of young minds. Thus, it would be difficult for me to calculate the amount of time and effort I spent for the sole purpose of attracting the right people as collaborators in research; to rouse and keep the interest of young psychiatrists in the work they had taken up; and to fill by adequate replacement the gaps left by those who tended away from their loneliness of country life.

Mitigation of some of these latter difficulties was provided by regular visits to London:

the lack of an adequate library, the urgent need for advice and discussion in technical matters and for encouragement were recurring features of my remote existence. All the undisturbed and restful contemplation of country-life would have been ineffectual without these journeys to the metropolis.

It is clear that the 15 years which he spent at Crichton Royal included long spells of disappointment and struggle such as would have

crushed the spirit of a less determined man; but Mayer-Gross's character and experience triumphed over many of the difficulties he encountered; his positive achievements were indisputable and impressive. Because of the intensive concern of the Heidelberg School in the study of psychotomimetic drugs, Mayer-Gross was prepared to take maximum advantage of the opportunity presented by the physical methods of treatment – induced hypoglycaemia, L.S.D., and what were at first chemically induced convulsions, soon to be replaced by electrical convulsions. During the ascendency of 'insulin shock treatment', Mayer-Gross, with the collaboration of a biochemist, set about investigating the relation of carbohydrate metabolism to brain function. Primitive movements, speech disorders, disturbances of consciousness, taste and choice of foods in mild hypoglycaemia, were investigated on the lines of an experimental psychosis. Likewise, evaluative follow-up observations were made of patients who had been subjected to a prefrontal leucotomy.

Concurrently with many of these investigations Mayer-Gross pursued work that he had been engaged in at Heidelberg and in London: agnosia, senile and pre-senile psychoses, and the focal disturbances in organic cerebral disease, recalling the earlier schema drafted up in conjunction with Guttmann. Other problems about which he published his findings were sleep and hypnagogic phenomena, depersonalization, spontaneous drawings as an approach to some psychopathological problems, biological rhythms and the depressive cycle, and the question of 'oneirophrenia'. A number of thoughtful papers on methodology (especially dealing with self-observation, self-report, and reaction types) were published. Outstanding among Mayer-Gross's later achievements was a textbook of psychiatry which he wrote in conjunction with E. Slater and M. Roth. First published in 1954, it has gone through several editions; a growing appreciation of the importance of social factors is evident in it. By comparing it with the textbooks currently in use in other countries (including the Anglo-American), one can see how it conveys the sober, empirical approach and execution which are characteristic of English psychiatry, with its distrust of subtlety, its disciplined longing for *terra firma*.

GENERAL ASSESSMENT

In a review of Mayer-Gross's total *œuvre* the reader is struck by evidence of a twofold purpose, namely to convey scientific findings, and to provide a clear and succinct account of the present state of knowledge in some disputed or intricate field of psychiatric enquiry, so that less erudite or less experienced psychiatrists may be helped. This generous and considerate trait was manifest throughout his career. In some instances it took the form of a review: the diagnostic status of schizophrenia and the extent to which its psychopathology entitled it to be divided into primary and secondary phenomena; the psychopathology of delusions; synaesthesias, hallucinations, and other forms of morbid perception; the predisposition of organic disease towards having a psychogenic overlay; the historic development of the artificial psychosis from the time of Kraepelin and Wundt, with especial regard to the experimental laboratory studies thereby facilitated; the psychology of pain; the psychosomatics of cardiac disease; the insufficiency of Kretschmer's techniques in determining his concept of constitution. As Mayer-Gross showed, for example, in the last of these items, he did not hesitate to engage in courteous but firm and reasoned contentions.

The judicial temper of his mind is well indicated in his expressed standpoint on psychoanalysis. For example, in 1955 he stated that

according to certain fashionable hypotheses nothing could be easier than the prevention of neuroses or even psychoses, the proper upbringing of children, education of mothers in the principles of motherly care, closer family ties and household coherence. After my travels to India two years ago...I became somewhat doubtful of these doctrines. However, the supposed influence of Western civilization on psychiatric illness, the hypotheses of the critical years in child development, the environmental contributory factors, undoubtedly present even in such mainly constitutional illness as schizophrenia, deserve fresh study and assessment in which research is combined with remedial treatment.

Finally, another topic in which observation and controlled studies should replace armchair interpretation, wishful thinking and premature theorizing, is the psychology of the group and its application in therapy. Our times have seen the misuse of the group spirit on an unprecedented scale and more suffering and degradation have been due to the psychological forces in the setting of the masses than have been seen for a long time in history. If we could tame some of these forces and reduce them to subjection for purposes of therapy we could probably dispose of many physical treatments and certainly dismiss prolonged psychoanalysis.

As Professor Richard Jung put it in his obituary notice of Mayer-Gross:

While he clearly attributed value to the phenomenological approach in psychiatry he remained an adherent in psychopathology and clinical studies of the unprejudiced description and analysis of psychic phenomena. He could not stand twisted phrases and artificial presentations, and he was strongly against pseudo-philosophical and existential generalities and semantics. At a psychiatric meeting where there was much lengthy hair-splitting about paranoid disorder, he brought the meeting to a quick conclusion by the following simple question: 'Why can this sort of psychiatry only be expressed in the German language?'

In keeping with the fair-minded, balanced view that appears in his lectures and writings, were the moderate claims that he made for his own work. Thus writing about his mental health survey he said: 'It is not claimed that psychiatric surveys can be compared with the broad and comprehensive social surveys previously mentioned (by Seebohm Rowntree, Caradog-Jones and others). The psychiatrist looks at the complex fabric of social life from one angle only. The facts he tries to assess are more subjective, less tangible and less definite. While he considers them essential and close to the roots of social conditions – good or evil – others may think of them as casual and unimportant.'

It is not easy to decide which of his major works contributed most of the firm reputation which Mayer-Gross earned; probably his masterly presentation of the symptoms, course and diagnosis of schizophrenia in the Heidelberg volume of the Bumke Handbuch. This last was a triumph of knowledge and sustained effort. No one would now attempt such a prodigious task or, if he attempted it, succeed as Mayer-Gross did. He had then, as always till the very end, a fund of vitality and confidence that denied obstacles, minimized impossibilities, and led him to tackle boldly every investigation that presented itself as an interesting quest to his fresh, resourceful, urgent mind. He had a sense of obligation towards his chosen branch of medicine and, more particularly, towards the young men who entered it and came under his influence: he spared no pains to train them well and to help their careers. His nature was generous and direct and entirely free from rancour. He made no secret of his opinions, neither on controversial matters nor on large issues when the occasion called for it: but he made no enemies, because his sincerity and goodwill were always manifest and he strove so steadily and buoyantly towards worthy ends.

His interests were many and varied. He enjoyed music and was a connoisseur of food and wines. When he came to London he always managed to go to a theatre or picture gallery. He was sociable and warm-hearted, and loved to be in the company of congenial friends. He was an enthusiastic gardener.

Mayer-Gross was elected a Member of the Royal College of Physicians of London in 1945; he was elected a Fellow of the College in 1951. He was President of the Section of Psychiatry of the Royal Society of Medicine in 1954. He delivered the Adolf Meyer Lecture to the American Psychiatric Association in 1958. He served as Consultant to the World Health Organization in drawing up its plans for the All-India Institute of Postgraduate Psychiatric Research and Training at Bangalore. He undertook this duty first in 1951 and 1952, although in 1949 he had had a coronary attack; he did not allow this to reduce his activities in the ensuing years. In 1958 he was Guest Professor in the Nerve Clinic at the University of Munich, and in 1960 took a similar guest professorship in the Psychiatric Clinic of the University of Hamburg. As it is stated in the biography of Mayer-Gross in Munk's Roll of the College of Physicians:

nature endowed Mayer-Gross with the physical capacities and the immense energies for remarkable productivity. On the intellectual side he was gifted with unflagging interest, enthusiasm and industry, with a sober realism devoid of preconceptions or sentimentality...He was very little troubled by doubts or hesitations, and he lost no energy or time in fighting himself. Such a dynamic temperament could easily have become dangerously ruthless, but for his warm natural kindliness, his good humour, his strong sense of fair play and his zest for all aspects of life.

Mayer-Gross died on 15 February 1961.

Psychiatry and the Jewish tradition[1]

AUBREY LEWIS[2]

Formerly of Institute of Psychiatry, London

SYNOPSIS The attitude to mental illness in early Jewish thought and the contributions of some modern Jewish workers to psychiatry are summarized. The possible associations of mental illness among Jews are discussed.

INTRODUCTION

In 1968 all members of the American Psychiatric Association received a circular inviting them to subscribe to a Journal of Existential Psychiatry. The Hebrew heading was without explanation or translation. It is taken from the second chapter of Exodus, where God says to Moses, 'I am that I am'. The quotation is apposite for a Journal of Existential Psychiatry but it is very unlikely that it would have been used, without explanation, unless it was going to be read by Jews in the main who could be expected to appreciate its relevance. I do not know what proportion of the membership of the APA is Jewish, but from casual inspection and many contacts and attendance at the APA congresses I should judge it to be high. I have had the same impression in this country where many senior figures in psychiatry are Jewish. In the pre-Hitler period in Germany and Austria, likewise, the proportion of psychiatrists who were Jews was high and distinguished.

FREUD AND HIS FOLLOWERS

I do not want to fall into either the congratulatory or the apologetic vein of discussion, but only to record my impression that a considerable number of Jewish doctors take to psychiatry as their specialty. It is not difficult to put forward conjectures why this should be so, but rather than offer facile generalization I would like to dwell on the outstanding case – Sigmund Freud

[1] The text of this paper has been adapted from the manuscript of a talk given by Sir Aubrey Lewis at the Leo Baeck College, London, in November 1968.
[2] Address for correspondence : Professor M. Shepherd, Institute of Psychiatry, De Crespigny Park, Denmark Hill, London SE5 8AF.

and his disciples. Psycho-analysis has had such a profound effect on psychiatry that in considering its founder we are exploring one of the most significant aspects of the problem.

In his Autobiographical Study Freud stated simply :

My parents were Jews, and I have remained a Jew myself . . . My father insisted that in my choice of a profession I should follow my own inclinations. Neither at that time, nor indeed in my later life did I feel any particular predilection for the career of a physician. I was moved, rather, by a sort of curiosity which was directed more towards human concerns than towards natural objects . . . My early familiarity with the Bible story . . . had, as I recognized much later, an enduring effect upon the direction of my interest.

He goes on to say that when he went to the University he found that he was expected to feel inferior and an alien because he was a Jew.

I refused absolutely to do the first of these things. I have never been able to see why I should feel ashamed of my descent or, as people were beginning to say, of my race.

He joined the B'nai B'rith and regularly attended its meetings every other Tuesday, and he read them several papers, on dreams and other psychological subjects.

He was, however, as is well known, irreligious. In the preface he wrote for the Hebrew version of his book *Totem and Taboo* he said that he had become estranged from the Jewish religion but that he was still Jewish in essence. In a letter to a Protestant pastor, Dr Pfister, he wrote 'The beauty of religion does not belong to the domain of psycho-analysis. . . . How comes it that none of all the godly people discovered psychoanalysis; why did they have to wait for a quite godless Jew ?'

Though religion was for him an area of psycho-analytic study but not of belief or practice, it was clear that his early upbringing had influenced his outlook greatly. He said to a Jewish friend who was worried about the religious upbringing of his son

If you do not let your son grow up as a Jew you will deprive him of sources of energy which cannot be replaced by anything else. He will have to struggle as a Jew, and you ought to develop in him all the energy he will need for that struggle. Do not deprive him of that advantage.

The logic is not impeccable, but the feeling behind it is undeniable. He had to struggle, as he wrote to the B'nai B'reth on his seventieth birthday:

it seemed to me [in the years after 1895] that I was like a man outlawed and shunned by everyone. In my isolation the longing arose in me for a circle of high-minded men who, regardless of the audacity of what I had done, would receive me with friendliness. Your society was a place where such men were to be found. That you were Jews was all the better, for I myself was a Jew.

His links with his family ensured some continuing contact with Judaism as a religion. Thus on his thirty-fifth birthday his father gave him the Bible he had used as a boy, and in a Hebrew inscription in it said

It was in the seventh year of your age that the spirit of God began to move you to learning ... You have seen in this Book the vision of the Almighty, you have listened willingly, you have tried to fly high on the wings of the Spirit.

The secular side of Judaism undoubtedly meant a great deal to Freud. He was a member of a Zionist society (Kadimah), and became a Governor of the Hebrew University of Jerusalem. His friendships were almost all with Jews.

In his earlier years Freud was on intimate terms with Joseph Breuer, Wilhelm Fliess, and Flaischl. These men were his seniors or contemporaries, and did not play quite the subordinate role inevitable in his psycho-analytic adherents. Breuer, twenty years older than Freud and firmly established as a research worker and physician of standing, was able to help him with advice and financial aid; and still more, by bringing to Freud's notice the extraordinarily interesting phenomena being manifested by a woman patient under hypnosis. As Freud always acknowledged, this had been a crucial event in the development of psychoanalysis. Breuer, incidentally, was the son of a prominent religious leader in the Jewish community of Vienna. Fliess was an even more potent factor in Freud's development. Freud wrote to him in 1896:

People like you should not die out, my friend; we others need the like of you too much. How much have I to thank you for, in consolation, understanding, stimulation in my loneliness, in the meaning of life you have given to me, and lastly in health which no one else could have brought back to me. It is essentially your example that has enabled me to gain the intellectual strength to trust my own judgment.

Fliess was, in fact, as Freud eventually realized, a crank, with unsupported theories about cyclic events in the body. His mystical ideas about numbers are reminiscent of Cabbalistic gematria: and are likely, as Bakan and others have suggested, to have encouraged Freud in interpreting some dreams and trivial acts on elaborate and laboured numerological lines. For example, he had written to a friend that he would not correct some proofs 'even if there were 2,467 mistakes': in a characteristic way Freud set about accounting for his choice of this number, 2467. It turned on an item in the newspaper which recalled to him his 24th birthday (24): 'then take the number that represents my age now, 43, and add it to the 24, and you get 67': so we account for this number 2467. This smacks, as other passages do, of 'gematria' and notarikon, and has been used to support the argument that Freud had imbibed enough mystic interpretation from his early Galician environment and from his parents for it to have had a large share in moulding psycho-analytic theory and method. This is rather a forced explanation of Freud's occasional style of playing with words and numbers in interpreting dreams and in the psychopathology of everyday life. But it is fair to conclude that he had a strain of mysticism which went far enough at times to recall passages in the Zohar and other Cabbalistic writings (which he had doubtless never read). The odd thing is that Freud believed

Jews to be free from mystical propensities. In a letter to Karl Abraham he said, apropos of the trouble with Jung, 'we Jews have an easier time, having no mystical element'. This indicated such a big scotoma that it must be regarded as a significant blunder, rather than a lacuna of knowledge. After all, we know from his own statement that his father came from a Chassidic milieu, and that his father's birthplace in Galicia was a famous Chassidic centre: his mother was born in Brody, likewise a Chassidic stronghold.

If we turn from Breuer and Fliess to consider the band of disciples whom Freud gradually gathered round him, the outstanding characteristic is that, with only two or three exceptions, they are all Jews. The exceptions were Jung and Ernest Jones. The others were Abraham, Stekel, Adler, Rank, Reik, Sachs, Ferenczi, Eitingon who steadily – or in some cases until they defected – were close to Freud. The innermost circle, romantically bound together by the Seven Rings, which was formed after the defection of Adler, Stekel and Jung, consisted of Rank, Ferenczi, Sachs, Eitingon, Abraham, and Jones, the only non-Jew. Jones made an interesting and amusing comment.

We were all free-thinkers, so there was no religious bar between us. Nor do I remember finding any difficulty from being the only Gentile in the circle. Coming myself from an oppressed race, it was easy for me to identify myself with the Jewish outlook which years of intimacy enabled me to absorb in a high degree. My knowledge of Jewish anecdotes, wise sayings and jokes became under such tutelage so extensive as to create astonishment among other analysts outside the small circle. . . . I will quote an amusing example, though it relates to a tragic situation. When the Nazis entered Vienna, they decreed that only an Aryan could be allowed to conduct the Psycho-Analytical Clinic. Unfortunately the only member of the Vienna Society answering to this description had just fled over the mountains to Italy. On hearing this I cried out 'Oh Weh, unser einziger Sabbath-goy ist fort.'

Freud was acutely – and perhaps excessively – aware that the great preponderance of Jews among the prominent advocates and practitioners of psycho-analysis could interfere with its spread and acceptance. When the dissension with Jung was approaching its climax, Freud asked Abraham to heal the breach, if possible. He wrote:

Be tolerant and don't forget that it is easier for you to follow my thoughts than for Jung since to begin with you are completely independent, and then racial relationship brings you closer to my intellectual constitution, whereas he, the son of a pastor, can only find his way to me against great inner resistances. His adherence is therefore all the more valuable. I was almost going to say it was only his emergence on the scene that has removed from psycho-analysis the danger of becoming a Jewish national affair.

In a subsequent letter to Abraham he wrote:

My opinion is that we Jews, if we want to co-operate with other people, have to develop a little masochism and be prepared to endure a certain amount of injustice . . . You may be sure that if my name were Oberhuber my new ideas would despite all the other factors have met with far less resistance.

To anyone familiar with English conditions in these matters, Freud's feelings must seem pathologically overwrought until the situation in Vienna is taken into account – the Vienna of which Lueger was Mayor and where violent anti-Semitic agitation was rife, going to the lengths of accusations of ritual murder. There was also the backwash of the Dreyfus affair. And it is not irrelevant to recall that Jung later expressed crude racist sentiments:

The Jew never has produced and presumably never will produce a culture of his own . . . The Aryan unconscious has a higher potential than the Jewish. Freud did not know the Germanic soul, any more than did his German imitators. Has the mighty phenomenon of National Socialism taught them better?

In England Jews played, at any rate at first, a very small part in furthering psycho-analysis, though it was David Eder who became secretary of the newly formed British Psycho-Analytical Society in 1913. David Eder was an active Zionist, a highly secularized Jew, and a devoted community doctor – a man of exceptionally unselfish character and moral strength.

I think that at first in the United States also there were, apart from A. A. Brill, few Jews who embraced psycho-analytic teachings and practice, but I have no firm evidence for this. At all events, the total wave of psycho-analysis which swept over the United States in the last two decades was partly the work of enthusiastic Jewish psychiatrists.

229

A prominent American psychiatrist, Walter Freeman, quotes the findings of a rough and ready check he made:

So many of my psychiatric colleagues are Jews that I selected two characteristic Jewish names, Cohen and Shapiro in the various directories and compared them with the Smiths. The American Psychiatric Association lists 44 Cohens and 26 Shapiros (70), together with 75 Smiths.

Among all the medical specialists in the USA 6% of these called Smith are psychiatrists, but 17% of those called Cohen or Shapiro are psychiatrists. Then Dr Freeman had a look at the members of the American Psycho-Analytic Association, and found five Cohens and five Shapiros, as against only two Smiths. He concludes, on a somewhat meagre and dubious sample, that psychiatry, and particularly psychoanalysis, attract Jewish physicians in the United States. There may be more satisfactory data, but I am unaware of them.

I mentioned earlier that Freud had an ambivalent attitude towards mysticism. He thought it alien to the spirit of Judaism, but at the same time followed modes of thought and interest which have made it possible for a psychologist, David Bakan, to make a reasoned case for supposing Freud to have been involved with the Jewish mystical tradition, partly of the messianic type to which Sabbathai Zevi gave form and substance, and partly of the Chassidian type harking back to Baal Shem. I think the argument is forced and weak but it is certain that he took an interest in such matters as Satanic poets. He wrote an article on demoniacal possession in the seventeenth century, making the paradoxical comment that 'the demonological theory of the Dark Ages has in the long run justified itself'. He elaborated the point and made it simpler in the following passage:

What in these days were thought to be evil spirits to us are base and evil wishes, the derivatives of impulses which have been rejected and repressed. In one respect only do we not subscribe to the explanation of these phenomena current in the Middle Ages; we have abandoned projecting them into the outer world, and we attribute their origin instead to the inner life of the patient in whom they are manifested.

230

THE BIBLE

Demonology has always had great interest for psychiatrists because of the similiarity, or more properly the identity of demonological reports with the hallucinations, delusions and other phenomena of psychoses. Jewish demonology has, like other forms of it, a long history. Thus we read that 'an evil spirit from the Lord tormented Saul', and in Josephus King Solomon is credited with the power to cast out demons; Josephus tells us also how he had himself seen a fellow-countryman free men possessed of demons, in the presence of Vespasian. Belief in evil spirits was of course universal in the Ancient World, and it is in a way surprising that there is so little mention of it in the Old Testament. The New Testament takes possession by evil spirits for granted in the numerous accounts of such happenings as the rush of the Gadarene swine into the sea. It is plain that in Galilee at that time belief in evil spirits causing disease was widespread, if not universal. But it was also recognized that madness could be feigned, as when David used the trick to deceive Achisch the Philistine; and that the prophetic rapture might be a form of madness: Zephania, you will remember, was reminded that it was his duty to supervise 'every madman who prophesies, to put him in the stocks and collar'. There can be no doubt that Isaiah, Jeremiah and other prophets experienced trances, visions, voices and other phenomena with which psychiatrists are familiar. Unlike lesser or earlier men called prophets, they did not use dances, music, intoxicating drinks or self-injuring frenzies to attain the trance state or ecstasy; and it would be presumptuous to equate the prophetic afflatus with the psychopathic disorders of consciousness to which it bears a resemblance.

In Biblical and Talmudic times the distinction between insanity and mental defect was not clearly made, though in the Mishna 'shoteh' mostly meant 'imbecile'. The causes of mental illness were twofold: personal shortcomings, and involuntary misfortunes, namely heredity, senility, and invasion by an evil or unclean spirit. The personal shortcomings might be sexual perversions, according to two or three passages in the Talmud. The public attitude towards the mentally ill seems to have been, on the whole, just and humane in intention, e.g. it is laid down that if a sane man's wife subsequently becomes insane, he should not divorce her; for mentally incompetent persons, a guardian must be appointed. The insane who were not violent were allowed to roam the streets, unless they belonged to well-to-do families, who looked after them at home, perhaps with a personal attendant. In a Midrash on Psalm 34 David asks God why he has put madness into the world – 'Master of the Universe, what profit is there for the world in madness? When a man goes about the market place and rends his garments, and children run after him and mock him, is this beautiful in thine eyes?' Resh Laqish, a third-century Amora, laid it down that no one commits a crime unless the spirit of madness has entered into him. Physicians were consulted when a man became deranged, as in the case of Herod the Great who lost his reason after murdering his wife Marianne.

Exorcism was practised, in dealing with the insane: Josephus describes the procedure. The affected person was given a ring to smell which had under its seal a scrap of Baar root. This drew out the demon through the patient's nostrils, while he recited incantations. As the demon retreated, he overturned a cup of water to prove he had left the man.

Although the belief in demons never became an essential feature of Jewish theology, it persisted, as superstitions do, and was developed into fairly elaborate forms. Ansky's Dybbuk is the most vivid reminder of how it continued to co-exist with more rational and fully sanctioned religious ideas and practices. It has, of course, died out in countries of Western civilization; and it illustrates the dictum of Abraham Joshua Heschel that 'today religious isolationism is a myth. For all the profound differences in perspective and substance, Judaism is sooner or later affected by the moral, intellectual and spiritual events within the Christian society, and vice versa.'

THE MEDIEVAL PERIOD

The medieval world, peopled with lurking demons capable of causing every kind of disease, must have been a terrifying place. Among Jews men like Nachmanides and Crescas adopted without question the prevailing demonology (though they never treated the demons as divine or semi-divine beings, nor gave Asmodeus, the most powerful of demons, the rebellious attributes of a Satanic figure). It was only Maimonides and Ibn Esra who denied that there were demons at all: and their scepticism could not prevail over the almost universal belief to the contrary. It is therefore no surprise that the Shulchan Aruch contains instructions for keeping the demons at bay. There were indeed very special and peculiar reasons why the author of the Shulchan Aruch should have believed that supernatural powers were about and around us.

In 1529 Joseph Caro, then Rosh Yeshiva in Adrianople, met Solomon Molcho, the Marrano mystic who was later burnt by the Inquisition. Molcho believed that a heavenly messenger, or Maggid, had come to guide him, and in accordance with an order from the Maggid he went to Palestine and then to Rome. Caro was greatly influenced by Molcho, embraced much of his Messianic and Cabbalistic teaching, and at the instance of his own Maggid went to Safed in 1536, to await the coming of the Messiah predicted for 1540. Safed was at that time a centre of Jewish learning and devotion: the people practised severe austerities, and made prayer and study the business of their lives. As Schechter said,

no place in Jewish history since the destruction of the Temple could point to so brilliant a gathering of men, so great in their respective branches, so diversified in the objects of their study, and so united by the dominant thought of religion as were attracted to Safed during the greater part of the 16th century.

In this fervid atmosphere of worship and Caballistic zeal, Caro prepared his immense codifying labours and composed the Shulchan Aruch, itself a synopsis, for the common man, of the more extensive and erudite codes he had compiled while in Adrianople. This was a sustained one-man effort, calling for great powers of organization and memory.

But at the same time as he was carrying through these exacting intellectual feats, which he continued until his death at the age of eighty-seven, he was the recipient of messages from a spirit guide, a Maggid who spoke through Caro's mouth, exhorting, enjoining, promising, praising, and expounding. Its pronouncements were bold, and claimed unquestionable authority. In a diary which Caro kept for fifty years (and which was published in 1646, seventy years after his death) these pronouncements were recorded. Some of the things said by the Maggid, through Caro as its medium, are psychiatrically significant. On one occasion the Maggid declared to him : 'I am the echo of your thoughts'; on another it explained that if Caro was perplexed about some knotty point in Talmudic exegesis, he should concentrate on the problem and wish to be helped by the Maggid who would then provide him with the answer. The Maggid also said : 'I speak through your mouth, not in a dream but as a man talks to a fellow man . . . I address you while your eyes are wide open, and your utterances are loud.' The visitations occurred oftenest on the Sabbath : of 135 of them dated with the day of the week, 109 occurred on Friday night. The Maggid took account of whether other people were present : if, while he was delivering himself of a message or homily, people came into the room where Caro was, the Maggid would cut short his remarks. He also now and then made comments on the political situation in Turkey and Russia. Now and then Caro heard the Maggid speaking to him through a lyre. The voice also uttered the strongest panegyrics on Caro: 'You are considered very eminent and lofty and sublime by the Holy One, Blessed be He, and the prophets, the tannaim, amoraim, geonim and codifiers in Heaven. Whatever you do, God will crown with success'; and, even, in detail: 'Maimonides is most pleased with the way you have elucidated Jacob ben Asher's Tur.' Sometimes the hyperbole of the Maggid's congratulation verges on blasphemy :

Whenever you go out into the street, my seven worlds and all their hosts escort you and proclaim before you 'Pay homage to the holy image of God' . . . numerous hosts, armies and worlds tremble at that proclamation . . . consider yourself as a king heading his army. I and all my hosts encompass you constantly, you are among us as a king among his troops. The worlds proclaim 'He is president of the grand Academy. He is God's beloved.'

In the latest entry in the Diary, 1572, the Maggid forbids him to cogitate 'over the dark world which Samuel places in your heart. If you only knew how many worlds suffer loss on account of your ceasing to meditate on the law [Torah] you would have preferred death to life.'

It requires no profound knowledge of psychiatry to recognize all this as an expanded, naïve version of the simple statement by the voice, 'I am the echo of your thoughts' – thoughts entirely in keeping with the milieu but expressing self-praise and other attitudes which could not decently be expressed in a direct form. There is a great deal more, of course, reflecting the ascetic preoccupations, the Cabbalistic symbolism, and the humdrum items which figure in the record (as an example of the humdrum: the Maggid says 'How can you wish me to talk to you after you have eaten horseradish. I have already told you about the mystery of good odours prevailing over bad odours.').

Inevitably the question will be asked : 'Were these visitations of the Maggid hallucinations, and what would be our diagnosis if such a condition came under our scrutiny today in some earnest Chassidic student of the Mishna and the Zohar ?'

The first part of the enquiry is easily answered : these were not in the least hallucinations, nor were there any delusions. Apart from the fastings and other austerities he subjected himself to, Caro lived a normal, busy, competent life, rearing several children, marrying three times, on one occasion entering into some commercial transaction, and producing his learned commentaries and legal or religious codes. There could be no question of schizophrenia here, nor of paranoid disorder (though he had his detractors and might have been excused for inveighing against them more than he did).

The Biblical parallel to his condition would be the witch of Endor (who was really a medium rather than a witch) : the dead Samuel spoke to Saul through her mouth. The classical parallel would, I suppose, be the Delphic sibyl, through whom Apollo pronounced his oracles : and in modern terms it would be someone like the medium Eusapia Palladino.

I would not like to equate Caro's experience with that of the prophets, like Isaiah. There is a world of difference between the enormous egotism of Caro and the universalistic passion and submergence of self in Isaiah or Jeremiah or

Amos. To enter into the complex questions raised by the prophetic utterances and behaviour would not be possible here, nor would I feel competent to do so. So far as Caro's Maggid is concerned, it can best be understood as an instance of mild dissociation, such as we nowadays encounter in hypnotic states and in a hysterical trance. But I would stress the mildness, the comparative normality of the experience, best shown by the clarity of consciousness, consistency of outlook with that of the non-dissociated state, and clear memory of what was said by the Maggid. I would therefore hesitate to call Caro's almost lifelong visitations pathological in any sense of the world. Taking his times, cultural setting and personal qualities into account, his conduct can be held as I have said, to be within the normal range. To bring about his dissociated state he used a technique which combined religious and hypnotic elements: he was instructed, for example, to picture the Tetragrammaton written with black ink on a parchment suspended before his eyes. This would correspond to the fixation used in inducing hypnosis, but Caro did not at any time, as far as we know, over all these years develop amnesia, catalepsy or any other of the cruder manifestations of the hypnotic state.

Caro paid tribute to the genius of that great codifier, Maimonides, but he had none of the rationalism of Maimonides. You will perhaps recall that in one of Maimonides' Responsa he wrote to Lunel that astrology was 'baseless foolishness', and that we accept only what is rationally proved and in accordance with the evidence of our senses, or based on trustworthy authority: 'let us never cast our reason backwards: our eyes are in front, not behind us'. While speaking of Maimonides, I would quote a modern sounding passage which shows this twelfth-century philosopher-physician in a 'psychosomatic' light. He wrote in his Aphorisms

The soul is subject to health and disease just as is the body. The health and disease of both undoubtedly depend on beliefs and customs which are peculiar to mankind. Wherefore I call senseless beliefs and degenerate customs diseases of humanity. Within the sum total of these diseases there is one which is widespread and from which men rarely escape. It varies in degree in different men. I mean this: that

everyone thinks he is cleverer than he is. This disease has attacked many an intelligent man . . . and he expresses himself on a science with which he is not familiar as if he were well versed in it. Especially if he meets with applause from persons of distinction he becomes a master and leader, and we have one more 'great man'.

The sardonic touch is understandable when one recalls the controversies in which he was engaged.

Belief in an animistic aetiology of mental illness can still be found among Jews who have lived in a relatively primitive society such as that of the Yemen: much of their notions of disease has been borrowed from their Arab neighbours. They classify mental disorders on simple lines: into fevers and non-fevers, and the afebrile conditions are either due to the evil eye, or to possession by a spirit, or to epilepsy. The conditions due to the evil eye are depression and anxiety: those due to spirits what we would mostly diagnose as schizophrenia or confusional states. For the former one should say the Shema, and make three parallel incisions on the patient's spine and throw cold water on him suddenly from behind. For a condition due to a spirit a metal object (often a red hot nail, i.e. cautery) is applied to the supposed site of the illness, and if this does not avail to drive out the evil spirit, an exorcism ceremony takes place in which the exorcist invokes the Master of the Spirits and says 'I request you to order the spirit who took possession of this man to leave his body immediately. If not, I will condemn all of you to eternal wandering.' Alternatively a dove or a sheep is revolved three times around the patient, and the exorcist then whispers to the spirits: 'I beg you to have mercy upon the man and take the sheep instead.' If the spirit then departs from the patient, a cup containing some fluid will seem to break. Amulets with magic formulae written on them are also used for exorcism in mental illness.

Some of all this reaches far back into the demonology of Babylon and Persia, or less remotely, to the Arabic of the Middle Ages. Its persistence among the Yemeni Jews is an outcome of their isolation over many centuries, and cannot last much longer now that they are living in Israel and adapting their mode of life and beliefs to the prevailing culture. The native healers have not disappeared from the scene yet however:

they fulfil an existing need. Those Yemenites who feel themselves strangers in a hostile Ashkenazi world turn to their 'moris' for comfort. It is those uncertain people who are sensitive and not sufficiently flexible to adapt themselves to the new environment who suffer most from the evil eye, and therefore turn to the 'mori' for assistance. Not only the older immigrants but also some of the younger ones, those who have failed in matters of love or business or are otherwise handicapped, seek his help.   [Hes, 1964.]

The moris, in fact, function much like our osteopaths and faith-healers. A patient treated effectively by a psychiatrist for a delusional condition may subsequently consult a mori for headaches or nightmares: there is much neurosis among the Yemenites, and much epilepsy.

There is a manifest continuity between this contemporary picture and Klausner's description of Galilee in the days of Herod. Wars, tumults and Roman oppression had multiplied the poor and the sick and neurotic: 'even educated people and those who had imbibed Greek culture, like Josephus, regarded these as cases of possession by an evil spirit and believed that certain men could cure them by miracles, driving out the unclean spirit'. What Klausner describes as 'some mystical force in certain men gifted with an inner life of spiritual strength, enabling them to influence nervous cases and especially hysterical women in what seems a miraculous cure', would now be accounted for in more familiar terms as a phenomenon of suggestibility or a placebo effect, robbed of its supernatural aura.

MENTAL ILLNESS AMONG JEWS

I have strayed a long way from my opening question: are Jewish doctors particularly prone to take up psychiatry? Returning to it by a somewhat hypothetical route, it is useful to look at a more tangible problem than Maggids and evil spirits present, namely the prevalence of psychiatric illness among Jews. There is a widespread belief that Jews are more prone than other people to develop nervous disorders and psychoses: and there is a widespread belief that the doctors who take up psychiatry as their specialty are themselves troubled by psychological problems which make the subject congenial or at any rate important and familiar to them. If both these assumptions are true, the original question admits of a simple answer. But I do not think the two assumptions are well substantiated. I shall not say anything further about the motives that lead doctors to specialize in psychiatry: it would lead too far, but the prevalence of psychiatric disturbances needs further consideration here.

If you look up the entry in the Jewish Encyclopedia on Nervous Diseases you find the following opening passage:

The Jews are more subject to diseases of the nervous system than the other races and peoples among which they dwell. Some physicians of large experience among Jews have even gone so far as to state that most of them are neurasthenic and hysterical . . . The Jewish population of Warsaw alone is almost exclusively the inexhaustible source for the supply of hysterical males for the clinics of the whole Continent.

That rather devastating statement came from a highly respected physician, Morris Fishberg, who was an authority on Jewish morbidity. In another entry, under the heading 'Insanity', he puts forward similarly pessimistic opinions about psychosis, e.g. 'in 1870 there was one insane among 1775 Catholics, while with the Jews it reached the alarming proportion of one insane in 384 of population'. He gives a table showing in Germany more than twice as high a proportion of Jewish insane as Catholics and Protestants, and in Denmark six times as high.

These statements represented the common opinion half a century ago. They were based on mental hospital statistics and the impressions of neurologists mainly. Such data as they relied on were of a sort that can be notoriously misleading. The number of patients admitted to mental hospitals in the course of a year depends on the number of available beds and the duration of stay, as well as on the reputation of the hospital, the procedures leading up to admission, and the criteria of acceptance: it is not a sufficient guide to the amount of mental illness in the population served. For this reason I would be reluctant to interpret the Preliminary Report on the Census of Mental Inpatients in Israel published by Dr Halevy in 1964. His figures show that there were 25 persons in hospital for every 10000 of population. Of the total patients in mental hospitals a fifth had been born in Israel. A quarter of the women were born in USSR or Poland, as were approximately a sixth of the men.

Contradictory assertions abound in this field. Thus American studies during the last forty years have run counter to the previously popular view. In 1925, for instance, first admissions to mental hospitals in New York City showed that the rate per 100000 of population was 42·7 for Jews, and 81·1 for non-Jews: for schizophrenia the rate was 16 per 100000 Jews, 23·5 per 1000000 non-Jews; for manic-depressive psychoses about the same in both populations.

An American investigation in 1954, directed not only at people admitted to hospital but embracing all persons under treatment for a psychiatric condition in the New Haven area, indicated that schizophrenia, the affective (manic-depressive) illnesses, and senile disorders were distributed in the same proportion as in the general population at risk, but neurotic disorder was 2½ times as frequent in the Jewish group. The authors account for this by assuming that Jews are more ready to seek and accept psychiatric help: 'they exhibit a high level of acceptance of psycho-analytical psychiatry, with a minimum of disturbance of their social values'.

In Germany before the advent of Hitler much interest was taken in the frequency of paranoid reactions in Jews, because it was thought that persecution and adverse discrimination would favour the widespread development of suspicious and morbid interpretation and projection, but, as Kehrer indicated in 1928, these paranoid features are, in unequivocal form, rare among Jews.

The most disputed area, in this context, is manic-depressive psychosis. Many textbooks (including Henderson & Gillespie) declare that Jews have an exceptionally high incidence of this condition, though some authorities modify this by saying that what is particularly common among Jews is a mixed condition showing not only manic-depressive but also schizophrenic and neurotic features.

A few years ago (1960) an Israeli psychiatrist reviewed the records of all manic-depressive patients admitted to Talbieh Hospital between November 1949 and December 1958. He found that the incidence was 40 per 100000, a figure appreciably lower than has been found in mental hospital data for the whole population in various areas of Europe and America: the basis for his calculations, however, was not very secure.

A more recent study was made in this country by Dr Fernando in 1966. He collected a random sample of British-born patients suffering from depression or anxiety living in East London and attending outpatient clinics, mostly at the London Jewish Hospital. He found no significant difference in degree of depression between Jews and non-Jews, but the Jewish patients showed slightly more hypochondriasis and less guilt than the non-Jewish. Apropos of hypochondriasis, it is noteworthy that Kenyon in his study of this condition in London found no preponderance of Jewish patients.

Depression may connote a heightened disposition to suicide. In the nineteenth century the statistics of most countries showed a lesser frequency of suicide among Jews than in the rest of the population: Germany was an exception. In this country the situation has been, for the most part, reversed, though statistics of suicide are far from trustworthy. In a recent analysis of the amount of suicide in Israel, Drabkin states that the crude average rate per 100000 Jews aged 15 and over for the period 1949–62 was 15, fluctuating annually between 12 and 20. This is lower than the rate for the corresponding period in Denmark, Austria, Switzerland and Hungary, but higher than for this country, the United States, Norway, Holland or Italy. Whereas in Western European countries the male suicide rate is three or four times the female rate, in Israel there is no such large sexual difference (men 17, women 13). Much has been written about suicide, including suicide among Jews of different countries, but there are still many obscure problems.

Before leaving the question of prevalence, something must be said about the allegedly high rate of neurosis among Jews. Light is cast upon this by the finding in a New York study that in that city the normal relation of numbers of patients in public and private hospitals is almost reversed:

Jews of all social classes indicated that it is the psychotherapist who is the most appropriate authority to turn to for help when psychological problems arise. Such a ready acceptance of psychiatric help by Jews from all walks of life minimises the significance of the allegedly higher rate of neurosis among Jews.   [Sanua.]

Moreover, the assessment of neurosis can be a highly individual, unreliable affair. Hence the wide divergencies in estimates of prevalence by different observers. Thus Hoch, who was aware of the pitfalls, found emotional disorder in 21% of the people living on a housing estate in Jerusalem. The diagnostic breakdown showed 2·6% of the population to be psychotic, 8·4% neurotic, 5·3% personality disorders, and 4·4% with psychophysiological disorders. It is hard to believe that one out of every five immigrants has one or other of these psychiatric troubles.

In welcome contrast to the disorders we have been considering are those which develop through alcohol. Every writer on the subject is impressed – or perhaps one should say has been impressed – by the great rarity of Jewish drunkards and Jews with alcoholic psychoses. It has been the subject of much conjecture for a long time. Immanuel Kant remarked upon it in 1798.

Women, clergymen and Jews do not get drunk, as a rule, because their civic position is weak. Their outward worth is based on the belief of others in their piety, chastity and separatist wisdom. All separatists, i.e. people who subject themselves not only to the law of the land but also to a special sectarian law, are exposed to the notice and criticism of the general community, and therefore cannot relax their self-control; intoxication would be a scandal for them.

Today the opposite view to this is widely held. Instead of supposing that risk of censure from others keeps Jews sober, it seems clear that their sobriety is imperilled or undermined by the example and pressure of the non-Jewish society to whose habits they tend to conform. Numerous observers have confirmed that if a sample, say, of university students in the United States is scrutinized, there is a clear gradation in drinking habits from the orthodox to the conservative, then to the Reform, and finally to the secular. Many writers connect this with the ritual use of wine – Kiddush, the four cups at Passover, Purim, and similar occasions for ritual drinking in great moderation. This is too summary an explanation. It is necessary to consider

the broad socio-cultural matrix within which drinking occurs . . . Where drinking is an integral part of social adjustment, where it is related to central moral symbolism and is used not for individual but for impersonal or communal purposes, sobriety is likely.

The situation in Israel is, as one might expect, neither stable nor simple. In a recent report (Shuval & Krasilowsky, 1964) it is made clear that mental hospital admissions for alcoholism made up, in the years between 1948 and 1960, 0·4% of all first admissions, but in 1962 it had risen to 3% of all first admissions, and there had been a corresponding increase in offences (especially traffic accidents and fatalities) attributable to alcohol. The socio-cultural background of the alcoholics admitted to the mental hospital varied from ethnic group to group. The men from Ashkenazie backgrounds had not established a stable family life, whereas the Sephardic and Oriental Jews were members of established families. Shuval & Krasilowsky believe that among the factors conducing to an increase in alcoholism in Israel is the economic advance: they are alarmed at the prospect:

as we try to be a 'society like all societies' it seems to us that it will become increasingly difficult to keep to the moderation in drinking pattern which was typical of the Jewish community isolated from interaction with groups with different cultural patterns, and values.

JEWS AND THE PSYCHOLOGICAL SCIENCES

It remains only to say a word about Jewish psychiatrists and Jewish psychologists. The psychiatrists are pretty diverse. Some of them are penetrated through and through with Jewish thought and Jewish learning. The most striking example of this that I know is Professor Henri Baruk of Paris. Early in the war, he tells us, he decided to learn Hebrew

and this study, begun in 1940 and continued without interruption ever since, took me into the world of Hebraic civilization, the Bible, the Talmud and that whole tradition which appeared to me, not only in the shape of a mere religious creed, as it is usually regarded, but as an extremely elaborate science, essentially experimental, a science of man, and more particularly a science of the factors which cause man to act.

He gave an impassioned account of what all this means to him in his lecture on Hebraic Civilization and the Science of Man, delivered in Edinburgh in 1960.

In striking contrast, so far as career and attitude to Jewish tradition go, was M. D. Eder: typically English in his education and outlook, utterly secular and, as he once told a Court, an atheist, he was at the same time a devoted and self-sacrificing Zionist, and he made on many people a permanent impression of moral force allied to a melancholy idealism. As Edward Glover put it,

Close friends could not fail to observe at times a certain sombreness in Eder's expression . . . It has sometimes been suggested that this sombre quality is characteristic of the Jewish people, and that it represents an ingrained reaction to the unusually traumatic history and traditions of the Jew . . . But we are on safer ground if we say that somewhere in the dark recesses of these melancholy types there dwells a deep sense of hurt, of baffled indignation, remorse or guilt.

If I had to pick another Jewish psychiatrist who could be regarded as conspicuously different from these two I would go on talking about the Italian, Cesare Lombroso, who did so much for criminology and anthropology, as well as for medicine.

But I think it would be better to finish by recalling what I said at the beginning about the adherents of Freud, who formed such a surprisingly Jewish company (apart from Ernest Jones). A similar group created Gestalt psychology: Kurt Goldstein, Kurt Lewin, Edgar Rubin, Max Wertheimer, David Katz, Adhemar Gelb, Zeigarnik, and perhaps the most distinguished of all, the philosopher Edmund Husserl. A. A. Roback, an American psychologist, writes vehemently on this concentration of Jewish talent in one branch of his subject and expresses his conviction that in the case of Jewish scientists,

religion may play a minimal part, but the culture of three thousand years may not be without its influence in shaping theories or systems. Whether there is a gene linking in this case, or a family tradition which, even in the most assimilated homes, has not been entirely eradicated . . . is not pertinent at this juncture when all that one demands is a recognition of the ethnic antecedent as a directive agency in the creative élan.

That is a fair enough pendant to the listing of Gestalt psychologists of note, and could apply to the psychiatrists too, though as Cecil Roth said in the preface to his book on the *Jewish Contribution to Civilization*, any sort of Jewish chauvinism is repellent.

REFERENCES

Bakan, D. (1958). *Sigmund Freud and the Jewish Mystical Tradition*. Van Nostrand : London.
Baruk, H. (1961). *Hebraic Civilization and the Science of Man*. World Federation for Mental Health : Geneva.
Becker, R. (1931). Die Geistesser Krankungen bei den Juden in Polen. *Allgemeine Zeitung für Psychiatrie* 96, 47–66.
Buber, M. (1931). *Jewish Mysticism*. London.
Fernando, S. J. M. (1966). Depressive illness in Jews and non-Jews. *British Journal of Psychiatry* 112, 991–996.
Fishberg, M. (1916). *Jewish Encyclopedia*. New York.
Freeman, W. (1968). *The Psychiatrist : Personality and Patterns*. Grune & Stratton : New York.
Freud, S. (1928). *The Future of an Illusion*. Hogarth Press : London.
Gordon, H. L. (1949). *The Maygid of Caro*. New York.
Halevi, H. S. (1964). *Mental Illness in Israel*. Jerusalem.
Herberg, W. (1959). *Judaism and Modern Man*. Meridian Books : New York.
Hes, J. P. (1964). From native healer to modern psychiatrist. Afro-Asian immigrants to Israel and their attitude towards psychiatric facilities. I. The road to the hospital. *Israeli Annals of Psychiatry* 2, 192–208.
Hes, J. P. & Wollstein, S. (1964). The attitude of the ancient Jewish sources to mental patients. *Israeli Annals of Psychiatry* 2, 103–116.
Heschel, A. J. (1966). *Graduate Journal* 7, 65.
Hobman, J. B. (ed.) (1948). *David Eder, Memoirs of a Modern Pioneer*. Gollancz : London.
Jacobs, L. (1962). *We Have Reason to Believe*. Vallentine : London.
Jones, E. (1957). *Sigmund Freud : Life and Work*, vols. 1–3. Hogarth Press : London.
Josephus, F. *Antiquities of the Jews*, book 8, chapter 2, para 5.
Jung, C. G. (1934). The state of psychotherapy today. (Translated from 'Zur gegenwärtigen Lage der Psychotherapie'. *Zentralblatt für Psychotherapie und ihre Grenzgebiete (Leipzig)*, VII, 1, 1–16).
King, A. R. (1961). The alcohol problem in Israel. *Quarterly Journal of Studies on Alcohol* 22, 321–324.
Knupper, G. & Room, R. (1967). Drinking patterns and attitudes of Irish, Jewish and white Protestant American Men. *Quarterly Journal of Studies on Alcohol* 28, 676–699.
Roback, A. A. (1952). *History of American Psychology*, chapter 24. Library Publishers : New York.
Rosen, G. (1968). *Madness in Society*, chapter 2. Routledge & Kegan Paul : London.
Roth, C. (1938). *Jewish Contribution to Civilization*. London.
Roth, L. (1960). *Judaism, a Portrait*. Viking Press : London.
Schecter, S. (1908). *Studies in Judaism*, second series. Black : London.
Shuval, R. & Krasilowsky, D. (1964). A study of hospitalized male alcoholics. *Israel Annals of Psychiatry and Related Disciplines* 1 (2), 277–292.
Sichel, M. (1908). Über die Geistesstörungen bei den Juden. *Neurologisches Centralblatt* 27, 351–367.
Snyder, C. R. (1958). *Alcohol and the Jews : a cultural study of drinking and sobriety*. Yale Center : Glencoe, Ill.

2-2

BIBLIOGRAPHY

1926

With CAMPBELL, T. D. The aborigines of South Australia: dental observations recorded at Ooldea. *Aust. J. Dent.*, **30**, 371–6.

With CAMPBELL, T. D. The aborigines of South Australia: anthropometric descriptive and other observations recorded at Ooldea. *Trans. R. Soc. S. Aust.*, **50**, 183–91.

1928

Traumatic pneumocephalus. *Brain*, **51**, 221–43.

1930

An investigation into the clinical features of melancholia. M.D. Thesis; Univ. Adelaide.

1931

Paranoid disorders. *Gen. Pract. Fr.-Br. med. Rev.*, **7**, 311–15.

Genetic problems in psychiatry: and their solution by the study of twins. *Eugen. Rev.*, **23**, 119–25.

1932

The experience of time in mental disorder. *Proc. R. Soc. Med.*, **25**, 611–20.

1933

Inheritance of mental disorders. *Eugen. Rev.*, **25**, 79–84.

1934

Melancholia: a historical review. *J. ment. Sci.*, **80**, 1–42.

Melancholia: a clinical survey of depressive states. *J. ment. Sci.*, **80**, 277–378.

The psychopathology of insight. *Br. J. med. Psychol.*, **14**, 332–48.

Mental reactions to bodily injury. *Med. Press*, **188**, 511–12.

Acromegaly in one of uniovular twins. *J. Neurol. Psychopath.*, **15**, 1–11.

German eugenic legislation: an examination of fact and theory. *Eugen Rev.*, **26**, 183–91.

Inheritance of mental disorders. In *The Chances of Morbid Inheritance*, ed. BLACKER, C. P. London: H. K. Lewis.

1935

Psychological syndromes in central nervous disease: a genetic interpretation. *Eugen. Rev.*, **27**, 213–15.

Neurosis and unemployment. *Lancet*, **2**, 293–7.
Prognosis in schizophrenia. *Lancet*, **1**, 339–41.
With MINSKI, L. Chorea and psychosis. *Lancet*, **1**, 536–8.

1936

Melancholia: prognostic study and case material. *J. ment. Sci.*, **82**, 488–558.
Prognosis in the manic-depressive psychosis. *Lancet*, **2**, 997–9.
Problems of obsessional illness. *Proc. R. Soc. Med.*, **29**, 325–36.
A case of apparent dissimilarity of monozygotic twins. *Ann. Eugen.*, **7**, 58–64.
Psychiatry and General Medicine. *Med. Press*, **192**, Symposium No. 2, 1–3.

1937

With SAMUEL, N., AND GALLOWAY, J. A study of cretinism in London
with especial reference to mental development and problems of growth.
Lancet, **1**, 1505–9 and **2**, 5–9.

1938

States of depression: their clinical and aetiological differentiation. *Brit. med.
J.*, **2**, 875–8.
The diagnosis and treatment of obsessional states. *Practitioner*, **141**, 21–30.
Some recent aspects of dementia. In *Festskrift tillägnad Olof Kinberg*, pp. 238–44.
Stockholm: Asbrink.
Paranoia and paranoid states. In *The British Encyclopaedia of Medical Practice* (1st
ed.), **10**, 292–301. London: Butterworth.
Alcoholic psychoses. In *The British Encyclopaedia of Medical Practice* (1st ed.), **10**,
332–41. London: Butterworth.

1940

With JACKSON, J. Psychiatric comparison of artificial menopause and the
effects of hysterectomy. *J. Neurol. Psychiat., Lond.*, **3**, 101–10.
Edward Mapother, M.D., F.R.C.P., Obituary. *Brit. med. J.*, **1**, 552–3.

1941

Psychological Medicine. In Price's *Textbook of the Practice of Medicine*, 6th ed.
(and subsequent editions). London: Oxford University Press.
Psychiatric aspects of effort syndrome. *Proc. R. Soc. Med.*, **34**, 533–40.
With JONES, M. Effort syndrome. *Lancet*, **1**, 813–18.

1942

Discussion on Differential Diagnosis and Treatment of Post-contusional
States. *Proc. R. Soc. Med.*, **35**, 607–14.
Incidence of neurosis in England under war conditions. *Lancet*, **2**, 175–83.
With SLATER, E. Neurosis in soldiers: a follow-up study. *Lancet*, **1**, 496–8.

1943

Social effects of neurosis. *Lancet*, **1**, 167–70.

Mental health in war-time. *Publ. Hlth., Lond.*, **57**, 27–30.

With GOLDSCHMIDT, H. Social causes of admissions to a mental hospital for the aged. *Sociol. Rev.*, **35**, 86–98.

1944

Depression (In 'Recent Progress in Psychiatry'). *J. ment. Sci.*, **90**, 256–65.

The psychological aspects of indigestion. *Practitioner*, **125**, 257–60.

With GOODYEAR, K. Vocational aspects of neurosis in soldiers. *Lancet*, **2**, 105–9.

1945

The industrial resettlement of the neurotic. *Labour Mgmt*, **27**, 40–3. Also in (1946) Suppl. to *Brit. med. J.*, **1**, 197–9.

Psychiatric investigation in Britain. *Amer. J. Psychiat.*, **101**, 486–93.

On the place of physical treatment in psychiatry. *Br. med. Bull.*, **3**, 22–4.

Psychiatric advice in industry, *Br. J. ind. Med.*, **2**, 41–2.

The treatment of alcoholism. In Interim Supplement to *British Encyclopaedia of Medical Practice*, pp. 11–12. London: Butterworth.

Sobre el lugar del tratamiento físico en psiquiatría. (i) *Revta. Asoc. méd. argent.*, **59**, 1235–7, and (ii) *Gac. méd. españ.*, **19**, 494–7.

1946

Early recognition of disease; mental disorders. *Practitioner*, **156**, 459–63.

Ageing and senility: a major problem of psychiatry. *J. ment. Sci.*, **92**, 150–70.

Memorandum to the Royal Commission on Equal Pay. Appendices IX and X to Minutes of Evidence taken before the Royal Commission on Equal Pay, pp. 130–4. London: H.M.S.O.

1947

The education of psychiatrists. *Lancet*, **2**, 79–83.

1949

Philosophy and psychiatry (Manson Lecture). *Philosophy*, **24**, 99–117.

Postgraduate study in mental health in Britain. *Br. med. Bull.*, **6**, 185–7.

With DAVIES, D. L. Effects of decamethonium iodide (C 10) on respiration and induced convulsions in man. *Lancet*, **1**, 775–7.

1950

Mental disorders. Section in *Chambers' Encyclopaedia*, **9**, 258–64. London: Newnes.

1951

Henry Maudsley: his work and influence (Maudsley Lecture). *J. ment. Sci.*, **97**, 259–77.

Social aspects of psychiatry (Morison Lecture). *Edinb. med. J.*, **58**, 214–47.

Medical psychology. In *A Century of Science*, ed. DINGLE, H. London: Hutchinson.

1952

Classification of schizophrenia. *Proceedings of the first World Congress of Psychiatry (Paris 1950).* Part 2. Paris: Hermann.

With SLATER, E. Psychiatry in the Emergency Medical Service. In *History of the Second World War: United Kingdom Medical Series. Medicine and Pathology,* ed. Sir Z. COPE, London: H.M.S.O.

Paranoia and paranoid states. In *British Encyclopaedia of Medical Practice* (2nd ed.), **10**, 362–70. London: Butterworth.

Alcoholic psychoses. In *British Encyclopaedia of Medical Practice* (2nd ed.), **10**, 394–402. London: Butterworth.

1953

Health as a social concept. *Brit. J. Sociol.,* **4**, 109–24.

Letter from Britain. *Amer. J. Psychiat.,* **110**, 401–5.

Hysterical dissociation in dementia paralytica. *Mschr. Psychiat. Neurol.,* **125**, 589–604.

Research in occupational psychiatry. *Folia psychiat. neurol. neurochir. neerl.,* **56**, 779–86.

Advances in psychological medicine. *Practitioner,* **171**, 403–12.

Contribution to Points of Research into the Interaction between the Individual and the Culture. In *Prospects in Psychiatric Research*, ed. TANNER, J. Oxford: Blackwell.

1954

With FLEMINGER, J. J. The psychiatric risk from corticotrophin and cortisone. *Lancet,* **1**, 383–6.

Aspetti psicosomatici della medicina clinica. *Recenti Prog. Med.,* **16**, 434–53.

1955

Philippe Pinel and the English. *Proc. R. Soc. Med.,* **48**, 581–6.

Mental aspects of ageing. *Ciba Fdn. Colloq. Ageing,* **1**, 32–48. London: Churchill.

The relation between operative risk and the patient's general condition: alcohol, other habits of addiction and psychogenic factors. *Sixteenth International Congress of Surgery, Copenhagen.* Brussels: Imprimerie Medicale et Scientifique.

1956

Sigmund Freud, 1856–1939. *Discovery,* **17**, 181–3.

Statistical aspects of suicide. *Can. med. Ass. J.,* **74**, 99–104.

Rehabilitation programs in England. In *The Elements of a Community Mental Health Program.* New York: Millbank Memorial Fund.

1957

Social psychiatry. In *Lectures on the Scientific Basis of Medicine,* 1956–7, **6**, 116–42. University of London: Athlone Press.

The offspring of parents both mentally ill, *Acta genet. Statist. med.*, **7**, 349–65.
Jung's early work. *J. analyt. Psychol.*, **2**, 119–36.
La enfermedad obsesiva. *Acta neuropsiq. argent.*, **3**, 323–35.

1958

Between guesswork and certainty in psychiatry (Bradshaw Lecturer). *Lancet*, **1**, 171–5 and 227–30.
Resettlement of the chronic schizophrenic. (i) *J. all-India Inst. mentl Hlth.*, **1**, 22–8; (ii) (1959). In *Report of the Second Internat. Congr. Psychiatry: (Zurich 1957)*. Zurich: Orell Fussli. **1**, 223–8.
J. C. Reil's concepts of brain function. In *The History and Philosophy of Knowledge of the Brain and its function*, ed. POYNTER, F. N. L. Oxford: Blackwell.
Fertility and mental illness. *Eugen. Rev.*, **50**, 91–106.
A psychiatrist looks at a layman. *Oxf. med. Sch. Gaz.*, **10**, 124–6.

1959

Families with manic-depressive psychosis. *Eugen. Q.*, **6**, 130–7.
The impact of psychotropic drugs on the structure, function and future of psychiatric services in hospitals. In *Neuro-Psychopharmacology*, eds. BRADLEY, P. B., FLÜGEL, F. and HOCH, P. Amsterdam: Elsevier Pub. Co.

1960

The study of defect (Adolf Meyer Research Lecture). *Amer. J. Psychiat.*, **117**, 289–305.

1961

Agents of cultural advance (Hobhouse Memorial Trust Lecture). London: Oxford University Press.
Amnesic syndromes; the psychopathological aspect. *Proc. R. Soc. Med.*, **54**, 955–61.
The chemical treatment of mental disorder. *Biology hum. Affairs*, **27**, 19–26.
Psychiatric education and training. In *Psychiatrie de Gegenwart*, eds. GRUHLE, H. W., JUNG, R., MAYER-GROSS, W. and MÜLLER, M., Band 3. Berlin: Springer.
Current field studies in mental disorders in Britain. In *Comparative Epidemiology of Mental Disorders*, eds. HOCH, P. H. and ZUBIN, J. New York: Grune & Stratton.
Psychiatry in Great Britain. In *Comtemporary European Psychiatry*, ed. BFLLAK, L. New York: Grove Press.

1962

Ebb and flow in social psychiatry (Bertram Roberts Memorial Lecture). *Yale J. Biol. Med.*, **35**, 62–83.
Inaugural speech of the scientific session. In *First Pan-African Psychiatric Conference 1961*, ed. LAMBO, T. A. Ibadan: Government Printer.
What are the foreigners up to? *Amer. J. Psychiat.*, **118**, 751–2.

1963

Medicine and the affections of the mind (Harveian Oration). *Brit. med. J.*, **2**, 1549–57.

Research and its application in psychiatry (Maurice Bloch Lecture). Glasgow: Jackson.

The psychoses. In *Cecil-Loeb's Textbook of Medicine*, 11th ed. (and 12th ed.), eds. BEESON, P. B. and McDERMOTT, W. Philadelphia: Saunders.

Symposium: Training for Child Psychiatry. *J. Child. Psychol. Psychiat.*, **4**, 75–84.

Demographic aspects of mental disorder. *Proc. Roy. Soc.*, B, **159**, 202–20.

Henry Maudsley. In *Grosse Nervenaerzte*, ed. KOLLE, K. Band 3. Stuttgart: Thieme.

1964

Health in 1984: changes in psychiatric methods and attitudes. *New Scient.*, **21**, 423–4.

Health. In *A Dictionary of the Social Sciences*, eds. GOULD, J. and KOLB, W. L. London: Tavistock.

Depression. In *Depression. Proc. Symposium, Cambridge, 1959*, ed. DAVIES, E. B. Cambridge: University Press.

1965

J. C. Reil: Innovator and Battler. *J. Hist. Behav. Sci.*, **1**, 178–90.

A note on personality and obsessional illness. *Psychiatria Neurol. Basel*, **150**, 299–305.

The Medical Research Council Social Psychiatry Research Unit. In *The Organization of Research Establishments*, ed. Sir J. COCKCROFT. Cambridge: University Press.

The Psychology of Shakespeare. In *Shakespeare: the comprehensive soul*, PRITCHETT, V. S. *et al.* London: British Broadcasting Corporation.

Man and Beast. *The Times Literary Supplement*, No. 3317, 817–8.

1966

Psychiatric dicta. *Lancet*, **1**, 974–5.

Survivance de l'Hystérie. *Evol. psychiat.* **31**, 159–65.

Cancer Country. *The New York Review of Books*, **VI**, No. 2, 24–6.

Analysing the Analyst. *The Times Literary Supplement*, No. 3346, 317–9.

1967

Problems presented by the ambiguous work 'Anxiety' as used in psycho-pathology. *Israel Ann. Psychiat. and related Disciplines*, **5**, No. 2, 105–21.

Empirical or rational? The nature and basis of psychiatry. (The Linacre Lecture, delivered in Cambridge). *Lancet*, **2**, 1–9.

1968

Periodicity. In *Symposium Bel-Air III Cycles biologiques et psychiatrie*, 1967 ed. J. DE AJURIAGUERRA, Geneva, Georg.

243

Cannabis: a review of the international clinical literature. In *Cannabis. Report by the Advisory Committee on Drug Dependence*, London: H.M.S.O.
Continuity in psychiatric training. In *Psychiatry in Transition*, ed. STOKES, A. B., University of Toronto Press for Clarke Institute of Psychiatry, Toronto.

1969

Medicine and Culture. In *Medicine and Culture*, ed. POYNTER, F. N. L., London: Wellcome Institute of Historical Medicine.
Introduction: Definitions and perspectives. In *The Scientific Basis of Drug Dependence*, ed. STEINBERG, H. London: Churchill.
Edward Mapother and the making of the Maudsley Hospital (The First Mapother Lecture). *Br. J. Psychiat.*, **115**, 1349–66.
Psichiatria sociale. *Recenti Progr. in Med.*, **47**, 267–78.

1970

Amphetamines, barbiturates, LSD and cannabis: their use and misuse. *Report on Public Health No. 124*. London: H.M.S.O.
Paranoia and paranoid: a historical perspective. *Psychol. Med.* **1**, 2–12.
Psychological factors in human fertility. Studies dedicated to *Erik Essen-Möller*. *Acta psychiat. scand.*, **46**, *Suppl. 219*, 109–17.

1971

'Endogenous' and 'exogenous'—a useful dichotomy? *Psychol. Med.*, **1**, 191–6.

1972

An indictment of Autonomous Man—Sir Aubrey Lewis on the idea of F. F. Skinner. *The Listener*, 23 March, 388–9.
'Psychogenic': a word and its mutations. *Psychol. Med.*, **2**, 209–15.
Classification and diagnosis in psychiatry: a historical note. In *Psychiatric Diagnosis in New York and London*, Cooper, J. E., Gurland, B. J., Sharpe, L., Copeland, J. R. M., and Simon, R. Maudsley Monograph No. 20, pp. 1–5. London.

1973

Manfred Bleuler's *'The schizophrenic mental disorders'*: an exposition and a review. *Psychol. Med.*, **3**, 385–92.
William Mayer-Gross. *Confrontations Psychiat.*, **11**, 109–25.

1974

Foreword to *Glossary of Mental Disorders and Guide to their Classification*. Geneva: W.H.O.
Psychopathic personality: a most elusive category. *Psychol. Med.*, **4**, 133–40.

1975

The survival of hysteria. *Psychol. Med.*, **5**, 9–12.

244

1976

A note on classifying phobia. *Psychol. Med.*, 6, 21–2.

1977

William Mayer-Gross: an appreciation. *Psychol. Med.*, 7, 11–18. (English original of article in *Confrontations Psychiatriques*, 1973—see above).

1978

Psychiatry and the Jewish tradition. *Psychol. Med.*, 8, 9–19.

In addition to signed work, there are numerous reviews and editorials.